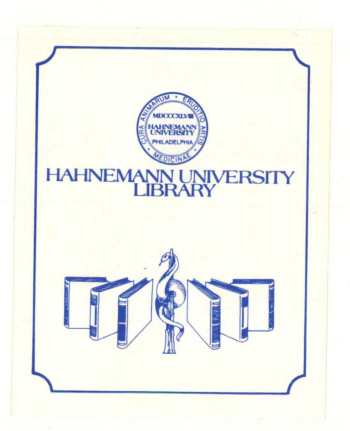

Invasive Cardiology

Invasive Cardiology

Principles and Techniques

edited by

Thomas M. Bashore, M.D.

Associate Professor of Medicine
Duke University School of Medicine
Director, Cardiovascular Laboratory
Duke University Medical Center
Durham, North Carolina

B. C. Decker Inc.   Toronto   •   Philadelphia

Publisher

B.C. Decker Inc
3228 South Service Road
Burlington, Ontario L7N 3H8

B.C. Decker Inc
320 Walnut Street
Suite 400
Philadelphia, Pennsylvania 19106

Sales and Distribution

United States and Puerto Rico
The C.V. Mosby Company
11830 Westline Industrial Drive
Saint Louis Missouri 63146

Canada
McAinsh & Co. Ltd.
2760 Old Leslie Street
Willowdale, Ontario M2K 2X5

Australia
McGraw-Hill Book Company Australia Pty. Ltd.
4 Barcoo Street
Roseville East 2069
New South Wales, Australia

Brazil
Editora McGraw-Hill do Brasil, Ltda.
rua Tabapua, 1.105, Itaim-Bibi
Sao Paulo, S.P. Brasil

Colombia
Interamericana/McGraw-Hill de Colombia, S.A.
Apartado Aereo 81078
Bogota, D.E. Colombia

Europe
McGraw-Hill Book Company GmbH
Lademannbogen 136
D-2000 Hamburg 63
West Germany

France
MEDSI/McGraw-Hill
6. avenue Daniel Lesueur
75007 Paris, France

Hong Kong and China
McGraw-Hill Book Company
Suite 618, Ocean Centre
5 Canton Road
Tsimshatsui, Kowloon
Hong Kong

India
Tata McGraw-Hill Publishing Company, Ltd.
12/4 Asaf Ali Road, 3rd Floor
New Delhi 110002, India

Indonesia
P.O. Box 122/JAT
Jakarta, 1300 Indonesia

Italy
McGraw-Hill Libri Italia, s.r.l.
Piazza Emilia, 5
1-20129 Milano Ml
Italy

Japan
Igaku-Shoin Ltd.
Tokyo International P.O. Box 5063
1-28-36 Hongo, Bunkyo-ku,
Tokyo 113, Japan

Korea
C.P.O. Box 10583
Seoul, Korea

Malaysia
No. 8 Jalan SS 7/6B
Kelana Jaya
47301 Petaling Jaya
Selangor, Malaysia

Mexico
Interamericana/McGraw-Hill de Mexico,
S.A. de C.V.
Cedro 512, Colonia Atlampa
(Apartado Postal 26370)
06450 Mexico, D.F., Mexico

New Zealand
McGraw-Hill Book Co. New Zealand Ltd.
5 Joval Place, Wiri
Manukau City, New Zealand

Panama
Editorial McGraw-Hill Latinoamericana, S.A.
Apartado Postal 2036
Zona Libre de Colon
Colon, Republica de Panama

Portugal
Editora McGraw-Hill de Portugal, Ltda.
Rua Rosa Damasceno 11A-B
1900 Lisboa, Portugal

South Africa
Libriger Book Distributors
Warehouse Number 8
"Die Ou Looiery"
Tannery Road
Hamilton, Bloemfontein 9300

Southeast Asia
McGraw-Hill Book Co.
348 Jalan Boon Lay
Jurong, Singapore 2261

Spain
McGraw-Hill/Interamericana de Espana, S.A.
Manuel Ferrero, 13
28020 Madrid, Spain

Taiwan
P.O. Box 87-601
Taipei, Taiwan

Thailand
632/5 Phaholyothin Road
Sapan Kwai
Bangkok 10400
Thailand

United Kingdom, Middle East and Africa
McGraw-Hill Book Company (U.K.) Ltd.
Shoppenhangers Road
Maidenhead, Berkshire
SL6 2QL England

Venezuela
McGraw-Hill/Interamericana, C.A.
2da. calle Bello Monte
(entre avenida Casanova y Sabana Grande)
Apartado Aereo 50785
Caracas 1050, Venezuela

Invasive Cardiology: Principles and Techniques

ISBN 1–55664–190–7

Library of Congress catalog card number: 89–51095

10 9 8 7 6 5 4 3 2 1

CONTRIBUTORS

Michael J. Barber, M.D., Ph.D.
Fellow, Division of Cardiology
Duke University Medical Center
Durham, North Carolina

Thomas M. Bashore, M.D.
Associate Professor of Medicine
Duke University School of Medicine
Director, Cardiovascular Laboratory
Duke University Medical Center
Durham, North Carolina

Mary Jo Chapman, R.N., B.S., B.S.N., R.C.V.T.
Clinical Coordinator, Cardiovascular Laboratory
Duke University Medical Center
Durham, North Carolina

Jack T. Cusma, Ph.D.
Assistant Medical Research Professor
Duke University Medical Center
Durham, North Carolina

Charles J. Davidson, M.D.
Assistant Professor of Medicine
Duke University Medical Center
Durham, North Carolina

J. Kevin Harrison, M.D.
Fellow in Cardiology
Duke University Medical Center
Durham, North Carolina

Katherine B. Kisslo, B.S., R.D.M.S.
Research Analyst
Duke University Medical Center
Durham, North Carolina

Mark Leithe, M.D.
Fellow in Cardiology
Duke University Medical Center
Durham, North Carolina

Thad Makachinas, B.S., R.C.V.T.
Cardiac Catheterization Laboratory
Duke University Medical Center
Durham, North Carolina

Mary Jane McCracken, R.N., C.C.V.T.
Technical Administrator
Duke University Medical Center
Durham, North Carolina

Paul Owens, R.N., R.C.V.T.
Cardiac Catheterization Laboratory
Duke University Medical Center
Durham, North Carolina

Thomas N. Skelton, M.D.
Assistant Professor of Medicine
University of Mississippi Medical Center
Division of Cardiovascular Diseases
Attending Physician
University Hospital
Jackson, Mississippi

Laurence A. Spero, B.S.E.
Analyst Programmer
Duke University Medical Center
Durham, North Carolina

PREFACE

We are in an era of unprecedented expansion of cardiac catheterization facilities. Cardiac catheterization involves a true team effort, with physicians and nonphysicians working closely together to obtain accurate and useful information for eventual patient management decisions. By addressing the needs of both physicians and nonphysicians in the cardiac catheterization laboratory, this book is meant to broaden the understanding of both groups. The physician will gain new insights into methodology and equipment, while the nurse and technologist will be given a broader view of analysis and interpretation. This interchange will be mutually beneficial.

Invasive Cardiology: Principles and Techniques presents the latest methodology in a "cookbook" fashion and includes chapters directly related to laboratory organization and patient flow. Other chapters review the basics of normal cardiac physiology and of abnormal cardiac disease states, with emphasis on interpretation. Specifics related to the efficient operation of both hemodynamic and radiographic equipment are outlined, and electrophysiology and interventional procedures are similarly described.

The list of contributors to this text includes a cross section of health professionals. The information herein is equally applicable to the training of resident physicians, nurse specialists, and technicians. Much space is devoted to helpful photographs and line drawings, but the reference list is intentionally limited to basic articles and reviews. It is anticipated that this textbook can be used to form the basis for a program of training personnel with widely divergent backgrounds in the proper performance of all invasive cardiovascular procedures.

Thomas M. Bashore, M.D.

To the diligent and compassionate staff of the Cardiac Catheterization
Laboratory at Duke University Medical Center

CONTENTS

CHAPTER 1

Introduction and Historical Perspective

Thomas M. Bashore, MD

The striking increase in the number of cardiac catheterizations being performed in the United States has resulted in a need for a reference source for the personnel who staff and operate cardiac catheterization laboratories and clinics. This book is meant to respond to that need. Rather than focus on detailed pathophysiologic mechanisms, this text is intended to provide a foundation for the understanding of the basic principles involved in performance of the various catheterization procedures in a practical manner. Although the text undoubtedly reflects bias toward the methodologic procedures as performed at Duke Medical Center, it is hoped that its content will be applicable to the performance of catheterization procedures at any institution.

This manual has been prepared specifically with the help of the many nurses and technicians in the Cardiac Catheterization Laboratory at Duke Medical Center. The text and figures are meant to provide guidelines for the performance of cardiac catheterization in an efficient and safe manner. Line drawings and schematics are used whenever possible to explain major concepts. The theoretical basis of the pathologic disease states studied are emphasized only to the degree that is necessary for the understanding of the results of these studies. This text is an outgrowth of a yearly training session that the personnel in the laboratory attend. These individuals provided both the inspiration and the perspiration needed to bring this manual together.

Historical Perspective

Modern cardiac catheterization and angiography are rooted in three major medical discoveries: the development of radiographic and appropriate imaging equip-

1

ment; the development of readily usable catheters and a safe means of cannulating the vascular system; and the discovery of a safe radiographic contrast medium. A brief review of these events may be of interest to the reader.

William Roentgen's discovery of the x-ray principle in 1895 quickly led to its application in humans. The first angiogram (of a human hand) was reported in 1896 by Haschek, and the beating heart was observed on fluoroscopy by Williams in 1896. It wasn't until the development of the 16-mm cinefilm camera by Stuart and colleagues in 1937 and the development of the modern film-roll changer in 1953 that cineangiography was able to develop. Most recently, digital angiography has started to be used in many of the laboratories around the country, and the future will undoubtedly see the routine use of the computerized storage of radiographic information in a digital format. It is equally likely that there will be a gradual shift from a cinefilm-based medium to a more computer-based digital-imaging format.

The first human catheterization procedure has been credited to Dr. Werner Forssmann in 1929. Over the protestations of his colleagues, Dr. Forssmann tricked an assistant, Nurse Gerda, into allowing him into the surgical suite, where she was able to provide access to the venipuncture instruments. He then inserted a urethral catheter into his own arm and walked to the basement of the hospital, where an radiograph was taken to demonstrate that the catheter was indeed in his heart.

By 1939, Klein and colleagues reported 11 human patients in whom cardiac output was measured using catheter techniques. Following this, the activity in catheterization suites during the 1940s dramatically increased, especially at the Bellevue Hospital in New York under the influence of Drs. Cournand and Richards. In 1956, Forssmann, Cournand, and Richards received the Nobel Prize in medicine for these efforts. Many advances occurred during the 1940s and 1950s. Left-heart catheterization provided the most formidable challenge. The left heart was first approached via left atrial puncture during bronchoscopy, by a posterior transthoracic puncture approach, by a suprasternal method, by a left subcostal technique, and via transseptal (transatrial septal) puncture. A practical method was finally devised by Seldinger in 1953 wherein a percutaneous needle was used to puncture the femoral artery, and the catheter exchanged over a guidewire. A modification of this method is in use today.

Cannulation of the coronary arteries, however, required the development of specialized catheter techniques. Radner, in 1945, is generally credited with being the first to visualize coronaries with radiographic contrast media. Sones and colleagues at the Cleveland Clinic described a practical method of selectively cannulating the coronary arteries in 1959. The Sones method utilized cutdown of the brachial artery for catheter insertion. Ricketts and Abrams, in 1962, suggested that a preformed catheter might be used from the femoral arterial approach. These catheters were subsequently modified by Judkins and Amplatz in 1967. Other modifications, such as those by Schoonmaker and King in 1974, are still in use. The Judkins approach is the most popular in the United States today.

In 1970, balloon-tip catheters were introduced that could be inserted without fluoroscopy by Swan et al. These catheters were then coupled to a thermal sensor so that thermodilution cardiac outputs could be measured along with pressures. Catheter designs changed only modestly in the 70s, until the advent of the interventional era. There is now a resurgence in catheter design and innovation.

The final step in the modern development of cardiac catheterization procedures required the development of a safe radiographic contrast agent. In 1931, Forssmann injected a bolus of Uroselectin into his right atrium and experienced only mild dizziness. Attempts at defining vascular structures using radiographic contrast have included the use of a variety of materials from the bizarre to the ridiculous, including buckshot, air, bismuth and oil, and potassium iodide. In the 1950s, a tri-iodinated benzoic acid contrast medium was developed that substantially reduced contrast reactions, diatrizoate. The 1980s has seen the introduction of nonionic and low-ionic media that have been shown to have even fewer side effects than the ionic diatrizoate compounds that have become standard.

The Future

The future of cardiac catheterization laboratories appears bright. Not only has catheter size been reduced and safety improved, but the innovative new designs in catheter function will allow for improvement in the current techniques of myocardial biopsy, angioplasty, and valvuloplasty. These innovations in catheter function provide hope that there may be an expanding role for laser technology to "vaporize coronary plaques," atherectomy devices to remove obstructing lesions, and stents to hold the vessels open.

We are probably only seeing the beginning of a marked improvement in our ability to utilize catheter techniques in the study and treatment of cardiac diseases. New catheters are also being developed for intraluminal angioscopy, two-dimensional echocardiography, and the measurement of flow velocity via either thermodilution, impedance, electromagnetic, or Doppler velocity methods. Intracardiac sensors are being placed on catheters to monitor metabolic changes, pO_2, or pH. We clearly are in an era in which the safety of catheterization has been well established, and we will see a marked evolution in techniques over the next two decades. The cardiac catheterization laboratory promises to be a dynamic setting for the study of patients with cardiac disease.

SELECTED REFERENCES

Amplatz K, Formanek G, Stanger P, et al. Mechanics of selective coronary artery catheterization via femoral approach. Radiology 1967; 89: 1040.

Brannon ES, Weens HS, Warren JV. Atrial septal defect: Study of hemodynamics by the technique of right heart catheterization. Am J Med Sci 1948; 210:480.

Brock R, Milstein BB, Ross DN. Percutaneous left ventricular puncture in the assessment of aortic stenosis. Thorax 1956; 11:163.

Cope C. Technique for transseptal catheterization of the left atrium: Preliminary report. J Thoracic Surg 1957; 37:482.

Cournand A. Cardiac catheterization: Development of the technique, its contribution to experimental medicine, and its initial application in man. Acta Med Scand [Suppl] 1978; S79:7.

Dexter L, Haynes FW, Burwell CS, et al. Studies of congenital heart disease: II. The pressure and content of blood in the right auricle, right ventricle and pulmonary artery in control patients, with observations on the oxygen saturation and source of pulmonary capillary blood. J Clin Invest 1947; 26:554.

Forssmann W. Experiments on myself: Memoirs of a surgeon in Germany. New York: Saint Martin's Press, 1974: 84.

Gorlin R, Gorlin G. Hydraulic formula for calculation of area of stenotic mitral valve, other cardiac valves and central circulatory shunts. Am Heart J 1951; 41:1.

Gruentzig A, Sennìg A, Siegenthaler WE. Nonoperative dilatation of coronary artery stenosis: Percutaneous transluminal coronary angioplasty. N Engl J Med 1979; 301:61–68.

Haschek E, Lindenthol O. Ein Beitrag zur proktischen Verwerthung der photographie noch Röntgen. Wien Klin Wochenschr 1896; 9:63.

Judkins MP. Selective coronary arteriography: I. A percutaneous transfemoral technic. Radiology 1967; 89:815.

Klein O. Zur Bestimmung des Zerkulatorischen Minutens Volumen nach dem Fickschen Prinzip. Munch Med Wochenschr 1930; 77:1311.

Mason JW. Techniques for right and left ventricular endomyocardial biopsy. Am J Cardiol 1978; 41:8874.

McKay RG. Balloon valvuloplasty for treating pulmonic, mitral and aortic valve stenosis. Am J Cardiol 1988; 61:102G.

Miller SW. History of angiocardiography. In: Miller SW, ed. Cardiac angiography. Boston: Little, Brown & Co., 1984:3.

Radner S. Attempt at roentgenologic visualization of coronary blood vessels in man. Acta Radiol 1945; 26:497.

Rashkind WJ. Transcatheter treatment of congenital heart disease. Circulation 1983; 67:711.

Ricketts HJ, Abrams HL. Percutaneous selective coronary cinearteriography. JAMA 1982; 181:140.

Rigler LG, Watson JC. A combination film changer for rapid or conventional radiography. Radiology 1953; 61:77.

Seldinger S. Catheter replacement of the needle in percutaneous arteriography: A new technique. Acta Radiol 1958; 39:368.

Schoonmaker FW, King SB III. Coronary arteriography by the single catheter percutaneous femoral technique. Circulation 1974; 50:731.

Simpson JB. Future interventional techniques. In: Califf RM, Mark DB, Wagner GS, eds. Acute coronary care in the thrombolytic era. Chicago: Year Book Medical Publishers, 1988: 392.

Sigwart V, Piel J, Mirkovitch J, et al. Intravascular shunts to prevent occlusion and restenosis after transluminal angiography. N Engl J Med 1987; 316:701.

Spears JR, Spokojny AM, Marais J. Coronary angioscopy during cardiac catheterization. J Am Coll Cardiol 1985; 6:93.

Stewart WH, Hoffman WJ, Ghiselin FH. Cinefluorography. Am J Roentgen 1970; 38:465.

Swan HJC, Ganz W, Forrester JS, et al. Catheterization of the heart in man with use of a flow-detected balloon-tipped catheter. N Engl J Med 1970; 283:447.

CHAPTER 2

The Cardiac Catheterization Suite

Mary Jane McCracken, RN, and Mary Jo Chapman, RN

Among the most important components of an efficient and smooth-running catheterization laboratory (or cath lab) are laboratory design, patient flow, and a well-trained and integrated staff. Other factors that enhance the operation of a cath lab are sufficient and well-placed technical components, technical backup, and an administrative network that will guarantee that the mission of the unit can be carried out with a minimum of stress to the patient and a maximum utilization of the expertise of the personnel. If these parameters can be met, the cath lab will be successful and its environment will be a pleasant and rewarding place in which to work. Efficient organization and personnel integration also make a clinical cath lab an excellent teaching vehicle for the training of medical, technical, and administrative staff.

Laboratory Design

At the center of activity and the focal point of information flow in the laboratory is a large, centrally located board that outlines the daily and hourly operation of the lab (Fig. 2–1). After the last patient has arrived in the cath lab suite and is prepared for catheterization, this board is prepared for the next day's caseload. As much information about the patient as possible is included on this scheduling board, including the patient's name, diagnosis, attending physician's name, cathing physicians' names (and that of the cardiovascular fellow assigned, if applicable), the patient's hospital room number, and hospital control number. Any deviation from the routine left-heart diagnostic procedure (e.g., left groin, right heart, transplant candidate, valvuloplasty, and so on) should also be written next

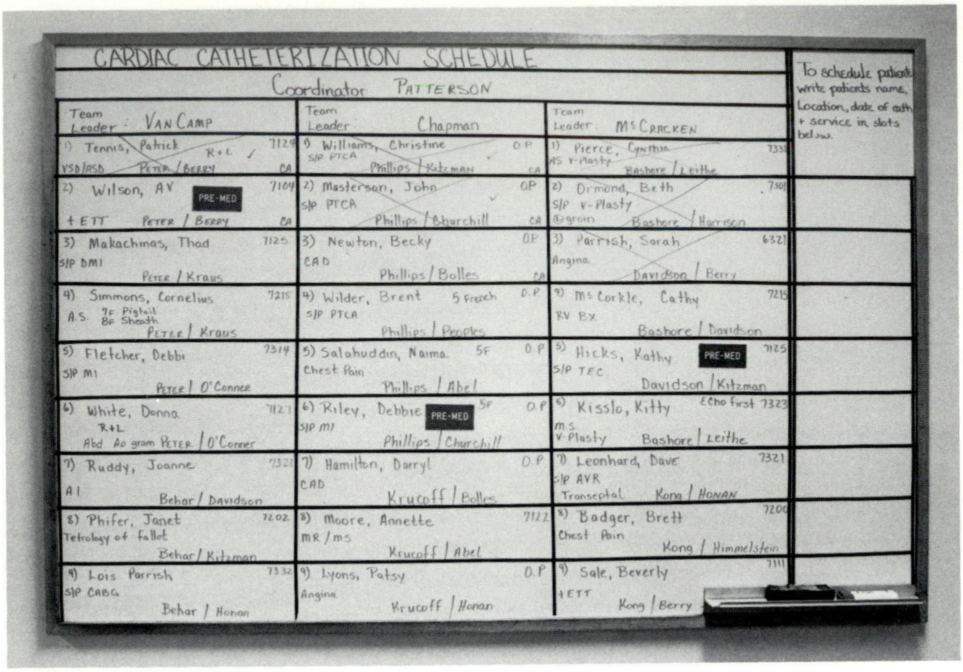

Figure 2–1. Representative scheduling board.

to the patient's name to alert the staff. This board should provide an up-to-the-minute status report on every patient as he comes through the lab. A cath-lab designate should control the board, updating it at every step in the patient's progress through the lab. Appropriate check marks or magnetic tags provide confirmation that the patient has been premedicated, has been sent for, has arrived in the lab, and has been discharged from the lab.

The cath-lab procedure itself is performed in a room with a functional area of at least approximately 750 square feet (minimum length is 25 feet and width 15 feet) (Fig. 2–2). Ancillary equipment (catheter racks, cabinets, shelf space, linen, sink, counter space, crash cart, and so on) is located around the perimeter of the room to allow for ease of movement around the angiographic table.

Control rooms that protect the technician from radiation exposure are now commonly in use in most institutions. Separate clear-glass shields may be used in the room to protect employees who must remain in the lab itself. Computer flooring in the control room is a valuable adjunct, as it raises the technician above the level of the procedure-room floor. The computer flooring allows for ready access to the myriad of cables and ducts that connect the control room to other areas of the cath lab. The control technician is in hard-wired headset communication with the physician at all times and monitors the patient's status during the procedure. He should be positioned so he has ready access to the x-ray console, the hemodynamic monitor, and the playback tape. The primary monitor-

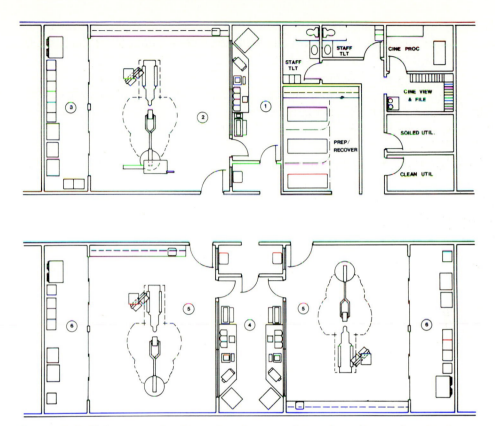

Figure 2–2. Representative floor plan for a traditional cardiac catheterization suite with single-plane x-ray equipment. A separate control room is shown in the top panel, and a shared control room is shown in the bottom panel. The need for a scrub area at the entrance to the control room is questionable nowadays; likewise, the reduction in the size of x-ray equipment makes large equipment rooms less necessary.

ing functions include keeping the procedure protocol, pressure recording, ECG monitoring, videotape playback, digital imaging control (if available), and x-ray control functions. The minimum area for a control room should be approximately 80 to 100 square feet.

From the standpoint of radiation safety, there are major advantages to having the control room isolated from the main cath lab and its x-ray equipment. A large leaded-glass window should be used to keep visual contact with the proceedings in the catheterization procedure room. In general, the physician should be on the opposite side of the table from the control room so that eye contact with the technician is possible. (This setup may not be feasible in some situations.)

The electronic switching cabinetry, generator, tetrodes, and so forth are best kept in a separate equipment room when possible, although recent advances have made these items less susceptible to heat and have somewhat reduced the need for separate cooling from the procedure room. Digital angiographic equipment also is best kept in an environmentally controlled room. All of these items produce considerable heat (Table 2–1).

The laboratory should also have adequate storage space for catheters, contrast media, film-processing supplies, manuals, and other extra equipment. The amount of storage is obviously dependent upon the volume in the cath lab. It is almost impossible to have "too much" storage space.

Whenever possible, film developing is best located within the catheterization area. This area should include space for viewing and splicing films and a darkroom for film development. Included in the darkroom is the film processor, an area for loading and unloading film, the chemistry for the processor, water feeds and drainage, and a silver recovery unit (these items are discussed in Chapter 4). A separate area for film storage should be close by with easy access. Some form of record to log the checkout of films should be provided to assist in what is one of the biggest headaches—the tracking of cinefilm location. In our own laboratory, a computer-generated name tag is used, and color-coded labels (changed each month) help prevent the misplacement of film in the wrong month's rack. Keeping track of cinefilm in a busy department remains a challenge for everyone.

Each laboratory should have a cinefilm viewing room. Both back-projection and screen-projection cinefilm viewers are available. This room frequently can double as a conference or teaching room or can be used for final dictation or entry of the report. In our institution, the reports are entered directly into a

TABLE 2–1
"Generic" Outline of Commonly Used X-ray Equipment, Their Weights, and the Amount of Heat Generated.

Item	Weight	Heat Generated (BTU/hr)
Control Room		
Bi-plane control desk	216 lb	850
Digital imaging viewing equipment	313 lb	5455
Physiologic monitoring equipment	1200 lb	3700
Data management system	500 lb	4200
Biplane Cath Lab		
AP gantry and x-ray	2646 lb	6169
X-ray table	700 lb	375
Quad monitor suspension	330 lb	1700
Lateral gantry and x-ray	1213 lb	480
Equipment Room		
Tetrode tank	1188 lb	3910
Transformer	1716 lb	1020
Rack cabinet(s)	300-816 lb	300-3060
Digital imaging interface rack cabinet	419 lb	3414
Digital imaging control cabinet	1544 lb	15365

computerized report-generating system, and the coronary tree is entered by the physician via a "touchscreen."

The final report can be generated through a variety of means. Although dictation is obviously the most common, one alternative is to have each step of the report entered as it is completed. For instance, the demographics and procedure can be entered by the technicians, the history and physical entered from forms filled out by the physicians and entered by data technicians, the ventricular volume and wall-motion analysis entered by a technician assigned that duty, and the final interpretation and description of the results entered by the physician. All of the these can be linked to a central computer system. The final report can then be output to a printer. Relevant data then become part of a permanent record that can be called up at any time. We have found such a system works well. A representative final report is shown in Figures 2–3 through 2–5.

Outpatient catheterization is a rapidly growing area of care for patients needing heart catheterization. This area will continue to expand in the near future, so it is important that an outpatient holding area be attractive and functional. It may be the patient's only contact with the hospital. The outpatient unit at our institution (Fig. 2–6) is designed to insure the maximum amount of tranquility and reassurance to the patient and his family. The area is painted in light pastel colors and has soft, indirect lighting. The minimal size of each cubicle should be 90 square feet. Certain rooms may provide monitoring if necessary. A crash cart, storage area, and work station for staff are kept close by. Outpatients are held from 1.5 to 3.0 hr after the procedure. A booklet outlining the catheterization is given to the patient and family prior to the procedure. The booklet (explained in greater detail in Chapter 3) also allows for the explanation of results and provides the patient with a permanent record.

Every effort must be made to make the patient's time in the cath lab a pleasant one. Remember, the patient is frightened, and while lying on his back has little to do except hear the voices of those around him. An atmosphere of efficient professionalism does much to alleviate the anxiety of the patient. Pleasant music is useful to pipe into the rooms when feasible. Everyone should be made to realize that each patient is unique and deserves everyone's full attention.

Personnel in the Catheterization Laboratory

The goal of the personnel in the cath lab is to safely perform diagnostic cardiac catheterization and other interventional techniques while ensuring the highest quality data and minimal psychological stress possible. In order to achieve this goal, certain criteria with regard to personnel and their responsibilities must be established.

Skilled and trained personnel are necessary for the smooth and efficient function of a laboratory. The members of the team may include some or all of the following: trained physicians, physicians' assistants (or PAs), monitoring or x-ray technicians, a laboratory administrator, patient-schedule coordinator, nurses,

```
CAD CARDIAC CATHETERIZATION

Reason for Catheterization
    Chest pain
    Congestive heart failure

Symptoms
    Date of onset: 03/??/89
    Typical angina present in last 6 wk
    Occurs with exertion or stress
    Relief by nitroglycerin
    Curent frequency: 14 episode(s) in the past 2 wk
    Course (last 6 wk): Progressing
    NYHA Class 3
    No ECG documentation of variant angina
    History of NYHA Class 3 CHF

Hospitalizations
    1 CCU admission(s) in last 6 mo for unstable angina
    Prior cardiac catheterization(s): 1

Medications
    Dipyridamole, 75 mg t.i.d.
    Insulin-NPH, 60 units
    Isosorbide dinitrate, 20 mg b.i.d.
    Nitroglycerin SL, 0.4 mg prn

Cardiovascular Risk Factors
    Hypertension
    Diabetes (type 2)
    Peripheral vascular disease
    Family history of premature heart disease
    Hyperlipidemia

PHYSICAL EXAMINATION
    HT: 162.5 cm       WT: 81.1 kg
    V/S:
      P: 75        BP: 150/60
    Lungs: No rales
    Heart:
      No S₃
      No S₄
    Pulses:
      Carotid: Right bruit and left bruit
      Dorsal pedis: Right absent and left absent
      Postib: Right absent and left absent
    Other:


A
```

Figure 2–3. A–C, Representative report from the catheterization procedure. Basic demographic data are presented in a tabular format for ease in review.

technical personnel, photography technicians, and a support staff that may include transporters, secretaries, nurse specialists, and specialized data technicians. Each member of the team must understand his role if the laboratory is to function in an efficient manner. A *physician director* must be on hand to assume primary responsibility for the operation of the laboratory.

In some institutions, *physicians' assistants* may perform some of the functions of the catheterizing physician. The PA can perform an initial history and physical exam, undertake patient preparation and teaching, obtain informed con-

LABORATORY FINDINGS
  Chest x-ray: Normal
  ECG: Normal sinus rhythm; right-axis deviation; anterior MI and inferior MI
  Other: Hematocrit—42; Bun—10; Creatinine—0.8

PROCEDURE   CINE #: 42607
  Premedication: Benadryl, 25 mg IV
  Anesthesia: 1% Xylocaine
  Arterial access site: RFA
  Diagnostic procedures performed:
    Left-heart catheterization
    Left ventriculogram
      Catheter(s) : 7 French pigtail
    Left coronary angiograms
      Catheter(s): 7 French 4-cm Judkins
    Right coronary angiograms
      Catheter(s): 7 French 4-cm Judkins
  Medications given: Normal saline, 75 cc IV; nitroglycerin SL, 0.12 mg; heparin, 2000 units IV
  X-Ray contrast: Hypaque (45 ml) and Omnipaque (130 ml)
  Patient condition: Stable
  Patient disposition: Returned to the ward

HEMODYNAMIC DATA
  LV: 150/6-16 mm Hg
  AO: 150/60 mm Hg; mean = 95 mm Hg
  BSA: 1.83 sq m

LEFT VENTRICULAR ANGIOGRAPHY (BIPLANE)
  Left ventricle:
    Chamber size: Mildly enlarged
    Mitral apparatus: Normal
    Overall contraction: Mild generalized hypokinesia

  Ventricular volume data (biplane):
    Ejection fraction: 41%

  Left ventricular-wall motion:
    Segment:
    Apical—severe akinesia
    Septal—severe asyneresis

  Mitral valve:
    Mitral valvular calcification: None
    Mitral Regurgitation: None

B

Figure 2–3 (continued).

sent, and initiate the actual procedure under supervision of qualified physicians. The PA can also function to complete the final report. Some have even proposed that the PA might be able to fill all of the roles generally assigned to a cardiovascular fellow in training. Medical-legal constraints in some locales, however, may limit the extent to which a PA may be able to perform certain aspects of the catheterization itself.

    The *laboratory administrator* is the nonphysician in charge of the laboratory. Duties include the development and monitoring of the annual budget, and the supervision of regular conferences and/or staff meetings. This person must act as liaison between the lab and other clinical departments and provide periodic staff evaluation (according to hospital policy). The supervisor is also an impor-

CORONARY ARTERIOGRAMS
    Dominance: Left
    SA node origin: Right
    AV node origin: Left

	Stenosis	Filling/Comment
Left Main Coronary artery:	Normal	
Left anterior descending:		
*Prox LAD	95%	
Mid AD	50%	
*Dist LAD	95%	
Left circumflex:		
*Marg 1 (large)	75%	
Right coronary artery:		
Prox RCA	95%	

* Denotes significant lesion.

FINAL IMPRESSIONS
    1. Significant ($> = 75\%$) two-vessel coronary artery disease:
            Left main: Normal
            LAD system: Subtotal stenosis
            LCX system: Subtotal stenosis
            RCA system: Subtotal stenosis and nondominant
    2. Mild generalized hypokinesia.
    3. Severe akinesia of the apical wall and severe asyneresis of the septal wall of the left
        ventricle.
    4. No evidence for mitral insufficiency.
    5. History of congestive heart failure.

Cardiac catherization performed by:

c

Figure 2–3 (continued).

tant link between the vendors and the laboratory. This person should have a solid
background in the functioning of each of the aspects of the cath lab and, preferably, should be someone who has actively worked in the laboratory prior to assuming this role. Depending on the size of the laboatory, the supervisor may
continue to work in an active clinical role. In a larger laboratory, it is generally
best that the administrator be full-time in that role.

If the lab supervisor is not in charge of patient flow, a separate *lab/
patient coordinator* may be used who is responsible for the day-to-day smooth
flow of patients through the lab. In addition to scheduling of procedures to be
performed, this coordinator must stay in touch with the schedules of the physicians, the changes in patient status that would influence catheterization orders,
staffing changes, or any other situation that may affect the flow of patients
through the lab.

In a large laboratory, we have found that there is an advantage to also
having a *clinical specialist*. This is a professional nurse with advanced cardiovascular training. The specialist uses this expertise to orient new personnel to conduct inservices, to act as a resource person for the staff, and to assist in emergency situations. By also functioning as a staff nurse, this individual provides an

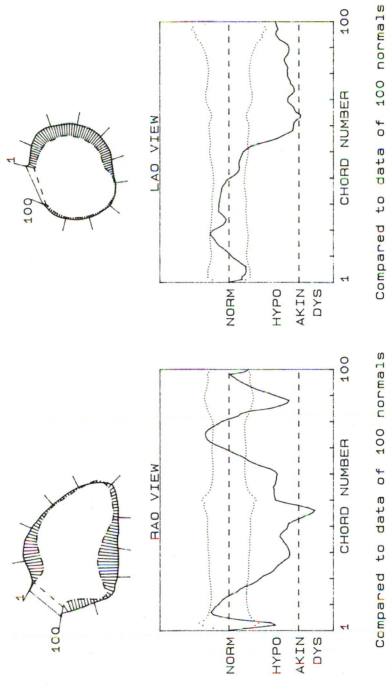

Figure 2–4. Representative ventriculographic report. The RAO view of end-diastole and end-systole is shown in upper left, and the LAO view is shown in upper right. One hundred chords are drawn around the ventricle and the amount of movement of each chord is plotted in the lower graphs. No motion is considered akinesia (AKIN); bulging or negative motion is dyskinesia (DYS); and less-than-normal motion is hypokinesia (HYPO). The dotted line defines a normal range of motion; each chord can thus be defined in terms of this normal range.

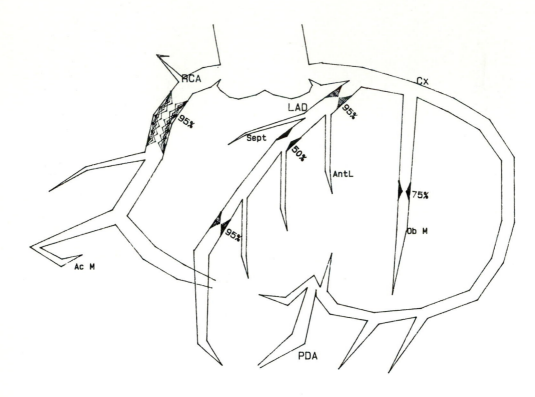

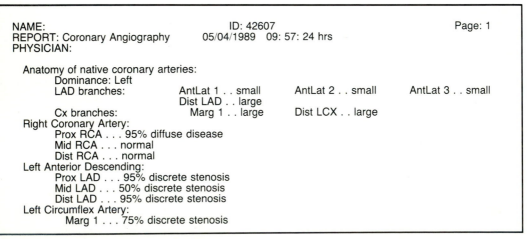

NAME: ID: 42607   Page: 1
REPORT: Coronary Angiography   05/04/1989   09: 57: 24 hrs
PHYSICIAN:

Anatomy of native coronary arteries:
    Dominance: Left
    LAD branches: AntLat 1 . . small   AntLat 2 . . small   AntLat 3 . . small
                    Dist LAD . . large
    Cx branches: Marg 1 . . large   Dist LCX . . large
Right Coronary Artery:
    Prox RCA . . . 95% diffuse disease
    Mid RCA . . . normal
    Dist RCA . . . normal
Left Anterior Descending:
    Prox LAD . . . 95% discrete stenosis
    Mid LAD . . . 50% discrete stenosis
    Dist LAD . . . 95% discrete stenosis
Left Circumflex Artery:
    Marg 1 . . . 75% discrete stenosis

Figure 2–5. Representative coronary-tree report generated by a computer touch screen. Each lesion and vessel is recorded both visually and in text mode for ready interpretation and recall.

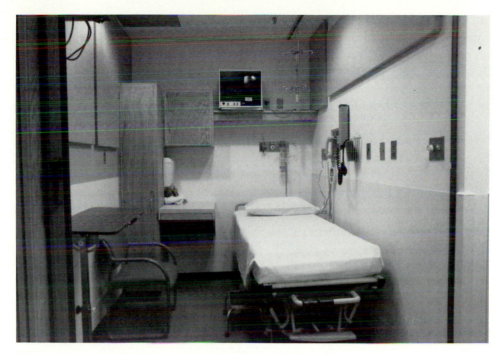

Figure 2–6. Representative outpatient holding room. Note monitor, oxygen and suction, BP cuff, locker for patient clothes, convenient counter, and comfortable but moveable bed. Buttons on the right wall are part of an emergency alarm system that alerts the main cath lab or nearby coronary care unit if a problem arises. A TV is mounted near ceiling on the left; wooden folding doors provide privacy.

important clinical liaison and can be especially valuable when new trainees are in the laboratory.

A thorough understanding of the instrumentation and radiographic technique is important for the position of *technician specialist*. In cooperation with individual service personnel, this specialist is responsible for routine care, maintenance, and trouble-shooting of the equipment used routinely in the lab. The individual provides the link between the laboratory and the company service representatives. In some institutions, there may be a single individual in this role for the entire cardiology department.

The *professional nurse* in the lab is primarily responsible for the ongoing assessment and care of the patient undergoing catheterization. A solid background and experience in intensive coronary care is beneficial. The nurse should be able to identify important ECG changes, have knowledge of the disease states being evaluated, and know how to respond to hemodynamic or electrophysiologic crises. Other duties include functioning as scrub nurse, maintaining the sterile field where appropriate, obtaining hemostasis after catheterization, and patient education.

Monitoring technicians constantly measure and appropriately record physiologic data during the procedure. Although it is preferable that these individuals have training as x-ray technicians, this is not possible in most locations. Most importantly, the technician must be alert to any change in patient status and any abnormal hemodynamic finding. Other duties include blood-gas evaluation, knowledge of sterile technique, entry of appropriate data into any record-keeping system, and familiarity with video recording systems.

The assurance of high-quality cinefilm processing is the responsibility of the *darkroom technician*. In smaller laboratories, this individual is usually one of the monitoring technicians as well. A thorough background in photographic technique is important. Calibration and maintenance of processing are essential, and development of a well-defined quality-control program should be a high priority.

Maintenance of catheterization equipment, storage, ordering, and sterilization may be the responsibility of one of the previously mentioned staff. In high-volume facilities, a separate position may be needed for these tasks.

In many labs, nurses and technicians cross-train in order to maintain a smooth-functioning lab when mandated by staffing patterns. In complex cases, however, it is necessary that the most qualified personnel be available to insure that patient needs are met. This is especially the case when interventional, pediatric, or electrophysiologic procedures are undertaken.

All staff members involved with patient care should maintain current cardiopulmonary resuscitation (CPR) certification. Advanced cardiac life support (ACLS) certification is also desirable.

Patient Flow

In a large-volume cath lab, a system that facilitates a steady, even flow of patients with a minimum of delay is necessary. Turnaround time in the laboratory must be kept to a minimum (less than 10 min). This can be best accomplished by having the next patient waiting in the catheterization lab area, by using disposable items, and by removing catheters in a holding room.

Inpatients should be evaluated by a physician or PA the day prior to catheterization or early enough the same day to assess laboratory data and make any necessary change in pretreatment. Routine precatheterization orders should generally be available to prevent overlooking important items (see Chapter 3). The patient should be transported to the lab with an attempt to minimize the waiting period after arriving in the lab. At all times, the patient must be in an area in which qualified personnel are readily available should the patient require assistance.

During catheterization, every effort should be made to insure the patient's comfort and safety. Explanation of unusual occurrences helps to decrease anxiety. Respect for patients' rights must be observed at all times.

Transfer to a post-catheterization holding facility enables labs to be utilized maximally. Catheters can be removed in the holding room by qualified personnel, and appropriate pressure to the catheter site can be applied, manually or mechanically, until hemostasis has occurred. In the holding room, one method of hemostasis that has been used with good success is the pressure clamp (see Fig. 3–4). The clamp should be applied as shown in Figure 3–5, with pressure maximally directed above the skin incision site and proximal to the arterial puncture. When properly applied, some blood flow should still be present, and distal pulses should be palpable. In general, the clamp should remain in place a full 10 min.

Patient education can be started in the holding area or once he is back on the floor. Instruction regarding maintenance of hemostasis by immobilization of the affected limb and direct pressure to the puncture site should be provided by the holding-room nurse. Any pertinent information about the patient's condition should be communicated directly to the nurse who is directly involved in follow-up care for that patient.

CHAPTER 3

The Preparation and Care of the Patient and the Laboratory

Paul Owens, RN, RCVT, and Thomas M. Bashore, MD

John Baker, a 54-year-old business executive, has been experiencing fatigue and tiredness. He has also noticed a squeezing feeling in his chest and neck during stressful business meetings. He decides to make an appointment with his family doctor. They discuss the possibility that heart disease is the cause of John's symptoms. John's exercise tolerance test is positive for myocardial ischemia. He also smokes one to two packs of cigarettes a day and is 20 lb overweight. His physician recommends that John undergo a cardiac catheterization. The catheterization shows severe three-vessel coronary artery disease. John is scheduled for coronary artery bypass surgery.

Sarah Jenkins, an 88-year-old retired schoolteacher, has been diagnosed as having severe aortic stenosis. Although in otherwise good health, she does not want to undergo open heart surgery. Her cardiologist recommends an aortic balloon valvuloplasty to relieve her worsening symptoms of heart failure. At heart catheterization, the peak-to-peak aortic gradient is 88 mm Hg, and the calculated valve area 0.5 cm^2. After the valvuloplasty procedure, the gradient is reduced to 40 mm Hg and the valve area increased to 1.0 cm^2. After a few days in the hospital, she is able to return home with a noticeable reduction in her symptoms, although she will need re-evaluation periodically because of the high rate of re-stenosis after these procedures.

Carol Sayer, a 54-year-old housewife, was admitted to the Coronary Care Unit with an acute myocardial infarction. Her physician administers streptokinase intravenously, with resolution of some of the electrocardiographic (ECG) changes. She is stabilized on intravenous nitroglycerine and intravenous heparin overnight, with no further chest pain. Her catheterization the next morning reveals a 95 percent blockage in her right coronary artery. Carol's physicians recommend that she undergo a percutaneous transluminal coronary angioplasty (PTCA) because of continued pain, and she agrees to the procedure. The procedure is performed electively the following day and without complications. The vessel diameter percent obstruction is reduced from 95 percent to 25 percent. Two days later, Carol goes home. She is soon able to resume her normal activities.

These examples illustrate the valuable information cardiac catheterization provides about the heart. With new invasive therapeutic procedures available, such as PTCA, alternatives to surgery and medical therapy can also be provided during catheterization.

Undergoing a cardiac catheterization is an obvious stressful experience for the patient. This stress can be reduced by providing information to the patient about what he is likely to experience during the catheterization, and why the catheterization is being done. This chapter is intended to provide an approach to the patient that has proved to be effective in our institution. It describes not only the care of the patient, but also of the laboratory itself.

Before Catheterization

Preparation of Patient

Although it is desirable that a nurse or technician from the catheterization department visit the patient beforehand, it is more likely that preprocedural teaching will be undertaken by the floor or CCU nurse. Many excellent audiovisual programs and information booklets are available. If you use these, check your hospital's protocols, because commerical products may differ substantially. Better yet, design and produce your own patient-education materials.

It is the physician's responsibility to inform the patient of the risks associated with the procedure, such as stroke, myocardial infarction, loss of pulse or circulation to the leg or arm, rhythm changes, allergic reactions, and even death. He will give a brief explanation of the procedure to the patient, and obtain the consent for the catheterization. Routine studies such as a complete blood count, electrolytes, coagulation studies, a lipid profile, chest radiograph, and a 12-lead ECG are frequently done prior to the procedure. Women of childbearing age should be asked about the possibility of pregnancy. A pregnancy test should be ordered when appropriate.

Patients are usually given nothing by mouth for about 6 hr or more prior to catheterization to prevent aspiration should nausea and vomiting occur during the procedure. An intravenous line should be started in the left forearm for access. The left arm is used because it is opposite the s'de of the physician during the study. Patients may receive intravenous hydration or medication through this intravenous line both before, during, and after the procedure. If the patient has a history of difficulty urinating or if the procedure is to be prolonged, a Foley catheter (or condom catheter, in men) should be inserted in the urinary bladder prior to the procedure.

The patient should bring both his dentures and glasses to the procedure. This allows his speech to be heard clearly and enables him to see what is going on in the room. The noise from the cine camera may interfere with a hearing aid, so you should ask the patient if loud noises (like a vacuum cleaner) drown out voices. If the patient does not know English, an interpreter should explain the procedure and be present at the catheterization or set up appropriate, recognizable signals (such as holding the breath, coughing, and so forth).

Ask the patient if he is allergic to seafood, iodine, tape, Betadine, radiographic contrast, or any other medications. The radiographic contrast contains iodine. If the patient is allergic, he has a fourfold greater chance of having a reaction than if he is not known to be allergic. Cimetadine (H_1) and Benadryl (H_2) blockers should be administered to the patient along with steroids (prednisone, or Solu-Medrol) prior to the study if contrast allergy is a concern.

If the patient is a diabetic on insulin, his insulin dose should be halved the morning of the study and D5/W used in the intravenous line. Patients with renal failure need hydration prior to and after the procedure to help keep the kidneys well perfused. Plasma expanders, such as mannitol, may also be used. Diuretics are frequently given in reduced dosage if the patient is not in heart failure, because the contrast agent will act as a diuretic following the catheterization. Prior to the procedure, the patient's groin and pubic area on the side to be used should be shaved over a large enough area to accommodate the drape opening.

The patient should be reminded that during the procedure, he will be asked to hold his breath in order to allow his diaphragm to move downward. This allows the heart to be better seen on fluoroscopy. He should be instructed to not bear down while holding his breath, because this will bring the diaphragm back into the picture. The x-ray room will be full of equipment, and it is kept dark so that x-ray screens can be seen. The room is also kept cool so that the equipment does not overheat. The x-ray equipment and table will also be moved around so that multiple views of the heart can be obtained. The patient should be aware of these situations.

Pre-catheterization orders are best standardized. Figure 3–1 shows the pre-catheterization orders used at Duke Medical Center. Your center may require modification of these.

Recent trends show a large increase in the number of catheterizations performed on an outpatient or same-day admission basis. The cardiologist's office will often send out an information booklet and information sheet for each outpatient. An example of such an information sheet is shown in Appendix 1. The patient should also bring with him any labwork or studies done recently by the local referring physician so that redundant studies are not done. Outpatients should be accompanied by a family member because they should not travel home alone after their procedure.

Patients who are being admitted to the hospital after the cardiac catheterization procedure need to arrive early enough to have their paperwork processed and any admission labwork or tests completed prior to catheterization. Spend

FORM
M05AA
Rev. 11-87

DUKE UNIVERSITY

MEDICAL CENTER

DOCTORS' ORDERS

PRE CARDIAC CATH ORDERS

(PATIENT IDENTIFICATION)

DATE	TIME	SEQ. ORD. #		DOCTORS' ORDERS	SINGLE AND STAT ORDERS CARRIED OUT	TIME GIVEN	DATE GIVEN/ INITIALS
				Cath scheduled for _____ .			
		1.		NPO past midnight except medications.			
		2.		Patient (may/may not) have light breakfast.			
		3.		Shave and prep (right/left) groin(s).			
		4.		18 gauge heparin lock in left forearm.			
		5.		IV Fluids (select one):			
			☐	a. None (Use heparin lock).			
			☐	b. 0.45% Normal Saline at _____ (rate).			
			☐	c. Other: _____ .			
				Begin fluids at _____ .			
		6.		Give to patient the Pre Cath Teaching Booklet.			
		7.		ON CALL TO CATH LAB:			
				a. Have patient void.			
				b. Pre-medication:			
			☐	1. None			
			☐	2. Benadryl 25mg IV			
			☐	3. _____			
				c. Dress in hospital gown only.			
		8.		Please have House Officer co-sign.			
				_____ M.D.			
				(Beeper # _____)			

FORM M05 B REV. 12/83
5 PART

Figure 3–1. Representative orders prior to cardiac catheterization.

time with these patients so that they have the opportunity to express their fears and anxieties. They will appreciate your taking the time to explain what they may expect during their catheterization.

All patients should have an identity bracelet with their name, date of birth, medical record number, and physician's name. A pre-procedure checklist should be completed according to your hospital policy. The chart and chargeplate should be sent to the catheterization laboratory with the patient. The patient should void prior to being transported to the cath lab.

The patient is generally transported by stretcher, wheelchair, or in bed. Stretchers (Surgilifts) (Fig. 3–2) are available that fit over standard hospital beds and standard radiographic tables and allow for minimal patient jostling during transportation. These stretchers use a sturdy pad, which is placed under the patient. Straps attached to the pad are then secured into the stretcher frame. The patient can then be easily lowered or raised with the minimum of effort for both patient and staff.

Patients who are receiving oxygen therapy, intravenous therapy, or cardiac monitoring require extra care during transportation. Make sure that portable oxygen tanks, infusion devices, and cardiac monitors are carried securely and safely, without causing discomfort or danger to the patient. Patients with supportive-care devices such as respirators or an intra-aortic balloon pump may require the assistance of specialized personnel, such as respiratory therapists, perfusion techs, and CCU nurses. Always have sufficient personnel to transport the patient and any necessary equipment safely.

Preparation of Cardiac Catheterization Room

The catheterization rooms, including the overhead equipment such as monitors and x-ray equipment, must be cleaned daily. Other equipment in regular use, such

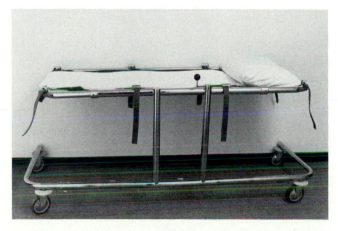

Figure 3–2. Stretchers (Surgilifts) allow transfer of the patient with minimal movement of the catheterization site.

as armboards, intravenous poles, injectors, stretchers and pads, x-ray shields, and so forth should be wiped down daily or when contamination by body fluids occurs. Your hospital's infection-control department can advise you as to the appropriate cleaning and disinfecting agents available.

Equipment in the room should be switched on and allowed to reach working temperature before the patient enters. Required self tests or calibrations should be run at this time, the fluoro and cine systems checked, and any film-quality assurance protocols performed before the first patient enters.

The emergency equipment should also be checked daily. If your cardiac-arrest cart is a sealed unit provided by the pharmacy department, these are often kept current by the pharmacists. If you have an open cart in the lab, then the drug expiratory dates, intravenous-fluid expiration dates, and the laryngoscope batteries and bulbs should be checked daily. This could be facilitated by keeping an expiratory date sheet. The defibrillator should be checked according to the manufacturer's instructions. It is a good idea to keep a sign-off sheet to document these daily checks. The cart must also have paddle gel or gel pads, ambubag and attachments, oral and endotracheal airways, and intravenous administration equipment.

If you have piped-in oxygen and vacuum, make sure you keep the attachments clean and operational. If you use portable oxygen tanks and portable suction units, make sure they are checked daily along with the emergency equipment. You should keep respiratory supplies in each room, including nasal cannula, connecting tubing, connectors, ventimasks, and two rebreather masks. You will also need connecting tubing, suction catheters, and suction handles. Some vacuum systems require disposable liners as well.

Trash cans kept in the rooms should be covered, as should the linen bin. Items for resterilization should be rinsed and stored for collection by the sterile-processing department. Trash and linen should be collected in a timely fashion by the environmental services department. Each room should have one or more containers for the disposal of sharp items such as needles, scalpel blades, and so forth.

In order to record the patient's name tag on cinefilm, you should tape the tag onto the image intensifier. It is best to lay a lead collar or gown across the tube to prevent x-ray overload. Imaging the name tag over the patient's body during the study results in unnecessary exposure to the patient.

The catheterization tray is set up prior to each case. Two people wearing scrub masks should open and prepare the tray. The person preparing the tray should also wear sterile gloves and, at most centers, a sterile gown. Scrub suits or uniforms are useful so that no loose or hanging clothing can come into contact with the sterile tray.

Care of Patient During Catheterization

The patient should be warmly welcomed on his arrival to the lab. Each member of the staff should introduce himself and explain his role in the laboratory. The armband should be checked again against the chart and cath-lab schedule. The chart and checklist can then be screened, and the cath-lab data sheets completed. The patient can be assigned a lab number that identifies the cinefilm and study data.

When taking the patient into the procedure room, remind him that it will be cooler. You can usually make patients feel more at ease by asking them about themselves—i.e., about their job, family, where they live, and so forth. Try and prepare the patient for each activity before it happens—"We're going to put some ECG patches on your chest now," or "I'm just connecting some IV fluid to your IV now." The patient will respond positively, and cooperate more fully. Do not ignore the patient and engage in unrelated conversations with other staff members. Maintain a professional decorum. Remember—the patient has little else to do while waiting than listen to your conversations. And listen he will!

Try to maintain the patient's privacy and safety when transferring him to the x-ray table. Use a stepstool for ambulatory patients, and support the patient while he gets onto the table. Patients brought to the lab on a standard stretcher or bed are usually brought into the room alongside the x-ray table. The brakes are locked, and the patient is assisted onto the table. A Surgilift device may be used to help transfer the patient. Some x-ray tables are quite narrow, and the patient will need help to get correctly positioned. Make sure the patient feels comfortable and secure. You may need to adjust the patient's pillow by doubling it over. Patients with heart failure may not be able to lie flat. A radiographic foam wedge can be used to elevate the patient's head enough for him to breathe more easily. Patients will not be able to sit up much higher than 20 to 30 degrees though, as this will interfere with the positioning of the x-ray camera.

You should check the intravenous site for signs of inflammation or infiltration or improper flow. It is important that the patient have a patent intravenous line during the procedure. If the patient arrives without a viable intravenous line, one should be started in the cath lab. Many hospitals require that personnel attend an inservice program and be certified before they can start intravenous lines.

Any further medications ordered by the physician can be administered through the Y-stoppers on the intravenous tubing, or through the stopcock. Several medications used often in the cath lab (e.g., Lasix) cause a burning sensation. Others (e.g., Benadryl, Ativan, Valium) cause drowsiness. You should tell the patient what to expect before you administer any medication.

The patient may come with several medications already infusing. The mixture of incompatible drugs can cause harm to the patient. The easiest way to avoid any incompatability problems is to have a separate intravenous line with only normal saline infusing through it and to use this line for administering drugs during the procedure.

The patient's heart rate and rhythm will be monitored throughout the procedure. Three to five electrodes are usually placed on the patient's upper body. If you use radiolucent electrodes and leads, they can be placed anywhere on the chest and abdomen. If you use metal electrodes, place them on the back of the shoulders and hips. A baseline ECG may be obtained at this time. Make sure the leads are positioned so that they don't interfere with cineangiography or get caught on the x-ray table. Mark the patient's distal pulses before the procedure and note their strength in case a problem in blood supply occurs after the procedure.

Any other medical equipment required to support the patient should be positioned so that, as far as is practical, it does not interfere with the range of movement of the x-ray table or the x-ray equipment. If personnel from other departments are required to stay with the patient during the procedure, make sure they are properly protected against radiation. Keep electrical cords out of traffic areas.

If the physician is using the femoral approach, the patient's genital area should be covered with a folded towel that is taped in place. This will protect this sensitive area from the prep solutions and provide privacy for the patient. Whether you are prepping the arm or the groin, swab from the center towards the perimeter.

Cleansing and sterilization of the site should be done with an antiseptic such as Betadine, Hibiclens, or isopropyl alcohol. Most laboratories use a prepackaged sponge kit. Remember to use an alternative to the iodine-containing prep solutions when you are with patients who are allergic to iodine.

The circulating person in the room should insure that the connections between the transducers and flush solution are adequately flushed and free of bubbles. The system is then zeroed to the level of the patient's right atrium. In practical terms, this is the midaxillary line. The room is then semidarkened. During ventriculography, the patient should be told that the power injections of contrast media will feel warm, and he may feel the sensation of urination. Check frequently with the patient. Let him know his approximate progress throughout the study.

Complications during catheterization are covered in detail in Chapter 6. If the patient complains of nausea, ask the patient to take slow, deep breaths. A cool washcloth across the forehead or an ice pack behind the neck may help (at least psychologically). Emesis basins should be readily available in the room, along with antiemetic drugs. Turn the patient's head to the side if he feels as if he is going to vomit. Offer the patient water or mouthwash to rinse his mouth with afterwards.

Arrhythmias can arise in the cath lab for a variety of reasons. Bradycardia is common when one is using ionic contrast for coronary injections. Coughing raises intrathoracic pressure, and this is translated to a rise in the arterial pressure that can maintain blood pressure even during ventricular fibrillation. Coughing allows for emergency equipment to be prepared or medications to be administered. The patient should practice coughing before coronary angiography.

Chest pain can occur during angiography. This usually resolves within a few moments after the coronary injection is completed. Prolonged chest or anginal pain should be appropriately treated.

The patient who is experiencing chest pain will be frightened and anxious. It is important to reassure the patient, and to explain any therapy or treatment and how it will help relieve the pain he is experiencing. Let the patient assign a number to the chest pain severity of between 1 and 10 (1 = barely noticeable, 10 = worst pain ever experienced) so that the effectiveness of any intervention can be measured.

Patients with a history of back problems may benefit from having an "egg-crate" mattress placed on the x-ray table. They may also require a strategically placed rolled towel or sheet under the small of the back or under the knees to help feel more comfortable. These patients may also require medication to help them relax and control pain.

Care of Patient Following Catheterization

At the end of the procedure, the patient should be given a brief preliminary report of the cath findings by the physician. The catheters are then removed, and pressure applied over the groin. It is more efficient if the catheters or sheaths are flushed with the heparinized flush solution and the patient transferred to a holding area, where the removal process can be performed. This allows for more rapid turnover of the main catheterization room.

Procedural documentation should be completed on a specific procedural data form. Be sure to include complications (a representative form is shown in Fig. 3–3). This will include amount of x-ray exposure time, amount of contrast used, amount of intravenous fluids administered, and any complications that occurred during the procedure. The time the patient leaves the room and any catheters or sheaths to be left indwelling are also recorded.

In the case of a Sones approach, a sterile pressure dressing is placed over the site, and the patient's arm is kept straight for at least 1 hr. The patient may be taken directly back to his room for observation. Using the femoral approach, either hand pressure or a clamp system (Fig. 3–4) should be applied just above the arterial skin-puncture site. Once the correct position has been obtained, enough pressure should be maintained to stop bleeding while permitting blood flow to the distal portion of the limb (Fig. 3–5). Direct pressure is usually applied for at least 10 to 15 min. Pressure is then released slowly, and the site is observed for any signs of bleeding. If bleeding continues, pressure should be reapplied for an additional 5 to 10 min. This is repeated until the bleeding has stopped. Bleeding that lasts for more than 30 min should be reported to the physician. If the patient was given heparin, an activated clotting time should be done. If the ACT is greater than 325, then protamine may be given to reverse the effects of the heparin. If no bleeding is observed, the site is cleansed, a topical antibiotic cream applied, and the site covered with a Bandaid or small sterile dressing. Some institutions will also place a pressure dressing over the site. This should be applied in such a way that the site can still be observed for bleeding or hematoma.

Should a hematoma form, the margins should be outlined in ink and a time recorded so that changes in the size of the hematoma can be assessed. Hematomas that continue to increase in size despite direct pressure should be re-

DUKE MEDICAL CENTER
CATHETERIZATION PROCEDURE FORM

DATE: ___ / ___ / ___   Consent Signed: Y N   Age: _____

A. Preliminary Data:

ROOM # _____   CINE FILM # _____   PREVIOUS DUKE CATH: Y   N

Patient Arrived at ___:___   12-Lead ECG at ___:___   *Known* Allergies _____

Lab Personnel: In Room _____   Control Room _____

                  Holding _____

Physicians: Attending _____   Fellow _____

Patient Data: Ht. _____   Wt. _____   BSA _____   Last Temp. _____   HR _____

                 BP _____ / _____

Pedal Pulses: (R) DP _____   PT _____   (L) DP _____   PT _____

                 Starting HR _____   Starting BP _____ / _____

LABS: PT _____   PTT _____   Platelets _____   Hgb _____   Hct _____   BS _____   K⁺ _____

         BUN _____   Cr _____   Triglyceride _____   Total Cholesterol _____   HDL Cholesterol _____

Premed: ( ) Benadryl _____ mg IM IV PO   ( ) Valium _____ mg IV IM   ( ) Other _____

Anesthesia: ( ) Xylocaine 1%   ( ) Other _____

B. Condition at Completion of Study:

Time Left Room ___:___   Time Left Holding Area _____

Transportation _____

Catheters Left in Place: ( ) None   ( ) Sheath-artery

                            ( ) Sheath-vein   ( ) Pacemaker   ( ) IABP

                            ( ) Arterial line   ( ) Swan-Ganz   ( ) Reperfusion catheter

Patient Returned to: ( ) Ward   ( ) CCU   ( ) Outpatient unit

Patient Transferred to: ( ) Ward   ( ) ICU   ( ) OR   ( ) ICC Lab   ( ) DCGH   ( ) EXP   ( ) ER

Patient's Condition: ( ) Stable   ( ) Other _____

C. Remarks Relevant to Future Catheterization:

_____

rev. 5/87

Figure 3–3. Procedural form (Part 1).

ported to the physician. With a small hematoma, a sandbag or pressure dressing may be applied. These simply tend to remind the patient to remain still, so one should not rely upon these methods to prevent further hemorrhage. One should still observe the site frequently for changes in size of hematoma. The site should be auscultated once there is no further bleeding. A bruit may imply either a pseudoaneurysm or arteriovenous fistula.

The most difficult type of bleeding to detect is called "retroperitoneal bleeding." There may be no directly observable signs of bleeding in the retroperitoneal space, although flank ecchymosis may occasionally be seen. Bleeding is

D. Protocol Data:

Heart Rate During Angio #1 _____

Angio #2 _____

Heart Rate During Fick _____

A.P.:   SID _____   Angles _____

LAT.   SID _____   Angles _____

Table Ht _____   Atrial Ht _____

Fluro Time: AP: _____   LATERAL _____

E. Contrast:

	Amount	Chamber	Flow Rate
Angio #1			
Angio #2			
Angio #3			

Total Renografin Used: _____   Lot # _____

Total Isovue Used: _____   Lot # _____

F. I.V. Fluids

Type   Amount

_____   _____

_____   _____

G. Medications:

Medication	Time	Dose	Route	Medication	Time	Dose	Route

H. Complications:

( ) None   Time   Time   Time

1. Arrhythmias

  ( ) Sustained VT __:__

  ( ) VF __:__

  ( ) Severe bradycardia (< 40) __:__

  ( ) Supraventricular __:__

  ( ) Heart block (2° or 3°) __:__

2. Hemodynamic

  ( ) Sustained hypotension __:__

  ( ) Pulmonary edema __:__

  ( ) Tamponade __:__

3. Ischemic

  ( ) Angina __:__

  ( ) Prolonged pain __:__

  ( ) Acute MI __:__

4. Vascular

  ( ) Coronary occlusion __:__

  ( ) Coronary dissection __:__

  ( ) Coronary embolus __:__

  ( ) Loss of pulse __:__

  ( ) Decreased pulse __:__

  ( ) Hematoma __:__

5. Allergic reaction

  ( ) Hives/urticaria __:__

  ( ) Bronchospasm __:__

  ( ) Anaphylaxis __:__

6. Neurologic

  ( ) Stroke __:__

  ( ) TIA __:__

7. Other

  ( ) Vomiting __:__

  ( ) Aspiration __:__

  ( ) Respiratory arrest __:__

  ( ) Clot on catheter tip __:__

  ( ) Clotted syringe __:__

  ( ) _____ __:__

8. Death __:__

Reviewed by: _____

Figure 3–3. Procedural form (Part 2).

detected indirectly by monitoring the patient's vital signs and hemoglobin and hematocrit. A patient who is bleeding will experience an increase in heart rate, a decrease in blood pressure, and increasing pallor. Similar symptoms can also occur as a result of contrast-induced diuresis, so this should not be confused with bleeding.

When the bleeding has been controlled and the site dressing applied, the patient can be transported back to his room. It is important to teach the patient the precautions that he should follow for the next several hours after catheteriza-

I. Procedures:

1. Arterial access site(s): _____

2. Venous access site(s): _____

3. Sheaths: _____

Procedures performed:	Time started	Catheter(s) (including gauge and size)
1. L. heart catheterization	___:___	
2. L. ventriculogram	___:___	_____
3. L. coronary angiograms	___:___	_____
4. R. coronary angiograms	___:___	_____
5. Bypass graft angiograms	___:___	_____
6. IMA angiograms	___:___	_____
7. R. heart catheterization	___:___	_____
8. R. ventriculogram	___:___	_____
9. PA arteriogram	___:___	_____
10. R. atrial angiogram	___:___	_____
11. L. atrial angiogram	___:___	_____
12. Oximetry run	___:___	
13. Fick cardiac output	___:___	
14. Thoracic aortogram	___:___	_____
15. Abdominal aortogram	___:___	_____
16. Ergonovine study	___:___	(dose) _____
17. Gastrograffin swallow	___:___	
18. Endomyocardial bx	___:___	_____
19. Transseptal cath.	___:___	_____
20. IHSS drug study	___:___	
21. Pulmonary HBP drug study	___:___	
22. Pacemaker insertion	___:___	_____
23. IABP	___:___	_____
24. Cardioversion	___:___	
25. Defibrillation	___:___	
26. CPR	___:___	
27. Intubation	___:___	
28. Balloon valvuloplasty	___:___	_____
		_____
		_____
		_____
		_____
		_____
		_____
		_____
29. Hemodynamic study	___:___	_____
30. PTCA	___:___	_____
31. RPC inserted	___:___	_____
32. Other _____	___:___	_____
33. Digital angiograms:	( ) Y ( ) N	

Figure 3–3. Procedural form (Part 3).

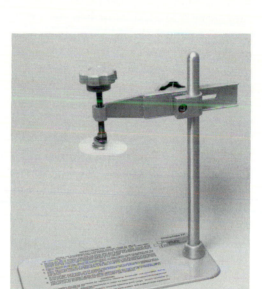

Figure 3–4. Clamp.

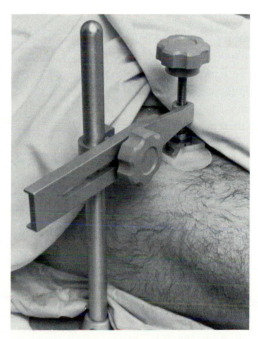

Figure 3–5. Clamp shown applied over the right femoral puncture site.

tion. Any activity that raises intra-abdominal pressure, such as coughing, sneezing, laughing, or passing urine into a urinal or bedpan, can cause bleeding to recur at the femoral site. The patient should be shown where to apply pressure to the groin and how firmly to apply pressure. If bleeding should recur at any time, the patient may feel pain or stinging at the site, or notice fresh bleeding. He should be told to apply pressure to the groin or arm and call for help. One should reassure the patient that direct pressure will be effective in controlling bleeding should it recur.

The patient's vital signs are monitored carefully in the post-procedural period. Routine post-catheterization orders are useful (Fig. 3–6). The vital signs should be monitored at least every 30 min for the first 3 hr, then hourly until the patient is allowed to get up. These checks should include pulse, blood pressure, catheterization-site distal pulses, color, temperature, and sensation.

Often patients with coronary artery disease also have peripheral vascular disease. In these patients, it is even more important to accurately document peripheral pulses prior to the catheterization study to establish a baseline. Patients with poor distal pulses may require the use of a Doppler stethoscope to determine the presence or absence of pulse. In the absence of a distal pulses, the patient's color, temperature, capillary refill, sensation, and movement (e.g., wiggling fingers or toes) should be carefully logged during the observational period.

The patient's head may be elevated 30 degrees for comfort. This makes it safer for drinking fluid and taking food and medications. After 2 hr or so, the patient may be turned from side to side (logrolled) to give skin care, change linens, and so forth.

Some patients experience difficulty passing urine while lying flat in bed. If bladder distension occurs, and the patient becomes uncomfortable, the physician should be notified. The doctor may order that a straight catheter or Foley catheter be inserted. The Foley catheter can be removed when the patient is ambulated.

The patient may be ambulated with assistance once the bed-rest time is up. For the newer catheters (5 or 6 French), the patient is usually ambulated in 3 hr, even when a femoral approach is used. It is a good idea to obtain sitting and standing blood pressures to rule out orthostatic hypotension. Most facilities ambulate patients 6 hr after the procedure when larger catheters are used.

Once the patient is up and feeling okay, encourage him to walk around in the room or in the hallway where he can be observed. Remind the patient to apply firm pressure over the site if he uses the bathroom. When standing, the patient should avoid any excessive bending or lifting for the next 24 to 48 hr. Showering should be avoided until the following morning. The site should be kept as dry as possible.

If sutures were used to close the skin incision following a Sones procedure, these are usually removed 4 to 5 days later. Suture removal may be done at the office of the patient's physician or in the outpatient clinic.

The care of the outpatient follows much the same routine, except that specific predischarge teaching and information on care of the catheterization site are given. Appendices 1 and 2 represent instructions given to outpatients at our

DUKE UNIVERSITY

MEDICAL CENTER

DOCTORS' ORDERS

(PATIENT IDENTIFICATION)

DATE	TIME	SEQ ORD #		DOCTORS' ORDERS	SINGLE AND STAT ORDERS CARRIED OUT	TIME GIVEN	DATE GIVEN/ INITIALS
				POST CARDIAC CATH ORDERS:			
		1		**VITAL SIGNS:** BP, pulse, and check			
				puncture site(s) (_____)			
				Q 15 min ×4, Q 30 min ×4, Q1 hr ×4			
				then resume routine vital signs.			
		2		**ACTIVITY:**			
				a. Strict bedside with leg(s) used for			
				cath straight until (_____)			
				b. May elevate head of bed up to 30 deg.			
				c. May log roll patient after two hours.			
		3		**MEDS:** Tylenol #3 2 tabs Q4H prn for pain			
				at cath site for headache.			
		4		**IV FLUIDS:** _____			
		5		**Call Cath Fellow (ID or ID 7606)**			
				for bleeding complications.			
		6		**Please have H.O. co-sign.**			
				_____M.D.			

FORM MO5 B REV. 12/83
5 PART

Figure 3–6. Representative orders after cardiac catheterization.

institution. If complications arise while he is traveling or after he arrives home, then he must have guidelines for the acute treatment of these complications or know where and how to seek help for more serious complications.

Other Issues of Quality Assurance

The following are major components of quality assurance that should be included in every catheterization laboratory:

1. Equipment and physical plant.
2. Patient care.
3. Staff training.

Equipment and Physical Plant

A program should be established that allows for periodic reporting of the status of the major equipment items in the cardiac cath lab. These items include the x-ray equipment, the hemodynamic-monitoring equipment, and the film-developing and cinefilm-projection facility.

In general, service contracts are obtained for all major items. Preventative maintenance schedules are available from the manufacturers and should be followed religiously.

The major in-house maintenance that is required on the equipment relates directly to film quality. Periodically, a line-pair phantom should be cined and the number of line pairs per inch counted to insure that resolution has not been degraded over time. These line-pair phantoms can be imaged with every film or on a daily or weekly basis, depending on the volume of cases. In addition, a sensitometry strip should be obtained at least once each day in the cinefilm-processing laboratory. A sensitometer is a small device that exposes a strip of film with a series of different light intensities. Thus, in a stepwise manner, a small strip of film is exposed with a range of different exposures. These different exposures are analyzed for film density using a densitometer. The plot of exposure versus density defines an S-shaped curve known as the H-and-D curve. The details of this are covered in Chapter 4.

The advantage of continuously monitoring the film exposure is that it allows one to know immediately whether changes in film quality are related to either the x-ray equipment or the cinefilm-processing equipment. If the H-and-D curve is altered, it implies that there has been a change in film processing. If cinefilm quality is poor, but the H-and-D curve has not been changed, then one assumes the x-ray equipment is at fault. The use of a simple line-pair phantom allows one to quickly observe whether resolution has changed. Using these two simple techniques, the film and x-ray system can be constantly monitored, and problems that might arise can be avoided before they impact on patient care.

Each hospital also has readily obtained guidelines regarding the quality assurance of major electrical equipment with the hospital, and these guidelines should be followed closely. In addition, each hospital has fire safety codes that are unique to individual hospitals. It should be understood that, although it is easy to stack equipment and carts in hallways when storage space is limited, clear access to the outside by two separate pathways is a universal fire code. The staff should be reminded that two corridors must always be clear. If a serious fire or other event arises that would require evacuation of staff or patients, a plan should be in place to effectively remove people from the premises. A periodic review of such a plan should be a regular part of quality assurance procedure.

Patient Care

Quality assurance of patient care is obviously of the utmost importance. It includes careful monitoring of the medical records and clinical reports, the appropriate input of financial data, and the use of an appropriate professional manner in the cath lab (reporting those invidivuals who are careless or inappropriate). For a cath lab to run efficiently, each member must feel part of a team; distractions resulting from horseplay or inappropriate conversations should be considered absolutely intolerable by every member of the staff.

Periodically, it is useful to monitor a series of patients to learn about their experience. We have found this particularly helpful when a new program, such as outpatient cardiac catheterization, is being established. A brief questionnaire should be sent to the patient to ask him directly about his experience. What generally occurs in this situation is that recurrent problems will be readily identified and can be addressed. In addition, many patients will be extraordinarily complimentary toward individuals, and these individuals should be similarly rewarded. Never underestimate the patient's perceptions of what is happening in the cath lab. Be aware that a patient who is being catheterized is always listening to the people surrounding him. His comfort and care are of the utmost importance. A periodic polling of patients with even a very simple questionnaire can be extremely revealing.

Staff Training

It is important that periodic educational courses be advanced for the staff. This creates numerous advantages. In particular, it alerts all of the staff to new procedures that are being performed and gives everyone a common ground from which to approach the problems that occur in the cath lab. We have found that a yearly course geared toward attempts at certifying everyone by a national certification board is very useful for providing general knowledge to the entire staff in the cath lab. This course not only focuses on new information but also reminds both the nurses and technicians in the laboratory of certain information that they may use less often. The credentialling boards provide a convenient goal for all of the technicians and nurses in the laboratory, and our hospital has provided financial incentive for the achievement of this goal.

In addition, it is important that periodic meetings of the staff take place with the supervisor and medical director. These should be scheduled meetings that occur at least weekly or biweekly. These meetings should be open season on the supervisor and medical director. Each staff member should feel at ease discussing problems that occur. The running of a laboratory of any size is substantially enhanced by having a continuing dialogue with administration and the physicians involved. Forums of this type allow problems to surface that can then be dealt with directly. These forums also allow for communication of any new problems or new procedures that may be instituted. This type of meeting should be held on a frequent basis and always at the same time. Scheduling this meeting at irregular intervals generally results in ineffective results. In a forum such as this, each staff member should be encouraged to discuss potential solutions. The meeting should end with definite decisions regarding each of the problems discussed.

Appendix I

Representative Outpatient Cardiac Catheterization Preparation Instructions

All of the staff and faculty in the Medical Center Cardiac Catheterization Laboratories welcome you. Accompanying this letter is a cardiac catheterization booklet that will describe in detail the catheterization procedures and what you should expect prior to, during, and following your heart catheterization. This booklet is yours to keep. On the last pages of the booklet are drawings of the heart that the physician may wish to use to explain the findings from the catheterization. Please familiarize yourself with this booklet, and feel free to ask questions about any aspect of your pending heart catheterization.

The Medical Center has been a national leader in the use of outpatient cardiac catheterization. We currently are performing over 25 heart catheterizations every day. About half of all of the cardiac catheterizations are performed on an outpatient basis. We have built an attractive outpatient area for you to stay in during your visit. This area is equipped with a comfortable bed, a television, and a phone should you desire to call home or your office. The nurses are specially trained in this area to assist you. The room will be your "home" while you are at the Medical Center. A locker is provided for you to store your clothes. The rooms are rather small, however, and there is only room for one family member other than yourself. We have provided a lounge in the main lobby of the Hospital for any other family members.

When you arrive at the Hospital, simply proceed to the main lobby. In the main lobby is an outpatient cardiac catheterization registration desk and the outpatient family waiting room. Go to the outpatient cardiac catheterization registration desk and check in. A member of the medical center staff will greet you and take down any information regarding insurance, etc. You may or may not need blood work prior to the catheterization procedure, and the forms for this will be filled out at this window also.

You will then be escorted to the outpatient cardiac catheterization suite, where you will be assigned a nurse and your own room.

In this room, the physicians and staff that will be participating in the cardiac catheterization procedure will greet you prior to the procedure. They will explain the procedure and results to you once the catheterization is completed. At 2 to 4 hr following the procedure, you will be asked to walk around to insure that no bleeding occurs at the site of the cath. You will then be discharged directly from the holding area.

At the Medical Center, we have now done several thousand outpatient cardiac catheterizations. We have found this to be a safe, efficient, and pleasant experience for the patient. Every effort will be made to make your stay comfortable. We appreciate the opportunity of caring for you, and fully realize our responsibility in providing optimal patient care. We understand that the evaluation of heart problems requires a team effort that involves both the staff and the patient. We feel we have the finest facility of its kind anywhere, and we want you to share our enthusiasm.

Appendix II

Representative Outpatient Cardiac Catheterization Instructions Following the Procedure

After the cardiac catheterization procedure has been completed, the attending physician will review the results with you. On occasion, complex results may not be completely available at the time you are ready to leave, and some arrangement will be made for you to receive these final results. You will be asked to walk around prior to going home to insure that no bleeding occurs at the site where the catheterization tubes were placed. On very rare occasions (approximately one in every 200 studies), bleeding will persist after the procedure, and you will require admission to the Medical Center overnight. Newer technology and new procedures have resulted in much less bleeding than in previous years, but you should be aware that occasionally this is a problem.

If bleeding occurs under the skin, discoloration and a large hematoma will form. These are generally not serious, but may be sore for several weeks after the procedure. The following is a checklist of recommended guidelines for you to follow after the catheterization:

1. If at all possible, it is best to have someone else drive you home. Although it is not uncommon that a patient drives himself home following the study, the risk of bleeding later on is increased, and it is preferable that someone drive you home.

2. While you are traveling home or to a local hotel, check the puncture site occasionally. If any oozing occurs or there is apparent swelling, firm pressure over the site will prevent further hematoma formation. You cannot hurt anything by pressing directly on the site. This pressure stops bleeding by allowing a small clot to form. If the bleeding continues after pressure has been tried for more than 30 minutes, proceed to the nearest Emergency Room, call your local physician, or notify the physicians listed below. If you notify your local physician or go to an Emergency Room, please have them call the doctor listed below so that we are aware that a bleeding problem has occurred.

3. If you should lose the feeling in your leg or foot after catheterization, it is equally important that you call the doctor listed below, proceed to the nearest Emergency Room, or contact your local physician. This might mean that a clot has formed in the artery to your leg, and this can be appropriately treated.

4. Pain at the site of the catheterization can generally be treated with a nonaspirin pain medication (such as Tylenol).

5. The cardiac catheterization x-ray material causes you to pass a considerable amount of urine. For that reason, you will be asked to drink plenty of liquids after the catheterization so that you do not become dehydrated.

6. To keep bleeding from occurring, you should also avoid heavy lifting or excess bending for at least 24 hours after the catheterization has been performed.

WHERE TO CALL IN CASE YOU HAVE A QUESTION OR THERE IS AN EMERGENCY:

Before 5:00 PM: Call the Cardiac Catheterization Laboratory at (XXX) XXX-XXXX and ask them to connect you with Dr. _____.

After 5:00 PM: Call (XXX) XXX-XXXX and ask the hospital operator to page Dr. _____ or the cardiac catheterization on-call physician. If you cannot reach anyone at these numbers, then you should call your attending physician at the Medical Center, Dr. _____, or the Director of the catheterization laboratory, (XXX) XXX-XXXX (beeper #XXXX).

We appreciate the opportunity of serving you in our outpatient facility. We are sensitive to your needs and concerns and want very much to let you know that your safety and well-being are our primary goal. If there is any problem that you wish to discuss or if you simply want to comment either positively or negatively about your experience in the outpatient cardiac catheterization laboratory, please don't hesitate to contact us. If you prefer to write, please write to:

Director, Cardiac Catheterization Laboratory
Box XXXX
The Medical Center, Your Town, Your State

CHAPTER 4

Angiographic Imaging Systems

Jack Cusma, PhD, and Laurence Spero, BSE

The X-ray System

The diagnostic information produced during the catheterization procedure is a result of the interaction between the x-rays used during image acquisition and the iodinated contrast material. The nature of the interaction between x-rays and the patient also determines the quality of the resulting images.

X-rays are a form of radiation known as electromagnetic radiation. Other types of electromagnetic radiation include radio waves, heat, visible light, and microwaves. Electromagnetic radiation is produced when charged particles are sped up or slowed down, resulting in the emission of waves traveling at the speed of light, which is 300,000,000 m per second. A diagram of a wave is shown in Figure 4–1. The wave appears as positions of alternating strong and weak intensity, all traveling to the right with velocity (v). The wave is characterized by its wavelength (λ), which is the distance in which the cycle repeats itself, measured in meters, and the frequency (f), which is measured in Hertz. The relationship between velocity, wavelength, and frequency is as follows:

$$\text{velocity (v)} = \text{wavelength } (\lambda) \times \text{frequency (f)}.$$

The electromagnetic spectrum is shown in Figure 4–2. The wavelengths corresponding to x-rays are in the range of 0.1 to 1.0 angstroms (A), where an A is 10^{-10} m.

In addition to being treated as a wave, an x-ray can be considered to be a particle traveling at the velocity mentioned previously. For most purposes encountered in diagnostic x-ray imaging, this view is sufficient for explaining the

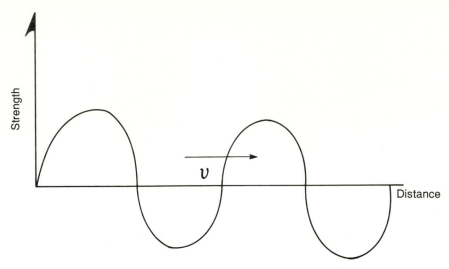

Figure 4–1. Diagram of a wave moving with velocity *v* showing the variation in strength as a function of position.

properties of x-rays. In this way, a single x-ray can be defined as a particle having an energy that is inversely proportional to its wavelength:

$$\text{energy} \, \alpha \, \frac{1}{\text{wavelength}} \, \text{m}.$$

The shorter the wavelength, the higher the energy. The energy is measured in units called "kiloelectron volts" (keV).

Production of X-rays

X-rays are produced when the speed of charged particles is changed. Diagnostic x-rays used in the catheterization laboratory are produced when fast-moving electrons collide with a tungsten metal target. As the electrons come to a stop, they give up their energy in the form of x-ray radiation. This process is termed *Bremsstrahlung*, which means "braking radiation." The energy of the x-rays ranges from 0 keV up to the entire energy of the electron before collision (e.g., 100 keV). Thus, the x-ray beam is called a "100 kVp beam" because its *peak* energy is 100 keV. This continuous range in x-ray energies is demonstrated in Figure 4–3, which shows a typical x-ray spectrum.

The entire process, which consist of speeding up the electron beam, slowing it down, and the emission of x-rays, takes place in an x-ray tube, which is shown schematically in Figure 4–4. The entire assembly is contained in a glass tube from which all air has been removed. If a vacuum did not exist, the electrons would collide with the air molecules and never reach the target.

The source of the initially slow electrons is called the "cathode," which

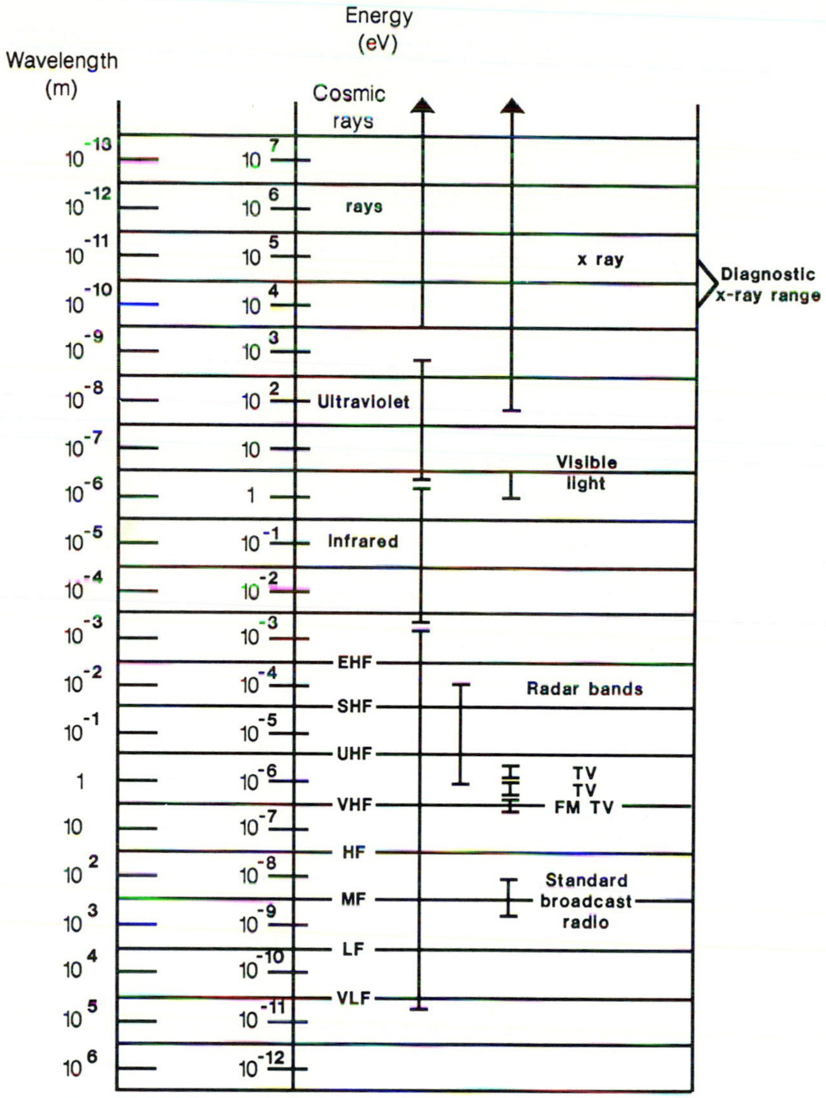

Figure 4–2. The regions of the electromagnetic spectrum.

consists of a wire filament made out of tungsten that is similar to the filament found in a standard light bulb. The heating of the filament to a high temperature results in electrons "boiling" off, ready to be drawn towards the target. The hotter the filament, the more electrons are available for the electron beam. The *number* of electrons flowing per second from the filament to the target is measured in milliamperes (mA).

Placing the filament at a negative voltage and the target at positive voltage causes the boiled-off electrons to be quickly pulled towards the target. The energy they have just before they collide with the target is just the voltage differ-

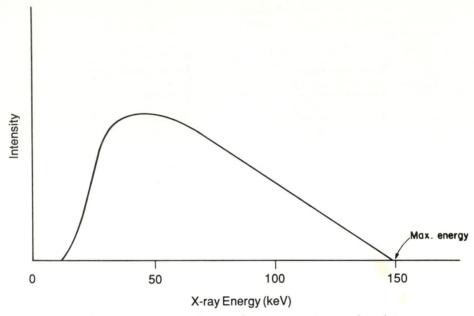

Figure 4–3. The continuous spectrum of x-ray energies produced in an x-ray tube.

ence between the filament and target (e.g., if the difference is 100,000 V [100 kV], the electrons have an energy of 100 keV). Electrons always flow in one direction (from the cathode to the target anode) because they are attracted to the positive voltage at the target.

Most x-ray tubes used in the catheterization laboratory actually have two filaments, one wire being smaller than the other. The small filament, which is about 0.6 mm in size, is used when sharper images are desired. Extensive use at the higher heating temperatures required to produce higher intensity beams, however, results in more rapid vaporization of the small filament. Thus, the larger filament, which is approximately 1.2 mm in size, is commonly used.

Two special features of the modern x-ray tube are apparent from Figure 4–5. First, it is apparent that the anode is tilted at an angle relative to the axis of the tube. This demonstrates the *line-focus principle*, which permits a larger area to be used to produce the x-rays while keeping the apparent size of the focal spot or x-ray source small. This is possible because of the tilt of the target to the axis by an angle of around 10 to 20 degrees.

Another feature of modern x-ray tubes is the fact that the target anode, made of tungsten as well, is actually much larger than the focal-spot area. The target is rotated at speeds of 3500 rpm to spread out the heat over a larger amount of material. Otherwise, if a single spot were used, that region would quickly become too hot and would limit the number of x-rays that could be continuously produced. A modern tube used in the catheterization laboratory would be expected, under normal use, to last approximately 2,000 hr.

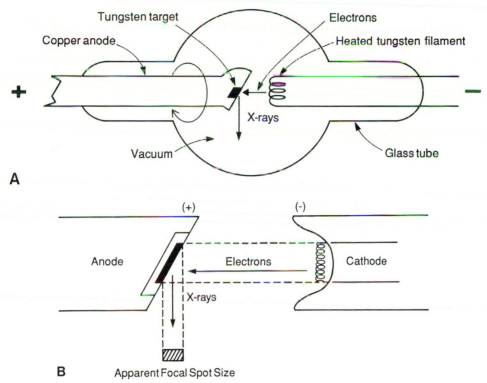

Figure 4–4. A, Schematic diagram of an x-ray tube. *B,* Example of the line-focus principle.

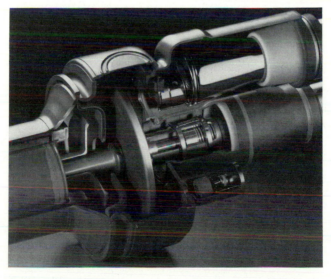

Figure 4–5. Cutaway view of a current design x-ray tube showing the target anode and cathode assembly. (Courtesy of Philips Medical Systems, Shelton, CT.)

X-ray Intensity

The x-ray intensity is a product of the number of x-rays that are produced by the target and the energy of each x-ray. To provide adequate diagnostic information, the intensity required must be high enough to produce enough x-rays passing through the patient to produce a large signal on an x-ray detector.

Several measures determine the x-ray intensity. The greater the number of electrons that collide with the target, the greater the number of x-rays produced. This number is the product of the number of electrons boiled off (mA) and the length of time, or exposure time, that the electrons are accelerated (measured in milliseconds). The product is measured in milliamperes. A doubling in the mA results in twice the number of x-rays being produced. Alternatively, the x-ray intensity can be increased by raising the voltage difference across the x-ray tube (kVp). This results in electrons with more energy, which then produce more x-rays when they collide with the target. In general, the automatic-exposure control used in modern catheterization laboratories varies both the mAs and the kVp to provide enough intensity to the film or other detector. Figure 4–6 shows how changing either the mA or kVp affects the intensity and wavelength of the x-rays in the beam. A change in wavelength corresponds to a change in energy of each x-ray.

X-ray Generators

The x-ray generator is the device that supplies the electrical power to the x-ray tube. This enables the x-ray tube to boil electrons off of the filament wire and then to accelerate the electrons towards the target. In most procedures encoun-

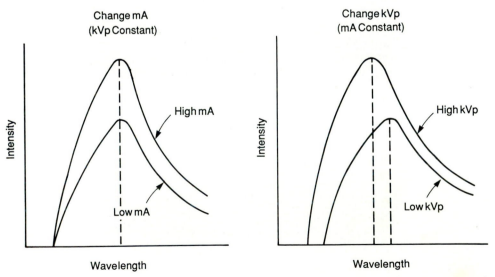

Figure 4–6. The change in x-ray intensity as a function of energy due to increased tube voltage or increased tube current.

tered in the catheterization laboratory, the generator also controls the exposure to the patient required to produce the desired film exposure.

In general, the x-ray factors that can be selected by the operator at the control panel are the exposure time for each pulse (measured in milliseconds); the voltage across the tube (kVp); and the tube current or the number of electrons in the beam (mA).

In cineangiographic procedures, a station is chosen where a specific pulse width (e.g., 3 msec) is chosen. The pulse width is simply how long x-rays are allowed to flow before they are shut off. The generator then varies the kVp and mA in order to obtain the desired exposure.

A particular x-ray generator-tube combination is specified by its rating. The limit on an x-ray tube that measures the maximum x-ray exposure that can be made safely is the tube rating. A single exposure is measured in *heat units*, which are the product of current, kVp, and exposure time. A procedure can also be limited by the total amount of heat that can be generated during a long series of exposures. This is because the target will heat up following many successive exposures. Modern x-ray tubes, for example, are capable of handling up to one million heat units.

X-ray Interactions with Matter

The type of diagnostic information that is obtained in angiography is determined by the way that x-rays interact with different materials such as patient tissues and contrast media. This interaction is referred to as the "attenuation" or "absorption" of the x-rays by material in the path of the x-ray beam. The relationship between the number of transmitted x-rays and a thickness of absorbing material is plotted in Figure 4–7 for the case where all the x-rays have a single energy. The amount of attenuation that is produced by an amount of material is characterized by its *absorption coefficient*. Keep in mind that the x-ray beam actually has a spread in energies. A particular value of interest is the *half-value layer* (HVL) for a material. This is the amount of material required to cut the number of x-rays in half, and it is represented by the following formula:

$$\text{half-value layer} = \frac{0.693}{\text{absorption coefficient}}.$$

Table 4–1 shows the thickness required for several materials to cut the x-ray intensity in half.

The value of the absorption coefficient for different materials in the body is different for the x-ray energies that are encountered in the catheterization laboratory. This, along with the different thicknesses of material in the human body, results in varying amounts of x-rays reaching the detector at different locations, and produces the familiar x-ray image of dark lungs, white bones, and intermediate brightness of other tissue seen on the final film images.

Additional diagnostic information is obtained by the use of iodinated

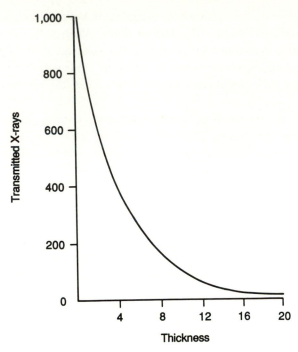

Figure 4–7. The number of x-rays transmitted by a changing thickness of material.

contrast material. The absorption coefficient of iodine is approximately four times that of bone, for example, so that it absorbs many more of the x-rays. The resulting white profile of the coronary arteries following injection with the iodinated contrast material is precisely the information used in the diagnosis of the extent of disease in the vessels.

A word should be said about scatter radiation. To this point, we have assumed that the only x-rays reaching the detector are those in the incident beam that were not absorbed by the tissue directly in line with the beam. That assumption lies behind the relationship between the detected x-ray signal and the tissue or contrast material in the beam. A contribution to the detected signal from other

TABLE 4–1
Thickness of Material Required for One HVL for an X-Ray Energy of 50 keV.

Material	HVL (cm)
Water	3.1
Plexiglass	2.8
Aluminum	0.7
Concrete	0.5
Copper	0.03
Lead	0.008

points in the patient is called "scatter radiation." This contribution, shown in Figure 4–8, results in an unwanted density on the films. It is also the source of most of the x-ray exposure to the laboratory personnel. The two main ways to reduce the scatter radiation reaching the film are (1) to increase the distance between the detector and the patient and (2) through the use of an antiscatter grid. The grid is a series of parallel lead-foil strips through which the primary radiation passes unaffected. Most of the scatter radiation is absorbed by the lead strips because the scatter radiation strikes the grid at sharper angles. Scatter grids are placed on the face of the x-ray detector (i.e., the image intensifier).

X-ray Detection

The x-rays that are transmitted through the patient cannot be seen by the human eye, so it is necessary to convert the image to a visible one. This is done by converting the energy of the x-rays into visible light, which can be used to expose film or can be viewed on a television monitor. A photograph of the equipment used in the conversion process is shown in Figure 4–9. Basically, the components consist of an image intensifier, a cinefilm camera, a television camera, and optical lens systems between the components.

The image intensifier, which was developed in the early 1950s, is the primary component in the image-formation process. The image intensifier, shown in Figure 4–10, converts the x-ray image formation to a corresponding image made of light in the visible spectrum. The x-rays that leave the patient strike an input phosphor screen made of cesium iodide (CsI) that ejects electrons when struck by x-rays. These photoelectrons are then accelerated and steered towards the output phosphor screen in a process similar to that used to accelerate the electrons in the x-ray tube. When these electrons strike the output phosphor screen, light is emitted. The number of light particles emitted at the output is much greater than the number of x-rays that strike the input screen owing to the extra energy given to the electrons during the acceleration process.

The resulting light output is then focused, using a series of lenses and

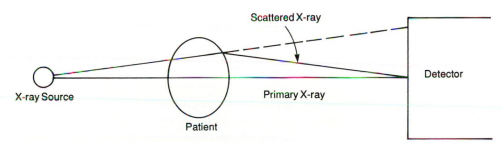

Figure 4–8. Schematic diagram of the effects of radiation scatter on the detected transmission image. The *dashed line* indicates the original direction of the scattered x-ray before deflection.

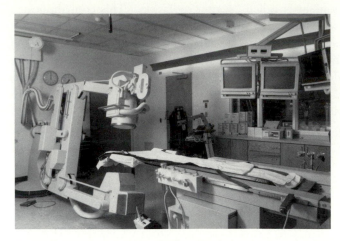

Figure 4–9. X-ray tube and image-intensifier assembly used for single-plane image acquisition.

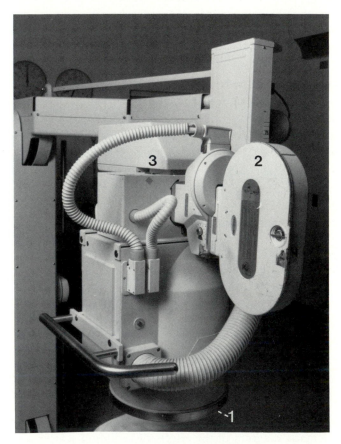

Figure 4–10. Image-intensifier assembly showing the input phosphor (1), the cinefilm camera (2), and the television camera (3).

mirrors that are shown in Figure 4–11. Following passage through a collecting lens, a beam splitter divides the light into two parts. One part is passed onto a television camera for display on a television monitor, and the other part is reflected towards a cinefilm camera for recording the procedure on film. We will return to the two cameras in more detail later in this chapter.

The maximum field size that can be detected by the image intensifier is simply the size of the tube, which is typically around 9 inches in diameter. Smaller field sizes can also be selected by the operator. Because the smaller field size at the input face of the image intensifier results in an output image of the same size, use of smaller fields (e.g., 6 inch or 4.5 inch) results in a more magnified image. Additional magnification is obtained by increasing the distance between the image intensifier and the patient, shown in Figure 4–12. The magnification is given by the ratio of two distances:

$$\text{magnification} = \frac{\text{source-to-image distance (SID)}}{\text{source-to-object distance (SOD)}},$$

where SID is the distance from the target in the x-ray tube to the image intensifier, and SOD is the distance from the target to the object plane of interest in the patient.

Film-Based Detection of X-rays

The process of recording angiographic images onto movie (cine) film is called cineangiography. This is the procedure used today in virtually all catheterization laboratories. As shown in Figure 4–11, a portion of the light output of the image

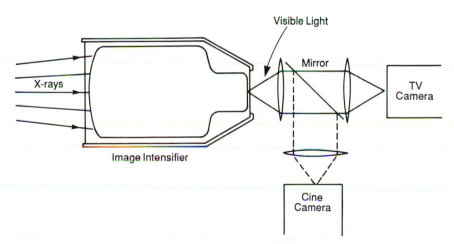

Figure 4–11. Schematic diagram of the image-intensifier assembly and the process by which input x-rays are converted to visible light.

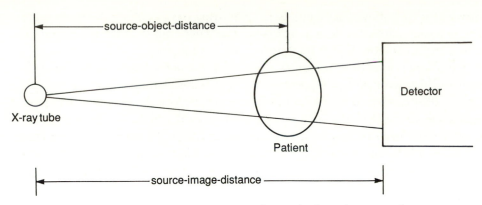

Figure 4–12. Diagram of the distances used to calculate the magnification in projection angiography.

intensifier is reflected towards the cinefilm camera. The camera size most often used is 35 mm, which is the size of each frame of the film. Thus, the initial image formed at the input to the image intensifier ends up reduced to an area that is at most 24 mm × 35 mm.

X-ray film is made of an emulsion that is coated onto both sides of a transparent plastic base. The light sensitivity of the emulsion is due to the presence of silver halide crystals, which undergo a chemical change when they are exposed to light. When light is absorbed by a halide crystal, which is a combination of silver iodide and silver chromide, it breaks up the crystal and leaves clusters of silver atoms. These clusters of silver crystals hold the latent image, which will become a visible silver deposit when the film is "developed." This results in dark areas on the film corresponding to bright areas of the image (i.e., a "negative" image).

Film development is the process by which the latent image pattern is converted to a pattern of silver metal. The entire processing sequence involves the following:

1. Development. The developer chemical is added to produce the chemical reaction that forms the silver metal.
2. Fixing. The silver halide crystals that were not exposed are converted to a form that is water soluble.
3. Washing. The film is washed with water to remove the chemicals used in the process.

Cinefilm is processed in many laboratories using an automatic processing machine that combines all the steps just described at a regulated temperature. The processors are self-contained so that they can operate under room light.

A particular film is characterized by the properties of speed, contrast, and grain. The exposure at the film is directly proportional to the x-ray exposure at the image intensifier, which, as described earlier, is measured in milliamperes. The more light exposure to the film, the more the film is darkened. A measure of this darkness is the film *density*, which is a number in the range of 0 to 1.0. The higher the density, the darker the film.

The relationship between total film density and light exposure, shown in Figure 4–13, is generally not a simple one. This S-shaped curve, known as the H-and-D curve, shows that the density is directly proportional to the *logarithm* of the exposure only over a portion of the curve. In particular, there is some film density at zero exposure, which is referred to as "fog," due to the development of unexposed silver halide crystals and a saturation point as the exposure increases.

The speed of a film is a measure of how much light is necessary to darken the film. This is determined by the exposure required to produce a density of 1.0. The contrast of the film is a measure of how well a film can differentiate between structures that absorb x-rays to only slightly differing amounts. The grain of the film is a measure of the particle sizes in the emulsion. In general, the finer the grain, the better the film will be able to record very small structures but the more exposure it will take to produce the same density. Thus, a tradeoff must be made between speed and fineness of detail.

The overall quality of the film image is measured in terms of the image contrast and the image sharpness or resolution. The contrast of the resulting image on film is the difference in film density. This depends on a number of factors.

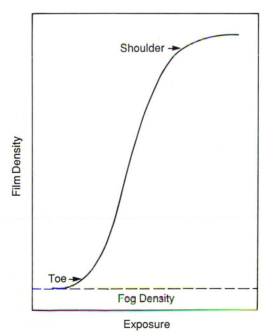

Figure 4–13. An example of a film-response curve showing the linear region along with the nonlinear portions of the curve.

First, the contrast varies within the patient owing to differences in thickness and density of material. This, in turn, is a function of the kVp of the x-rays used. Low kVp will provide higher contrast between, for example, bone and tissue and iodine. It will also be absorbed more by the patient, so that not enough radiation is transmitted to darken the film, forcing an increase in the kVp. A rise in the kVp used will, however, decrease the contrast and result in noisier, or grainier, images. Finally, the contrast is dependent on the type of film and processing used.

The sharpness of the system is the ability to define edges that are close together. Many factors cause a reduction in sharpness. First, motion in the patient during the exposure can produce blurring of objects, such as the edges of the coronary arteries. Second, the focal spot of the x-ray tube can cause blurring because the x-rays do not come from a single point but are actually spread out over an area. Additional blurring can take place in the image intensifier and lens system. Finally, the film used, grain size, and so forth can be a factor in determining the sharpness of the image. The final measure of sharpness of the image is the system resolution. Figure 4–14 shows a series of line patterns used to evaluate the resolution of an imaging system. The smaller the spacing that can be seen before the lines blur together, the higher the resolution of the system.

Viewing

Following development of the cinefilm, it is necessary to view it. The most commonly used method is by means of a cinefilm projector such as that shown in

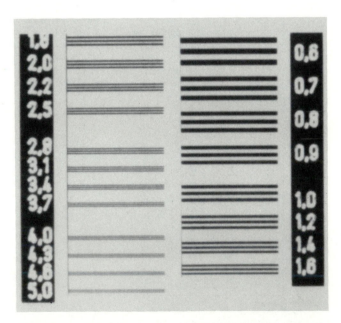

Figure 4–14. Radiograph of a resolution pattern indicating the measured resolution in line pairs per millimeter. The numbers represent how many line pairs can be distinguished per millimeter. The greater the number, the better the resolution.

Figure 4–15. The film is displayed on a large screen, and the film is played forward or backward and stopped for viewing single images.

Fluoroscopy

As described earlier, the image intensifier allows for the conversion of the transmitted x-ray intensity to a form that is visible to the human eye. In the previous section, the way in which this light image was recorded onto film was described. The light output of the image intensifier can also be displayed as a television image on a monitor or for recording onto videotape. This allows the physician to view the images that are being recorded on film as the contrast material is injected and passes through the heart. It also permits the positioning of the patient in the field before injection of the contrast. This dynamic display of x-ray images is referred to generally as "fluoroscopy." In the catheterization laboratory, the term is customarily applied to the use of television display of the patient during positioning of the patient and of the catheters in preparation for the acquisition of the diagnostic sequences. During this mode of display, the x-ray tube is operated at a much lower tube current (around 0.5 to 5.0 mA) than that used during the actual cineangiographic acquisition (100 to 1,000 mA). This reduces the x-ray exposure, because the total time of operation during the preparation stage is usually much greater than that during the cineangiographic sequences themselves.

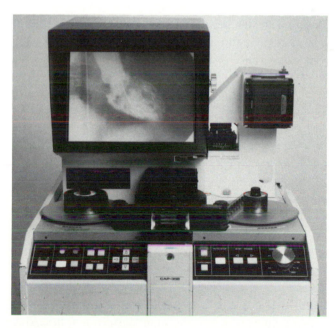

Figure 4–15. Cinefilm viewer used to display 35-mm cinefilm.

The operation of the x-ray tube during fluoroscopy has been described earlier. The only major difference is that the tube current is lower and the automatic exposure control during fluoroscopy must be calibrated for the lower x-ray intensity that reaches the image-intensifier face. In most laboratories, the x-rays are being produced continuously during fluoroscopy, but in newer facilities, the fluoroscopic image is formed from pulsed exposures of the x-rays. This technique, called "pulsed fluoroscopy," requires a different form of television display system. In all methods, a timer is used to sound an alarm when fluoroscopy has been on for a 5-minute interval.

Television Display

The output light signal from the image intensifier is split into two components, as shown in Figure 4–11. One part is used to expose the cinefilm, as described earlier, and the remainder is focused onto the input face of a television camera. The television camera performs the next function in the fluoroscopic imaging chain—to convert the light signal to an electrical signal that can be displayed on a monitor and recorded with a videotape recorder.

The basic operation of a television camera in x-ray imaging is similar to that used in commercial television. The light incident on the camera target produces an electrical signal on the target that is proportioned to the amount of light. A high velocity beam of electrons then moves across the target to measure the electrical signal at every point. Figure 4–16 shows a diagram of the camera target and the lines traveled by the scanning beam of the camera. The standard television image consists of 525 horizontal lines that are divided into two fields of 262½ lines each. This is called an *interlaced scan* of the image because adjacent lines belong to different fields. The first field is read in 1/60th second, followed by the second field, so that the entire image, or *frame*, is read in 1/30th second. This is done to avoid an appearance of flicker, because the human eye will notice

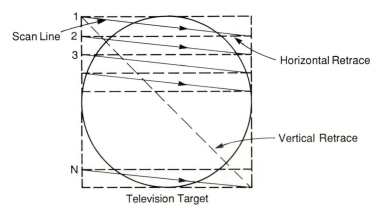

Figure 4–16. Pattern of scan lines on the target of a television camera. In most cases, the same pattern is followed on the display monitor.

changes occurring at 1/30th second, but it cannot detect the changes occurring 1/60th second apart. Another method in which the camera target is read one line after the other without alternating in the 1/30th second is called "progressive," or "sequential" scanning. This method is used when pulsed fluoroscopy is available, and its display is such that no flicker occurs.

The electrical signal produced by the television camera is amplified and is then fed to a monitor that is similar to a home television set. At the monitor, the signal itself is converted into an electron beam that scans the inside surface of the picture tube. Magnets are used to steer the electron beam within the picture tube so that the position on the screen corresponds to the original position on the camera target. The target end of the tube is coated with a fluorescent material that emits light in direct proportion to the number of electrons, producing the familiar visible-light output.

The same electrical signal that is fed to the monitor for display can also be used as the input to a videotape recorder. This permits recording of the images displayed on the monitor during the cinefilm sequences and allows for a quick review of the sequence without waiting for film to be developed. It also provides a backup of the examination in the event that the cinefilm results are not of good quality or destroyed.

Flicker

Let us consider what is seen on the monitor during acquisition of the cinefilm images. The cinefilm-camera shutter is opened at regular intervals; most often, 30 frames per second is used. The x-ray image is formed during a short pulse of x-rays (say, 3 to 5 msec) before the opening of the shutter. Pulses of x-rays are used to "freeze" the motion of the moving vessels during the exposure and thus avoid blurring. This results in a stationary image at the output of the image intensifier when the shutter of the cinefilm camera opens for exposure and produces a stationary image on the television camera target. If interlaced scanning is used, half of that image is read in the first 1/60th second and displayed on the monitor. The process of reading the first field also reduces the electrical signal at the adjacent lines belonging to the next field. No new light is input to the camera target, and that reduces the signal in the second field being displayed. To the eye looking at the monitor, the bright field is much more visible and the eye detects its changing at a rate of 30 per second. During "regular" fluoroscopy without acquisition of cinefilm images, x-rays are continuous, and the image on the camera target is constantly being refreshed, so that no brightness difference exists between fields; thus, no flicker is detected. During cineangiography, flicker becomes evident whenever the framing rate is < 50 frames per second.

Digital Cardiac Imaging

An alternative method for the formation and storage of cardiac angiographic images has been available since the early 1970s with the development of *digital radiography.* This field, which was made possible by the combination of digital computers and traditional radiographic equipment, first received widespread acceptance in computed tomography (CT). Whereas standard radiographic and angiographic methods resulted in images recorded on film, digital imaging produces a collection of numbers that can be stored in a computer, recalled for display, and altered in order to form new images. Although CT images provided images of different slices in the patient, they could not provide the dynamic sequences of images required in angiography. The development of digital angiography required development of additional computer equipment to meet these faster requirements.

A digital angiography system closely resembles the standard cineangiography apparatus shown earlier with a few modifications, which are shown in Figure 4–17. The same television camera can be used for fluoroscopy and digital angiography, but, in general, digital imaging requires a better-quality camera that has low electrical noise and low lag (i.e., some of the images on the camera target remain on the target after being scanned by the electron beam). The output signal from the television camera, which was described in the previous section, is fed to a specialized computer or *digital-processing unit.*

It is the function of the digital processor to convert the electrical signal to an array, or matrix, of numbers. Because the memory size of a computer is limited in the quantity of numbers that can be stored, it is necessary to *sample* the image at regular intervals. Figure 4–18 is a diagram demonstrating how an entire image is sampled and converted to 16 individual picture elements, or *pixels.* In most digital angiographic studies, the image displayed on the monitor is sampled and stored in a matrix of 512 rows, each having 512 pixels, for a total of 262,144 pixels. Also used are matrices of 256 × 256 and 1024 × 1024. An example of a digital coronary angiogram is shown in Figure 4–19 for matrix sizes of 512 and 32.

During the sampling process, the electrical signal is converted to a *digital* number that can take on only whole values. For example, the brightest spot in an image is given a value of 255, and complete darkness is assigned a value of 0, with possible intermediate values of 1,2,3,......, 253,254. Such a conversion is said to result in 256 different *grey levels,* or it represents the image brightness using eight binary digits or bits. This format of assigning values is exactly that

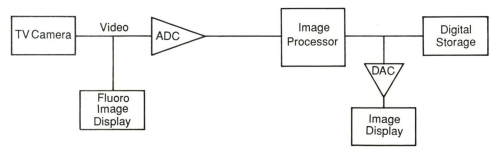

Figure 4–17. Schematic diagram of the digital-imaging process showing the additional equipment required to convert the TV signal to a digital image.

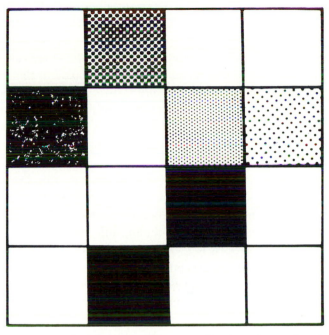

Figure 4–18. Schematic diagram of a 4 × 4 matrix of pixels in which the intensity in each entire pixel is assigned a number. This number is then defined in terms of increasing "greyness." The most intense pixels become the darkest.

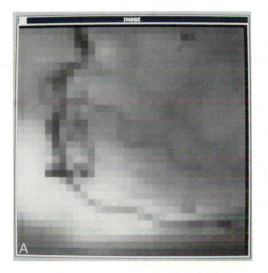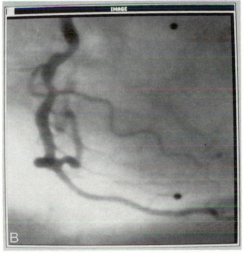

Figure 4–19. An example of the effect of changing the pixel matrix on the image resolution. A coronary angiogram is shown comparing a 32 × 32 image matrix (*A*) with a 512 × 512 matrix (*B*).

used in every kind of computer for storage of numbers. Because angiographic images are typically acquired at a rate of 30 frames per second, acquisition of images in a 512×512 matrix requires at least 8 million such operations every second.

The digital-processing computers must control the image acquisition, store the images, make changes to them, and control display of the resultant images. Some digital systems control exposure factors and the television camera, whereas others synchronize to the existent system and just convert the images and store them as they come in. In all of them, the images are stored in the memory, which must be at least large enough for one image and, in many cases, for two or three images. Images can then be transferred to long-term storage devices.

The two primary advantages of digital imaging are the elimination of the need for film and its processing and the capability of modifying or processing the images. Because conversion of the images occurs instantly, the images can be recalled immediately for viewing at the end of an injection sequence. During this procedure, the conversion process is reversed and the pixel value is converted into an electrical signal to drive the television monitor. One example of useful processing is the method of *widowing and leveling* during display. This permits the viewer to change the brightness and contrast of a displayed image to visualize some features preferentially over others. This is performed on the pixel values before they are displayed, but it does not alter the original image stored in memory.

Another example of processing of digital images is the technique called *digital subtraction angiography* (DSA). In fact, digital angiography was originally developed for the purpose of producing subtraction images of contrast-filled blood vessels, shown schematically in Figure 4–20. In particular, with the technique of temporal subtraction, an image acquired before the injection of contrast, called the "mask image," is subtracted from images obtained following the contrast injection. The result is an image of only the iodine-filled vessels, because the other structures are subtracted out by the image processor.

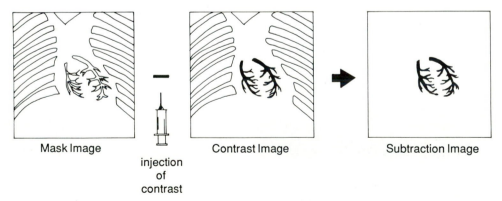

Mask Image   injection of contrast   Contrast Image   Subtraction Image

Figure 4–20. Schematic diagram of temporal subtraction of a preinjection mask image from the later contrast image.

The use of temporal subtraction with selective injection of contrast has resulted in good-quality images in the catheterization laboratory. To obtain such images in the heart, it is necessary to acquire the two images at the same point in the cardiac signal. This is done by *gating* the acquisition to the electrocardiographic (ECG) signal of the patient. As can be seen in Figure 4–20, the use of subtraction increases the visibility of the coronary artery by eliminating the background structures. An additional advantage is the ability of DSA to provide good-quality images even with reduced concentrations of contrast material. One should recall that, because the computer stores all the images, the unsubtracted images are available even if a good subtraction cannot be made.

The use of digital images also makes it possible to perform many other processing operations, including measurement of ventricular volume and ejection fraction, measurement of coronary stenosis, and determination of blood-flow parameters.

Several factors still limit the widespread use of digital angiography in the cardiac catheterization laboratory. The acquisition of images in a pixel format means that there is an ultimate limit to the smallest vessel that can be seen—the size of a single pixel. For a 15-cm field of view and a 512 x 512 matrix, this results in a pixel size of 0.22 to 0.30 mm, but if one uses a 1024 x 1024 matrix, it is reduced to 0.1 to 0.15 mm. Although this seems significantly larger than what is possible, theoretically, with cinefilm, the situation is not so simple. The elimination of background structures through subtraction improves the visibility of small vessels in digital images. In comparison, the motion of vessels, the overlying structures, and variations in film processing can mean that the results obtained with cinefilm are often worse than what one would theoretically expect.

At this time, an inexpensive, long-term storage medium for digital images is not widely available. The fast digital disks used during acquisition can store roughly one patient's worth of data, but the images must be transferred to another device so that new images can be acquired with the disk. Examples of such devices are low-speed and high-speed digital magnetic tapes and optical disks that use a laser beam to record the numbers that make up the image information. The availability of a suitable storage medium will permit the long-term storage of angiographic results without the need for film, and it will also permit the viewing of the images at any location to which the image data can be sent over computer or phone lines. At the destination, the numbers can be converted back to brightness levels for display and processing.

Radiation Exposure

A complete description of the x-ray imaging procedure in the catheterization should include an awareness of the biological effects of x-ray radiation and possible risks to the laboratory personnel. In this section, therefore, the basic principles and definitions will be presented for the purpose of increasing the awareness and knowledge of the lab personnel.

Units of Exposure

The most commonly used measure of *radiation exposure* is the *roentgen*, or R, which is a measure of x-rays per unit area. A second unit that is sometimes used is the *rad*, which is the unit of absorbed dose or the energy actually absorbed by tissue. A third unit that measures the biological effect of radiation on a human being is the *rem*. For most purposes, when one is using diagnostic x-rays, the approximation

$$1 \text{ R} = 1 \text{ rad} = 1 \text{ rem}$$

is valid.

Because the R is the unit encountered most often, the discussion will be in terms of exposure. For procedures in the cath lab, the amount of exposure, say for each pulse during a cinefilm sequence, is much less than 1 R and is measured in units of milliroentgens, or mR, where

$$1 \text{mR} = \frac{1}{1000} \text{ R}.$$

Typical Exposure to the Patient

As we discussed earlier, the number of x-rays produced by the generator is measured in terms of the mA, where mA is the product of the tube current in mA and the exposure time in seconds. The amount of x-ray exposure actually produced also depends on the kVp used, as shown in Table 4–2, where the value of exposure at a point 50 cm from the tube is calculated for a range of kVp.

The relationship between exposure and distance is referred to as the "inverse square law" because the exposure is proportional to the inverse of the distance squared. In other words, if the exposure at a distance of 50 cm is 40 mR, then the exposure at a distance of 100 cm is given by

$$E = 40 \text{ mR} \times (50/100)^2 = 10 \text{ mR}.$$

TABLE 4–2

X-ray Exposure at a Distance of 50 cm from the X-ray Tube as a Function of Peak Tube Voltage.

Tube Voltage (kVp)	Exposure (mR)
60	16
70	24
80	32
90	40
100	48

Exposure to Personnel

Because the primary x-ray beam is restricted by lead collimators to be directed at the patient, the exposure to laboratory personnel is due to x-rays scattered from within the patient into the room. This is reduced from the primary beam typically by a factor of approximately 500 near the table to a dropoff of over 10,000 beyond the extent of the table. For quick calculations, one can assume that the scatter radiation dose is 1/1000th of that to the patient. Again, the inverse square law is useful in judging the decrease in dose as a function of distance.

Shielding

Although the x-ray factors used are those chosen to be the lowest necessary and the personnel are instructed to remain a safe distance from the primary source, additional shielding is required to further reduce the exposure to nurses and technicians. Examples of commonly used shielding are lead-lined aprons, lead barriers, and leaded glass. The effectiveness of shielding is measured in terms of HVLs. The HVL is the thickness of lead required to reduce the exposure by a factor of one-half (see Table 4–1). The HVL for lead ranges from 0.15 mm at 70 kVp to 0.27 mm at 125 kVp. The total amount of dose reduction is determined by multiplying by one-half for each HVL. A 0.5-mm thick lead apron, for example, is around 3 HVLs for 70 kVp x-rays, resulting in a reduction of $(1/2) \times (1/2) \times (1/2) = 1/8$ of the incident exposure.

Measurement of Exposure (the Radiation Badge)

The commonly used method for monitoring exposure to radiation is the use of thermoluminescent dosimeter, or TLD, badges. These badges have the property that after being exposed to radiation, they glow when heated; the amount of light they produce is related to the radiation exposure. The TLD badge should be worn on the collar outside a lead apron in order to monitor the possible radiation to the lens of the eye if it is not shielded. Badges are collected at regular intervals to keep track of exposure of personnel.

Dose-Limit Recommendations

The average annual exposure to various types of radiation experienced in the United States is in the range of 140 to 300 mrem. National and international organizations have made recommendations for the maximum allowable radiation exposure. This limit for members of the general public is equal to 500 mrem, or 0.5 rem. The recommended limit for individuals who are exposed to radiation during employment is equal to 5 rems for whole-body exposure. When broken down by organs, the maximum limits range from 75 rem for hands to 5 rem for the eyes and gonads.

Of special concern is the maximum recommended limit to the fetus;

which is 0.5 rem for the 9 months of gestation. The greatest sensitivity to radiation is from the second through ninth week after conception. In determining the dose to the fetus, it should be kept in mind that this will be less than the mother's skin dose and will generally be less than one-half of the skin dose.

SELECTED REFERENCES

Bushong SC. Radiologic science for technologists. St. Louis: CV Mosby, 1988.

Curry TS III, Dowdey JE, Murry RC Jr. Christensen's introduction to the physics of diagnostic radiology. Philadelphia: Lea & Febiger, 1984.

Johns HE, Cunningham JR. The physics of radiology. Springfield: Charles C Thomas, 1983.

Shapiro J. Radiation protection. Cambridge: Harvard University Press, 1981.

Indications for Cardiac Catheterization

Thomas M. Bashore, MD

With very few exceptions, diagnostic cardiac catheterization is indicated in virtually all adults undergoing cardiac surgery. Certainly it is inappropriate for the cardiothoracic surgeon to be expected to confirm the severity of valvular or coronary lesions with visual inspection or palpation. All decisions regarding the performance of catheterization, however, should be based on an appropriate risk-benefit ratio. Overall mortality from adult diagnostic cardiac catheterization is in the 0.1 percent range in most laboratories; therefore, there are few patients who can't be studied safely if proper techniques are followed. Cardiac catheterization is rapidly evolving, and over the next 10 years, it will likely evolve in two broad directions. At one extreme, hemodynamically unstable patients are being studied during acute myocardial ischemia. At the other extreme, there is a rapid trend toward more and more patients being studied in the outpatient setting. This has expanded the indications for diagnostic cardiac catheterization to include both ambulatory and critically ill patients. This expansion is unprecedented in cardiology.

Cardiac catheterization should be considered a diagnostic test to be used in concert with other complementary diagnostic tests. It provides anatomic information, but rarely provides functional information, and it should not be considered the sole study required for the complete assessment of cardiac disease in any one patient. Cardiac catheterization in valvular or congenital heart disease is clearly best performed with full knowledge of echocardiographic and other functional studies, because these data may markedly simplify and shorten the catheterization by preventing redundant data from being obtained.

The general indications for cardiac catheterization are described in the following sections. Those particularly pertinent to the electrophysiology laboratory are described in Chapter 14. Because of the rapidly expanding indications for interventional techniques, only a superficial effort will be made to describe patients in whom these techniques are to be used. The proliferation of newer devices in interventional catheterization will likely vary the types of patients and lesions that are appropriate.

Coronary Artery Disease

There is no better means for the identification of the presence or absence of coronary artery disease than coronary angiography. The improvement in the catheterization procedure and the reduction in the mortality and morbidity associated with catheterization has made the diagnosis of coronary artery disease by noninvasive methodology much less desirable or appropriate. Anatomic disease does not necessarily correlate with functional disease, however, and the role of pharmacologic or exercise stress in defining functional disease should not be forgotten. In addition, the variability in our ability to accurately and reproducibly assess the severity of a coronary angiographic lesion, and the dynamic nature of certain coronary artery disease states (e.g., spasm, thrombosis, plaque rupture, and so on) make it clear that too much reliance on coronary angiography alone is unwarranted. In this era of active intervention in the coronary artery disease process, many centers have taken an aggressive approach to the identification of the presence of coronary artery disease. The aggressiveness of individual centers in approaching patients during acute myocardial infarction, for instance, is dependent upon local philosophies and facilities.

Clearly, if the identification of coronary artery disease is a primary concern, catheterization should be performed in all cases. This information may be crucial to the care of patients with a variety of chest pain syndromes or in anyone in whom the presence of coronary artery disease needs to be appropriately excluded. Coronary angiography remains the gold standard for identification of the presence of coronary disease despite difficulties in its ability to accurately quantify the extent of this disease. Table 5–1 outlines the recently published AHA/ACC guidelines on those who should undergo coronary angiography (J Am Coll Cardiol 1987; 10:935). New guidelines are currently being developed that will address the indications for cardiac catheterization in not only the inpatient setting, but also in the outpatient facility, the free-standing laboratory, and the mobile laboratory.

Myocardial Disease

Catheterization procedures provide useful information regarding the hemodynamic status of patients with primary disease of the heart muscle, but these procedures may not always be required for appropriate diagnosis. Echocardiography can describe wall thickness and chamber sizes. Radionuclide angiography can provide information regarding the ejection fraction. Catheterization can identify the etiologic role of coronary artery disease in patients with diffuse myopathy, detect active myocarditis by myocardial biopsy, define the extent of valvular regurgitation, and provide data regarding the responsiveness of heart and lung pressures to acute drug therapy. The pulmonary vascular resistance is a necessary measurement before cardiac transplantation is contemplated since high pulmonary vascular resistance effectively eliminates the procedure as an option.

Valvular Heart and Congenital Heart Disease

Catheterization provides information that both confirms and complements clinical and noninvasive data in patients with valvular heart disease. Only rarely should patients undergo cardiac valvular surgery without cardiac catheterization, despite recent controversies suggesting that it is perhaps unnecessary in many cases. The risk-benefit ratio of preoperative catheterization is heavily weighted in favor of the procedure. In certain clinical situations, such as patients with atrial myxoma or young patients with endocarditis, acute mitral regurgitation, acute aortic insufficiency, or a secundum atrial septal defect, catheterization may not add sufficient additional information to warrant its use. The majority of adult patients should undergo cardiac catheterization and coronary angiography prior to surgical intervention. Children frequently can be operated on safely with noninvasive information only, but one should consider the importance of pulmonary pressure and the possibility of missing anomalies such as anomalous venous connections before one decides to rely solely on noninvasive data.

Indications for Percutaneous Transluminal Coronary Angioplasty

Indications for balloon angioplasty are dependent on a number of factors, including the type of lesion, the location of the lesion, the amount of myocardium in jeopardy from the lesion, the presence or absence of collaterals from other arteries into the lesion area, the patient's symptomatic status, and the availability of appropriate "tools" (catheters) for approaching the lesion.

Balloon angioplasty is now a well-established procedure; more than 200,000 angioplasties are performed yearly in the United States. The procedure requires the appropriate seating of a guiding catheter in the orifice of the coronary, then the insertion of a balloon-tipped catheter, usually with a steerable wire in its nose, or a guidewire, over which a balloon catheter will eventually be placed. This means that the lesions chosen and the location of the lesion make a major difference regarding success rates. Recently, guidelines have been established that provide a basis for understanding which patients are currently felt to benefit from PTCAs (J Am Coll Cardiol 1988; 12:529).

Lesions that are long (>20 mm), tortuous, located on a sharp bend, or have an angle within them are poor candidates for angioplasty. Lesions with thrombus or marked calcification also do poorly. Lesions at the origin of the right coronary artery or left anterior descending (LAD) artery are particularly prone to

TABLE 5–1
Indications for Coronary Angiography

KNOWN OR SUSPECTED CORONARY DISEASE (Known: prior MI, CABG, or angioplasty. Suspected: abnormal ECG with stress or other evidence for ischemia).
  Asymptomatic Patients
    Definite indications:
      1. Evidence for high risk for serious CAD on exercise testing.
      2. Individuals in high-risk occupations (airline pilots, bus drivers, etc.).
      3. Following successful resuscitation from cardiac arrest.
    Possible indications:
      1. Any positive exercise test.
      2. Multiple risk factors for CAD.
      3. Prior myocardial infarction.
      4. Following cardiac transplantation.

  Symptomatic Patients
    Definite indications:
      1. Medical treatment "failure."
      2. Unstable angina.
      3. Printzmetal's or variant angina (spasm).
      4. Angina associated with the following:
        a. Positive exercise test.
        b. Side effects of medical therapy.
        c. Occupational or lifestyle "need to know."
        d. Episodic pulmonary edema.
      5. Before major vascular surgery.
      6. After resuscitation from cardiac arrest.
    Possible indications:
      1. Angina in the following groups:
        a. Female patients < 40 yr with positive exercise tests.
        b. Male patients < 40 yr of age.
        c. Patients < 40 yr of age with prior MI.
        d. Patients requiring major nonvascular surgery.
      2. Class 3 or 4 angina (angina with less than normal exertion or angina at rest).
      3. Patients in whom CAD cannot be excluded by noninvasive means owing to arthritis, vascular disease, etc.

ATYPICAL CHEST PAIN OF UNCERTAIN ORIGIN
    Definite indications:
      1. When noninvasive stress test reveals high risk for CAD.
      2. Suspected coronary spasm.
      3. Associated with abnormal LV function or failure.
    Possible indications:
      1. Patients in whom CAD cannot be excluded by noninvasive studies.
      2. Severe symptoms despite negative noninvasive tests.

ACUTE MYOCARDIAL INFARCTION
  Acute, evolving MI (< 6 hr)
    Definite indications:
      1. None yet agreed upon.
    Possible indications:
      1. Within first 6 hr in patients who are candidates for revascularization therapy.
      2. After IV thrombolytic therapy with persistent symptoms.

  Completed Myocardial Infarction (> 6 hr)
    Definite indications:
      1. Recurrent episodes of ischemia.
      2. Suspected myocardial rupture or acute mitral regurgitation with symptoms.
      3. Suspected left ventricular pseudoaneurysm.

TABLE 5–1
(continued)

Possible indications:
1. Following thrombolytic therapy.
2. CHF or hypotension during intensive medical therapy.
3. Recurrent VT or VF.
4. Cardiogenic shock.
5. Coronary embolism suspected.

Convalescent Myocardial Infarction (up to 8 wks)
Definite indications:
1. Class 3 or 4 angina.
2. Presence of CHF.
3. Positive exercise study.
4. Non–Q-wave infarction.
Possible indications:
1. Mild angina.
2. Less than 50 yr of age.
3. Need to return to unusually active or vigorous activity.
4. Previous history of MI or angina for > 6 mo before current MI.
5. Thrombolytic therapy given.

VALVULAR HEART DISEASE
Definite indications:
1. Prior to valve surgery in an adult with chest pain.
2. Prior to valve surgery in a male patient > 35 yr of age.
3. Prior to valve surgery in postmenopausal women.
Possible indications:
1. During cath in men < 35 yr of age or women > 40 yr of age when valve surgery is being considered.
2. Multiple risk factors for CAD.
3. Reoperation for valve or heart surgery.
4. Endocarditis (if evidence for coronary embolization).

CONGENITAL HEART DISEASE
Definite indications:
1. Symptoms of angina
2. Suspected coronary anomaly
3. Male patient > 40 yr of age or postmenopausal woman.
Possible indications:
1. In presence of a congenital lesion with high frequency of coronary anomalies.

MISCELLANEOUS
Definite indications:
1. Disease of the aorta that has high incidence of CAD.
2. LV failure of unknown cause.
3. Angina associated with hypertrophic cardiomyopathy at risk for CAD.
Possible indications:
1. In dilated cardiomyopathy.
2. Recent blunt chest trauma.
3. Male patients > 35 yr of age and postmenopausal women to undergo other cardiac surgery (i.e., pericardiectomy).
4. Prospective transplant donors.
5. Kawasaki's disease (coronary aneurysms).

Modified from Ross J, Brandenburg RO, Dinsmore RE, and members of the subcommittee task force on coronary angiography of the AHA/ACC. J Am Coll Cardiol 1987; 10:935.

restenosis. Very proximal left circumflex or LAD arterial lesions may not be good candidates because the balloon may occlude the left main artery during inflation. Total obstructions present their own unique problems. When performing the procedure, one must assume a "worst-case" scenario (i.e., what will happen to the patient if the vessel is totally occluded and a heart attack occurs in the distribution of the vessel). If there has been previous heart damage and the patient's life is dependent upon the vessel under consideration, it is generally prudent to exclude that lesion from consideration for angioplasty. Bypass grafts (especially distal lesions) can also be approached in certain instances but the results, especially for proximal graft lesions, have been disappointing. Left main arterial lesions should not be attempted. Diabetic patients appear particularly prone to restenosis and this should be kept in mind when considering angioplasty. Patients with dynamic stenosis or thrombus (i.e., unstable angina or acute MI) may also be poor candidates. Thus, there are both patient-related and lesion-related factors that must be considered when PTCA is contemplated. Table 5–2 outlines the lesion-related factors.

Newer devices, such as atherectomy, laser, rotobladors, or combination

TABLE 5–2
Characteristics of Type A, B, and C Lesions

Lesion-Specific Characteristics	
Type A Lesions (high success, > 85%; low risk)	
Discrete (< 10 mm in length)	Little or no calcification
Concentric	Less than totally occlusive
Readily accessible	Not ostial in location
Nonangulated segment, < 45 degrees	No major branch involvement
Smooth contour	Absence of thrombus
Type B Lesions (moderate success, 60 to 85%; moderate risk)	
Tubular (10 to 20 mm in length)	Moderate to heavy calcification
Eccentric	Total occlusions < 3 mo old
Moderate tortuosity of proximal segment	Ostial in location
Moderately angulated segment, > 45 degrees, < 90 degrees	Bifurcation lesions requiring double guide-wires
Irregular contour	Some thrombus present
Type C Lesions (low success, < 60%; high risk)	
Diffuse (> 2 cm in length)	Total occlusion > 3 mo old
Excessive tortuosity of proximal segment	Inability to protect major side branches
Extremely angulated segments, > 90 degrees	Degenerated vein grafts with friable lesions

From Ryan TJ, Faxon DP, Gunnar RM, and members of the subcommittee task force on PTCA of the AHA/ACC. J Am Coll Cardiol 1988; 12:529; with permission.
*Although the risk of abrupt vessel closure is moderate, in certain instances the likelihood of a major complication may be low, as in dilation of total occlusions less than 3 months old or when abundant collateral channels supply the distal vessel.

devices may eventually have specific indications. At this time, these devices remain investigational, and their role yet to be defined. The importance of the endothelium in preventing restenosis may limit the use of devices that are designed to remove it.

The indications for cardiac catheterization and interventional procedures will continue to evolve. It cannot be overstressed that catheterization data should always be used in conjunction with other historical and functional data to provide the most complete anatomic and functional assessment of any cardiac lesion. Visual angiographic interpretation generally underestimates the severity of the lesion and provides little understanding regarding disease significance. The whole patient should be treated, and not just the lesion.

The use of cardiac catheterization in nontraditional facilities, such as the free-standing laboratory, will likely cause the cardiology community to rethink indications for cardiac catheterization. Clearly, many patients, including young children, can be studied in an outpatient facility. The issue of which patients are appropriate for study in such facilities (especially those without surgical backup) is currently being addressed by the American College of Cardiology and the American Heart Association. At no time should either convenience or monetary savings be used as the sole justification for potentially putting a patient at unnecessary risk for cardiac catheterization.

SELECTED REFERENCES

Ross J, Brandenburg RO, Dinsmore RE, and members of the subcommittee task force on coronary angiography of the AHA/ACC. J Am Coll Cardiol 1987; 10:935.
Ryan TJ, Faxon DP, Gunnar RM, and members of the subcommittee task force on PTCA of the AHA/ACC. J Am Coll Cardiol 1988; 12:529.

CHAPTER 6

Complications of Cardiac Catheterization

Thomas M. Bashore, MD

Diagnostic Cardiac Catheterization

The risk from cardiac catheterization is evolving as rapidly as are the procedural methods and indications. The majority of information available is derived from two large multicenter trials and from two large surveys. These trials were reported in the late 1960s and 1970s, and so may not be completely relevant today. The two large multicenter trials include the American Heart Association (AHA) cooperative study of cardiac catheterization and the Society of Cardiac Angiography Registry. The AHA cooperative study evaluated 16 laboratories over a 2-year period and was published in 1968. The Society of Cardiac Angiography Registry evaluated 66 laboratories over a 14-month period. The study included 53,581 patients, and was published in 1982. These two studies were performed at a time when coronary angiography was not routinely obtained.

The two studies most often quoted regarding the risk of coronary angiography are those by Adams, Fraser, and Abrams (1973), in which 46,904 patients were reported, and the report from the Coronary Artery Surgery Study (CASS), which included 7,552 prospectively studied patients (Davis et al, 1979). Table 6-1 outlines the major complications reported in each of these studies.

Death from cardiac catheterization ranges from 0.14 percent to 0.75 percent depending on patient population and era. The patients at highest risk are those adult patients with left main arterial disease and poor left ventricular function. In addition, the extremes of age and the presence of associated valvular heart disease (especially aortic stenosis or mitral regurgitation) increase the observed risk of mortality. The risks of myocardial infarction vary from 0.07 percent to 0.6 percent; cerebrovascular accidents, from 0.03 percent to 0.2 percent;

TABLE 6–1
Complications of Cardiac Catheterization

	Overall Coronary Angiography			
	Cooperative Study	SCA Registry	Adams Survey	CASS Study
Year reported	1968	1982	1973	1979
No. patients	12,367	53,581	46,904	7,553
Death	0.75%	0.14%	0.45%	0.2 %
Myocardial infarction	NA	0.07%	0.61%	0.25%
Stroke	0.2 %	0.07%	0.23%	0.03%
Vascular	0.3 %	0.56%	NA	0.7 %
Arrhythmias	1.3 %	0.56%	0.77%	0.63%

Abbreviations: SCA = Society of Cardiac Angiography.
CASS = Coronary Artery Surgery Study.
NA = not available.

and significant arrhythmias, from 0.56 percent to 1.3 percent. Reports of local artery problems have varied widely with most series, suggesting a slightly greater incidence of complications when the brachial artery approach is used versus the femoral artery method. Vascular complications appear to occur more commonly in women, perhaps owing to their smaller vessel size. Local complications such as thrombosis, hematoma, recurrent bleeding, and pseudoaneurysm formation are seen with variable frequency.

Systemic reactions can vary from mild vasovagal ("fainting") reactions to severe vagal discharges that can lead to death. Hypotension may occur as a result of vasovagal reactions, vasodilation due to ionic contrast medium or diuresis after the procedure, cardiac tamponade, or acute myocardial ischemia, and reduced cardiac stroke volume. Acute anaphylaxis may also occur in reaction to the x-ray contrast medium. Less common complications include the precipitation of pulmonary edema, the showering of cholesterol emboli (blue toe syndrome), and injury or dissection of the pulmonary or coronary arteries.

Following the procedure diuresis is common, and hypotension may occur with late dehydration. Protamine sulfate is often given to reverse the effects of heparin and may result in profound vasodilatation and hypotension. The use of nonionic contrast media clearly reduces the acute adverse hemodynamic and electrophysiologic problems observed with the use of ionic contrast media. The high cost of nonionic contrast media has prevented its routine use in many situations, however. Acute renal injury may occur following administration of either the ionic or nonionic contrast media agents.

Based on the available literature, a high-risk profile can be generated that describes those patients at greater risk. This is presented in Table 6–2. With the advent of outpatient cardiac catheterization and even mobile catheterization facilities, decisions regarding the appropriate setting for performance of catheterization will become a major issue. This table provides some guidance. Patients at greatest risk should not be studied in settings without immediate cardiovascular

TABLE 6–2
High-Risk Profile for Mortality from Cardiac Catheterization

Overall mortality	0.14%
Age-related mortality	
< 1 yr	1.75%
> 60 yr	0.25%
Coronary artery disease	
One vessel	0.03%
Three vessel	0.16%
Left main	0.86%
Congestive heart failure	
NYHA FCI or II	0.02%
NYHA FC III	0.12%
NYHA FC IV	0.67%
Valvular disease	
All valvular disease patients	0.28%
Mitral valve disease	0.34%
Aortic valve disease	0.19%

Other definite high-risk subsets for morbidity and mortality
    Unstable angina
    Acute myocardial infarction
    Renal insufficiency
    Significant ventricular ectopy
    Congential heart disease
        Arterial desaturation present
        Pulmonary hypertension

Other potential high-risk subsets for morbidity or mortality
    High risk for vascular complication
        Morbid obesity
        Severe peripheral vascular disease
    Prosthetic valve patients
    General debility or cachexia
    Poor ejection fraction (< 30%)
    On anticoagulation or having a bleeding diathesis
    Uncontrolled systemic hypertension
    Diabetes mellitus that is difficult to control
    Chronic steroid usage
    Prior contrast allergy
    Severe chronic obstructive lung disease

backup.

The treatment of emergencies during cardiac catheterization is covered in Chapter 12.

Coronary Angioplasty

Coronary angioplasty presents a unique set of potential complications over and above those observed with diagnostic cardiac catheterization. The number and type of complications with PTCA are clearly related to the type of patient under-

TABLE 6–3
Complications Associated with Coronary Angioplasty

Total patients = 20,417

	n	%
Any complication	3112	15.2%
Hospital death	212	1.0%
Emergency surgery	980	4.8%
Myocardial infarction	369	1.8%
Prolonged angina	684	3.4%
Coronary occlusion	534	2.6%
Hypotension	452	2.2%
VF/VT	941	4.6%
Local vascular injury	583	2.9%
Excessive blood loss	291	1.4%
Neurologic events	200	1.0%

From the Society for Cardiac Angiography, 1988.

going angioplasty as well as the operator experience and the type of device being used to perform the procedure. Of the two large studies that review these complications, the NHLBI PTCA Registry was comprised primarily of patients with single vessel disease in whom early PTCA equipment was used. In 1988, the Society for Cardiac Angiography Registry reported a larger number of patients and provides a more contemporary experience. Table 6–3 outlines data from this report. Overall complications during PTCA occur in about 15% of the patients. Many of these complications, however, are relatively transient and without residual. Death occurs in only around 1% and emergency surgery is required in about 5%. As more and more anatomically difficult patients are being attempted, these numbers have not apparently risen dramatically. This suggests that the technical improvements in the procedures have had substantial impact on the risk of coronary angioplasty.

Electrophysiological Procedures

Complications related to electrophysiological procedures are surprisingly small when one considers that many of these patients have serious underlying cardiac disease. In addition, it is rather remarkable that major problems do not occur frequently when the end point of many of the studies is the induction of serious arrhythmias. Most electrophysiological studies are not monitored hemodynamically, so that the true incidence of certain complications, such as hypotension, is likely underestimated. The majority of the catheterization is via the venous structures, however, and this prevents major complications related to arterial injury.

Table 6–4 outlines complications of electrophysiological studies from a review of 8545 electrophysiological studies in 4015 patients. The survey was conducted at six university centers from January of 1979 to December of 1983 (Horowitz, 1986). Overall the risk of death is about 1 in 1000, and the risk of

TABLE 6–4
Complications Associated with Electrophysiological Studies

Total patients = 4015		Total procedures = 8545	
Complication	*n*	*% of studies*	*% of patients*
Death	5	0.06	0.12
Cardiac perforation	19	0.22	0.5
Major hemorrhage	4	0.05	0.1
Arterial injury	8	0.1	0.2
Venous thrombosis	20	0.23	0.5

From Horowitz LN. Safety of electrophysiologic studies. Circulation 73:11–28, 1986.

cardiac perforation is 1 in 2000. Further discussion regarding electrophysiological studies can be found in Chapter 14.

SELECTED REFERENCES

Adams DF, Fraser DB, Abrams HL. The complications of coronary angiography. Circulation 1973; 48:609.

Braunwald E, Swan HJC. Cooperative study on cardiac catheterization. Circulation 1968; 37 (Suppl 3): 1.

Davis K, Kennedy JW, Kemp HG, et al. Complications of coronary arteriography from the collaborative study of coronary artery surgery (CASS). Circulation 1979; 59:1105.

Hildner FJ. Registry Committee Annual Report, Society for Cardiac Angiography, chap. 3. Risks of cardiac catheterization. In Pepine CJ, Hill JA, Lambert (eds). Diagnostic and Therapeutic Cardiac Catheterization, Baltimore: Williams and Wilkins, p 27; 1989.

Horowitz LN. Safety of electrophysiologic studies. Circulation 73:11–28, 1986.

Kennedy JW. Complications associated with cardiac catheterization and angiography. Cathet Cardiovasc Diagn 1982; 8:13.

CHAPTER 7

Basic Anatomy and Physiology of the Heart

Thomas M. Bashore, MD, and Mary Jo Chapman, RN

An understanding of the basic anatomy and physiology of the heart is of obvious relevance for proper acquisition of data in the cardiac catheterization laboratory. Each member of the catheterization team should appreciate the fundamental goal of the catheterization procedure and should understand what methods are required to obtain clinically relevant data. As the catheterization proceeds, each member should be aware of where the catheters are located by noting the position of the catheters on the fluoroscopy monitor and by the pressure waveforms displayed.

This chapter describes the basic anatomic features of the heart and outlines the most important physiologic principles involved. The chapter concludes with representative catheter positions and pressures from each chamber in a manner similar to that which would be expected during a routine hemodynamic cardiac catheterization.

Overview of Anatomy

The heart is generally described in terms of the right heart (responsible for pumping blood from the venous system to the lungs) and the left heart (responsible for pumping blood from the lungs to the periphery). Right-heart structures include the superior vena cava, inferior vena cava, right atrium, tricuspid valve, right ventricle, pulmonic valve, and pulmonary arteries. Left-heart structures include the pulmonary veins, left atrium, mitral valve, left ventricle, aortic valve, and the aorta with its branches.

Figure 7–1 illustrates the basic structures observed in the anteroposterior

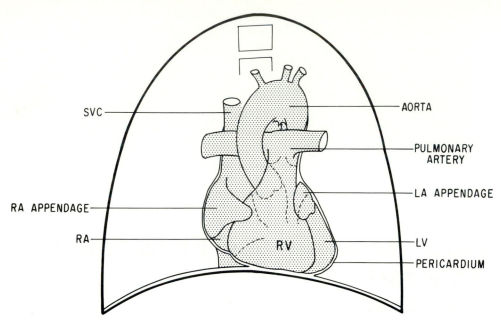

Figure 7–1. Anteroposterior schematic view of the heart. The shadow of the heart is bounded by the superior vena cava (SVC), right atrium (RA), diaphragm, left ventricle (LV), and left atrial (LA) appendage, in counterclockwise order. The mediastinum shadow includes the pulmonary artery (PA) and aorta.

view of the heart; this view is similar to what one might see fluoroscopically. Figure 7–2 outlines similar structures in the lateral view. Several clinically important features are noteworthy. Although the heart can be thought of as a right- and left-sided structure, it is actually more of an anterior (right atrium [RA], right ventricle [RV]) and posterior (left atrium [LA], left ventricle [LV]) structure. As shown in the figures, the RA and RV are anterior and lie below the sternum. The pulmonary artery and pulmonary valve lie in front of the aortic valve. The LA and LV lie behind the right heart, with the apex of the LV peeking out from behind the RV to form the left lateral border of the heart in the anterior view.

Figure 7–3 is a cross-sectional view of these structures. It reveals that the interventricular septum slants toward the anterior chest wall, resulting in the RV being the anterior ventricle and the LV being the posterior ventricle. Behind the LA lies the esophagus and spine. On both sides of the heart are the lungs.

Specific Anatomic Structures

Blood is returned to the heart from the venules. It passes through veins of increasing size and empties into the vena cavae and ultimately into the RA.

The major veins utilized during cardiac catheterization are the femoral veins, the brachial veins, the jugular veins, and the subclavian veins (Fig. 7–4).

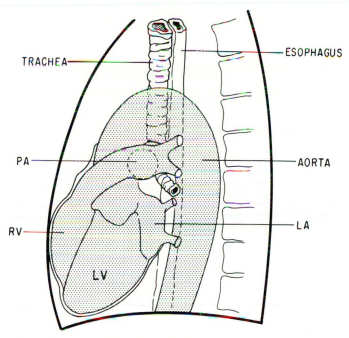

Figure 7–2. Lateral schematic view of the heart. In the lateral view, the right ventricle (RV) is anterior and the left ventricle (LV) posterior. The left atrium (LA) lies against the esophagus. PA = pulmonary artery.

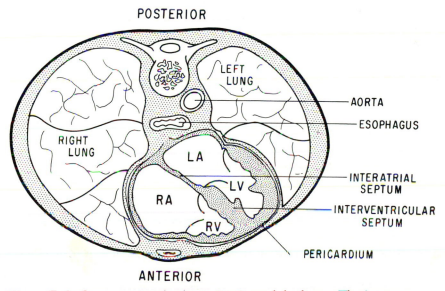

Figure 7–3. Cross-sectional schematic view of the heart. The interventricular septum slants toward the chest wall. The right ventricle (RV) is anterior to the left ventricle (LV). RA = right atrium. LA = left atrium.

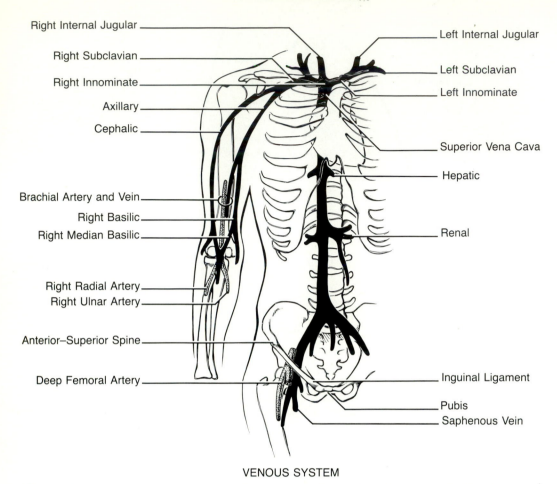

Right Internal Jugular

Right Subclavian

Right Innominate

Axillary

Cephalic

Brachial Artery and Vein

Right Basilic

Right Median Basilic

Right Radial Artery

Right Ulnar Artery

Anterior–Superior Spine

Deep Femoral Artery

Left Internal Jugular

Left Subclavian

Left Innominate

Superior Vena Cava

Hepatic

Renal

Inguinal Ligament

Pubis

Saphenous Vein

VENOUS SYSTEM

Figure 7–4. Major venous system pertinent to cardiac catheterization. (Modified from Anthony CP, Thibodeau GA. Textbook of anatomy and physiology. St. Louis: CV Mosby, 1983: 454; with permission.)

Arterial access during cardiac catheterization is achieved using the femoral and brachial arteries (Fig. 7–5).

The normal heart weighs from 220 to 280 g in women and from 280 to 340 g in men. It is about the size of an individual's fist. The RA (Fig. 7–6) receives venous blood from the superior and inferior vena cavae. Its wall is about 2 mm in thickness and has an average capacity of 50 cc. It is divided into two parts: (1) the RA appendage, and (2) the main body of the atrium. The RA appendage, a "dog-eared" projection, has no known function. It is lined with a mesh-like series of muscle bundles called "pectinate muscles." Its pocket-like nature is taken advantage of to cradle atrial pacing wires when atrioventricular (AV) sequential pacing is required.

The body of the RA has smooth walls, as does the interatrial septum that separates the LA and RA. The fossa ovale, an oval depression in the septum, is a

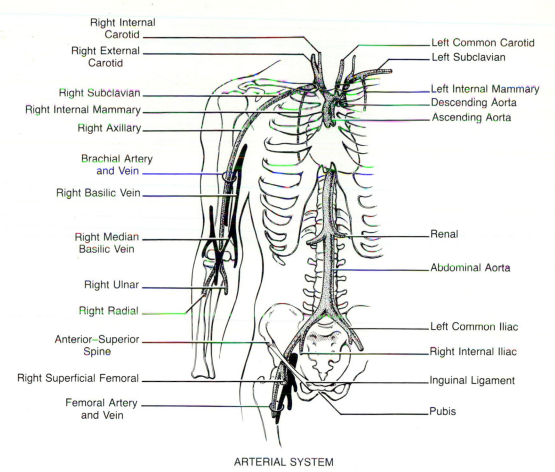

Right Internal Carotid
Right External Carotid
Right Subclavian
Right Internal Mammary
Right Axillary
Brachial Artery and Vein
Right Basilic Vein
Right Median Basilic Vein
Right Ulnar
Right Radial
Anterior–Superior Spine
Right Superficial Femoral
Femoral Artery and Vein

Left Common Carotid
Left Subclavian
Left Internal Mammary
Descending Aorta
Ascending Aorta
Renal
Abdominal Aorta
Left Common Iliac
Right Internal Iliac
Inguinal Ligament
Pubis

ARTERIAL SYSTEM

Figure 7–5. Major arterial system pertinent to cardiac catheterization. (Modified from Anthony CP, Thibodeau GA. Textbook of anatomy and physiology. St. Louis: CV Mosby, 1983:438; with permission.)

remnant of the foramen ovale—an important structure during fetal development that allowed blood to pass from the RA to the LA and bypass the lungs. In 20 to 25 percent of adults, a "probe-patent" foramen exists, in which the flap on the LA side of the foramen can be pushed open. This is rarely functionally significant because LA pressure is usually higher than RA, and the flap is held shut against the foramen.

The coronary sinus contains blood that has circulated through the coronary arterial system. It drains into the right atrium between the inferior vena cava and the tricuspid valve. The eustachian valve is a fold of membranous tissue in the floor of the RA and is located near the orifice of the inferior vena cava. It plays an important part in fetal circulation, diverting blood from the inferior vena cava toward the interatrial septum and through the fossa ovale. In adults, it has no functional significance.

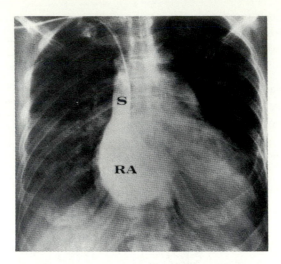

Figure 7–6. Angiography of the superior vena cava (S) and the right atrium (RA). (From Wenger NK, Hurst JW, McIntyre MC. Cardiology for nurses. New York: McGraw-Hill, 1980:22; with permission.)

The RV is a crescent-shaped chamber with walls thinner than those of the LV. The RV functions to pump a large volume of blood against a low resistance, whereas the LV is of smaller volume and is designed to pump a high pressure against a high resistance. For that reason, the RV is larger and has thinner walls than the LV (Fig. 7–7). Blood flows from the RA, into the RV, and then to the pulmonary arteries. To do this, the blood must take a turn greater than 90 degrees. The blood-flow pattern can be represented by a teapot wherein blood must flow into the base of the spout and then out the end of the spout (Fig. 7–8). A stout band of muscle, the moderator band, often traverses the RV chamber near the apex. The moderator band contains a branch of the right bundle branch from the electrical conduction system of the heart.

Between the RA and RV is the tricuspid valve, which has three indistinct leaflets. Strings (chordae tendinae) anchor the tricuspid valve to the RV via multiple sites. Unlike the mitral valve, the tricuspid valve chordae attach both to papillary muscles and to the RV wall (Fig. 7–9).

Within the RV, there is a line of demarcation between the inflow area of the RV, which is the trabeculated portion, and the outflow tract, or infundibulum, which is smooth. It consists of a ridge of muscular tissue that is called the "crista terminalis." The location of ventricular septal defects (VSD) is often classified in relation to this ridge. An RV angiogram is shown in Figure 7–10.

As blood flows from the RV to the pulmonary artery (PA), it passes across the pulmonic valve, a trileaflet structure. The right main PA reaches across the heart to the right lung and is, therefore, longer than the left main PA (see

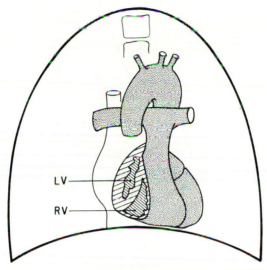

Figure 7–7. Right ventricle (RV) versus left ventricular (LV) thickness and orientation. The RV is much thinner and is designed to handle volume loads. The LV is thick and designed to pump high pressure.

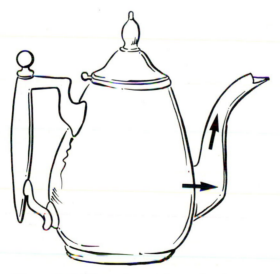

Figure 7–8. The teapot reflects the shape and flow of blood through the right ventricle.

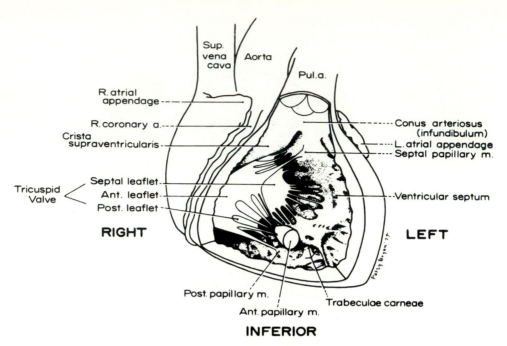

Figure 7–9. The shape of the right venticle is shown. In addition, the multiple attachments of the tricuspid valve to the right ventricle are evident. The three leaflets of the tricuspid valve include the anterior, posterior, and septal leaflets. (From Wenger NK, Hurst JW, McIntyre MC. Cardiology for nurses. New York: McGraw-Hill, 1980:27; with permission.)

Figs. 7–10 and 7–11). Blood flows through the pulmonary beds and returns to the LA via four major pulmonary veins (Fig. 7–12).

The LA lies posteriorly and is similarly divided into a smooth body and heavy trabeculated atrial appendage. The LA appendage wraps around the RV outflow tract and forms part of the left border of the heart (see Fig. 7–1). The relationship between the atria and ventricles in a cross-sectional view of the heart is shown in Fig. 7–3. In the anteroposterior view, the LA is posterior to the RV and central to the LV (Fig. 7–13).

The LV is an ellipsoid, somewhat bullet-shaped chamber, with walls two to three times thicker than the RV. The LV needs to generate high pressure. The increased wall thickness allows the generation of these higher pressures at the lowest possible wall stress in accordance with the law of Laplace:

$$\text{wall stress} \propto \frac{\text{chamber radius} \times \text{pressure}}{\text{wall thickness}}$$

This law is used often in cardiovascular medicine to show the interrelationship between wall stress and chamber size, pressure and wall thickness. Normally, the heart compensates for increased intracardiac pressure or volume by

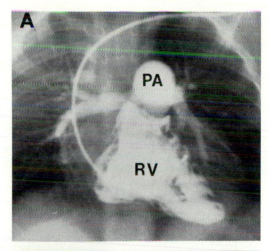

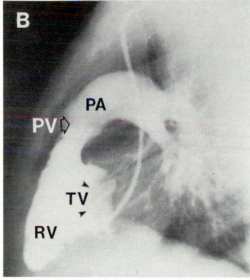

Figure 7–10. The right ventricular (RV) angiogram reveals the triangular shape of the RV in the pulmonary arterial (PA) view (*A*) and the lateral view (*B*). The RV is a "pancake" shape. The arrows in *B* point toward the tricuspid valve (TV). (Modified from Davies ML. Cardiac roentgenology: Shadows of the heart. Chicago: Year Book Medical Publishers, 1981:52; with permission.)

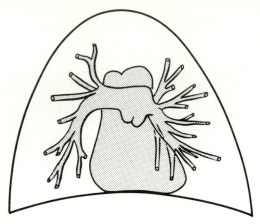

Figure 7–11. Pulmonary arterial pattern.
The right main pulmonary artery is
longer than the left. The arteries radiate
from the hilum on the chest radiograph,
and this pattern helps distinguish them
from the pulmonary veins on the chest
radiograph.

wall hypertrophy (or thickening), thus keeping wall stress at a minimum. If
either the radius or pressure rises, the wall stress can be reduced by increasing wall thickness. Because peripheral resistance to flow is so much higher
(by a factor of 10) than pulmonary resistance, the LV walls are required to
be much thicker than the RV walls (see Fig. 7–7). Thus, the LV is particularly

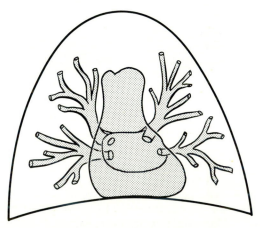

Figure 7–12. Pulmonary venous pattern.
The four pulmonary veins drawn into
the posteriorly located left atrium. Veins
tend to be vertical in the upper lobes
and horizontal from the lower lobes.
This helps distinguish them from pulmonary arteries.

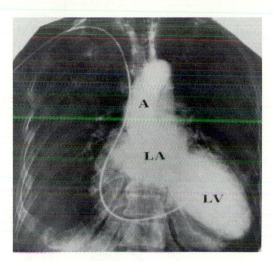

Figure 7–13. The angiographic relationship between the left atrium (LA) and left ventricle (LV) in the AP view. A = aorta. (From Wenger NK, Hurst JW, McIntyre MC. Cardiology for nurses. New York: McGraw-Hill, 1980:23; with permission.)

suited to be a pressure-generating chamber, whereas the RV is considered better suited to volume work. The interventricular septum is muscular except at its uppermost portion, where it is thin and membranous. In general, the septum is considered to be part of the LV rather than the RV.

Blood entering through the mitral valve must take an almost 180-degree turn before leaving the LV and entering the systemic circulation (Fig. 7–14).

The mitral valve has two major leaflets—the anterior leaflet (triangular in shape) and the posterior leaflet (rectangular in shape) (Fig. 7–15). Chordae tendinae from both leaflets attach to two large LV papillary muscles (the posteromedial and anterolateral). This arrangement is important for proper function of the mitral leaflet (Fig. 7–16).

The LV outflow tract is composed of the interventricular septum on one side and the mitral anterior leaflet on the other. This relationship is important in certain disease states in which the anterior leaflet may play a role in LV outflow obstruction (such as in hypertrophic cardiomyopathy) (see Fig. 7–15).

The aortic valve is a trileaflet structure with three cusps of approximately equal size. The pockets in these leaflets are called "sinuses of Valsalva." The aortic valve is located deep within the heart posteriorly to the RV outflow and adjacent to the interatrial septum (Fig. 7–17). This relationship has particular relevance when attempts at puncture of the interatrial septum during transseptal catheterization are performed.

The pulmonic and aortic valves are referred to as "semilunar valves." The tricuspid and the mitral valves are called "atrioventricular valves." The pulmonary and aortic valves are similar in size; the tricuspid valve, however, is considerably larger than the mitral valve. The valves are attached to a fibrous skeleton

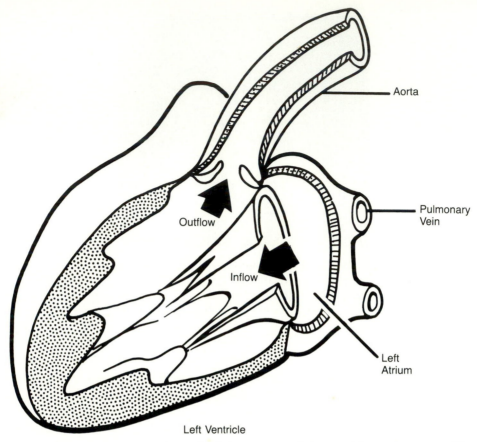

Aorta

Outflow

Pulmonary
Vein

Inflow

Left
Atrium

Left Ventricle

Figure 7–14. Flow pattern from the left atrium to left ventricle to the aorta. Note the sharp turn the blood must take out of the left ventricle in order to enter the aorta.

made of collagenous material. A central fibrous body exists to provide support for not only the valvular tissue, but also for the attachments of the atrial and ventricular chambers as well. Included in this fibrous structure are rings that encircle the valves of the heart. "Annulus fibrosis" is a name given to the connective tissue around the mitral and tricuspid valves. The membranous portion of the interventricular septum also attaches to the central fibrous body (Fig. 7–18). The electrical system of the heart passes through this area as well.

The entire heart is enclosed in a fibrous sac called the "pericardium." The pericardium can be thought of as a balloon, with the heart being a fist pushed into the balloon. The pericardium has two surfaces: the visceral pericardium, which is the portion that lies on the surface of the heart, and the parietal pericardium, which lies against adjacent mediastinal structures. The inside of the pericardial sac contains a small amount of fluid that acts as a lubricant. The pericardium functions to maintain a frictionless environment, to isolate the heart and to prevent overdistension of the heart.

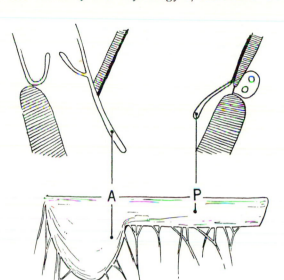

Figure 7–15. The mitral leaflet. The anterior (A) leaflet is triangular in shape, and the posterior (P) is rectangular. In the upper panel, note that the aortic outflow tract is made up of the anterior mitral leaflet on one side and the interventricular septum on the other. (From Kalmanson D. The mitral valve: A pluridisciplinary approach. Acton, MA: Publishing Services Group, 1976:35; with permission.)

The coronary arteries arise from the right and left cusps above the aortic valve (Fig. 7–19). The left main coronary artery almost immediately divides into the left anterior descending (LAD) artery and the left circumflex (LCX) artery. After dividing, the LAD artery continues down the interventricular septum and around the LV apex. The main branches of the LAD artery are diagonal branches (called "anterolaterals" in some institutions) and the septal perforators. The diagonals are so called because of their diagonal course along the LV free wall. Usually, three to five diagonals are evident during angiography. The septal branches, or septal perforators, arise at approximately a 90-degree angle from the LAD artery and supply the interventricular septum. A large first septal perforator is usually a readily identifiable landmark on coronary angiography.

The LAD artery supplies blood to the anterior two-thirds of interventricular septum, the anterior portion of LV and RV, the anterior papillary muscles of both ventricles, as well as the right bundle branch and the anterior portion of the left bundle branch of the conduction system.

The LCX artery departs from the left main at a sharp angle, running along the AV groove, giving off two to five obtuse marginal branches that supply the lateral LV and posterior LV and the LA. In 40 percent of the population, the

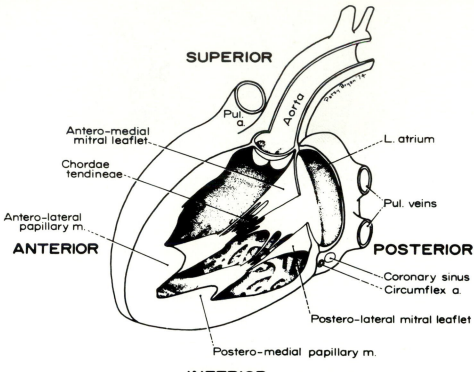

SUPERIOR

Pul. a.

Aorta

Antero-medial mitral leaflet

Chordae tendineae

Antero-lateral papillary m.

ANTERIOR

L. atrium

Pul. veins

POSTERIOR

Coronary sinus
Circumflex a.

Postero-lateral mitral leaflet

Postero-medial papillary m.

INFERIOR

Figure 7–16. The mitral apparatus. There are two major papillary muscles in the left ventricle (posteromedial and anterolateral). Chordae tendineae attach to both leaflets of the mitral valve from both of the papillary muscles. (From Wenger NK, Hurst JW, McIntyre MC. Cardiology for nurses. New York: McGraw-Hill, 1980: 29; with permission.)

sinus node is also supplied by the LCX artery. In approximately 10 percent of people, the posterior descending branch, which runs along the inferior portion of the interventricular septum, is also supplied by the LCX artery. When this occurs, the coronary anatomy is considered to be left dominant. A large branch may also be present between the origin of LAD and LCX arteries. This branch is referred to as a "ramus intermedius" (or optimal diagonal).

The right coronary artery (RCA) originates from the right coronary cusp of the aortic valve. It travels down the right AV groove and continues past the acute margin of the RV to the posterior AV groove; it has branches going to the posterior interventricular septum toward the apex and to the diaphragmatic (inferior) surface of the LV. The RCA supplies blood to the RA, RV, and the inferior third of the interventricular septum. In 60 percent of people, it supplies the sinus node, and in 90 percent, the AV node of the conduction system. A right-dominant system is one in which the RCA supplies the posterior descending to the interventricular septum. Further branches to the LV lateral wall are called "posterolater-

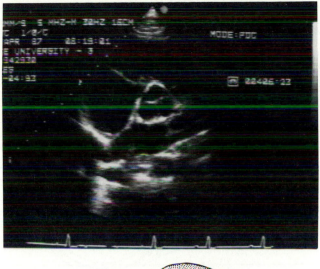

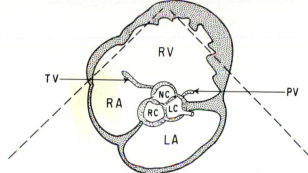

Figure 7–17. Relationship of aortic valve and the left atrium (LA) in cross-sectional echocardiographic view. The two-dimensional echocardiogram is shown at the top, and a schematic outlining the structure is shown on the bottom. RV = right ventricle. TV = tricuspid valve. PV = pulmonary valve. RA = right atrium. RC = right coronary. LC = left coronary. NC = noncoronary.

als." If the RCA ends in the posterior descending with no posterolateral branches to the LV, then the system is called "codominant" (Fig. 7–20).

The epicardial coronary arteries lie in the fat along the surface of the heart. Branches from the epicardial coronaries are sent into the heart and branch out throughout the myocardium (Fig. 7–21). These smaller branches are not well seen on angiography. Blood flow to the epicardial (outer) portion of the heart can vary considerably from blood flow to the inner portion (endocardium). Once supplied to the myocardium, blood returns through the coronary venous system, with almost 90 percent returning to the RA via the coronary sinus (Fig. 7–22).

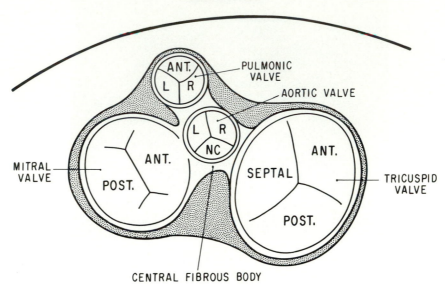

Figure 7–18. Relationship of each of the four valves to each other and to the fibrous skeleton of the heart. The trileaflet pulmonic valve is anterior and to the left of the aortic valve. The fibrous skeleton includes the mitral and tricuspid annuli and the central fibrous body. Ant = anterior. Post = posterior. NC = noncoronary.

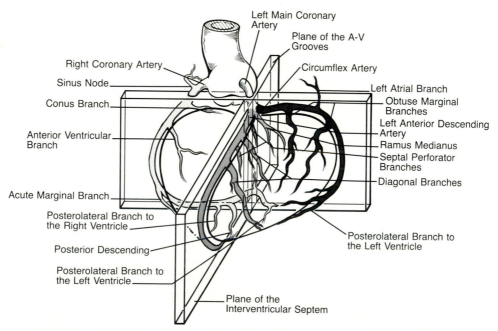

Figure 7–19. The two planes that define the location of the coronary arteries. The right and left circumflex arteries lie in the same plane, while the left anterior descending travels perpendicular to that plane. Branches from each vessel are shown. The left circumflex artery is outlined in black, the left anterior descending in gray, and the right circumflex in white.

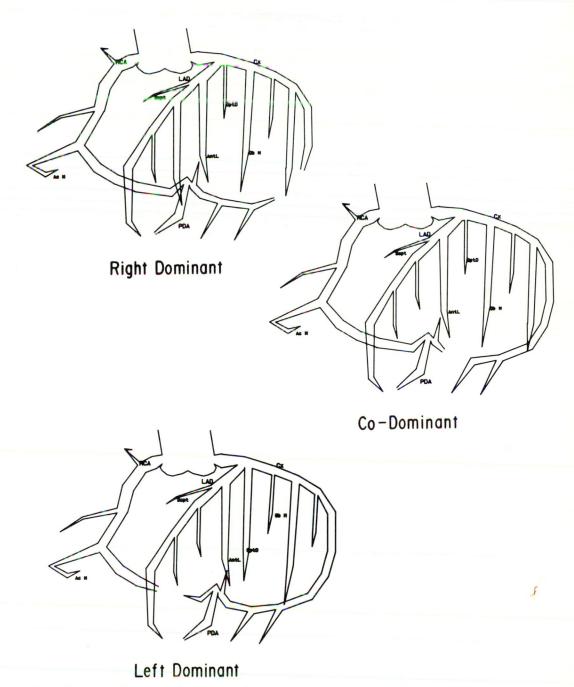

Right Dominant

Co-Dominant

Left Dominant

Figure 7–20. Definition of coronary dominance. The posterior descending artery (PDA) defines dominance. If the PDA arises from the right coronary artery (RCA) and has branches to the left ventricle (LV), the vessel is right dominant. If the RCA ends in the PDA, the system is codominant. If the PDA arises from the left circumflex (LCX) artery, then the system is considered left dominant. (From Sabiston DC, Spencer FL. Gibbons's Surgery of the Chest. 5th ed [in press].)

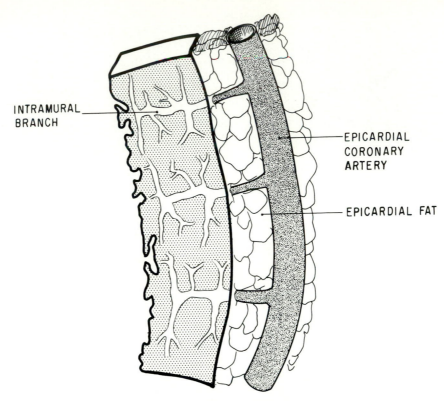

Figure 7–21. The epicardial coronary artery sends branches into the myocardium, with intramural branches to the epicardium and to the endocardium.

The remaining 10 percent of coronary venous return goes directly into the respective heart chambers via Thebesian veins. A small anterior cardiac vein also drains the RV conus into the RA. The anterior interventricular vein drains the anterior surface. Once it reaches the A-V groove, it becomes the great cardiac vein. As drainage enters from the lateral and inferior walls of the heart, the structure becomes the coronary sinus. The boundary between the coronary sinus and the great vein is the remnant of the left SVC, the oblique vein of Marshall. Coronary flow occurs primarily in early diastole, when the pressure between the ventricular chambers and the aorta is the greatest.

Conduction System

The electrical conduction system of the heart is a pathway of specialized cells that facilitate the movement of an electrical impulse through the heart, resulting in depolarization of the heart cells and, ultimately, a systematic contraction of the heart.

The "pacemaker" of the heart is the sinus or sinoatrial (SA) node, located essentially on the surface of the heart at the junction of the superior vena

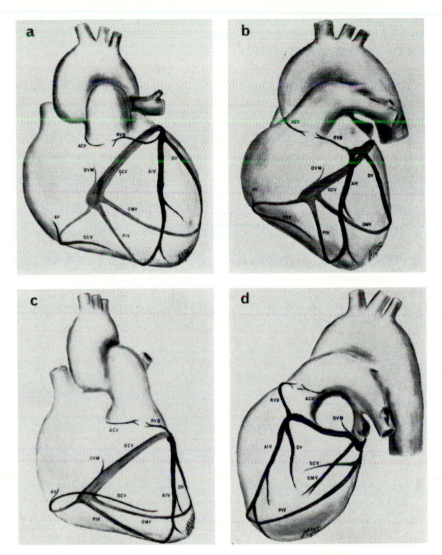

Figure 7–22. The coronary venous system. The views shown are the anteroposterior (a), the left anterior oblique (b), the right anterior oblique (c), and the left lateral (d). The major veins include the anterior interventricular (AIV), the great cardiac vein (GCV), the oblique vein of Marshall (OVM), and the anterior cardiac vein (ACV). The coronary sinus begins at the OVM. (From Gensini GG, et al. Anatomy of the coronary circulation in living man: Coronary venography. *Circulation* 1965; 31:780; with permission.)

cava (SVC) and RA. It is only 1 to 2 mm below the epicardial surface of the RA. The SA node spontaneously and rhythmically depolarizes and sends an impulse to the RA and LA, causing the atria to contract. The impulse then is slowed by a special area (AV node) located between the atria and ventricles. This "brake" allows atrial contraction to be completed before the onset of ventricular contraction. As the electrical impulses traverse the atria, a P wave is displayed on the surface electrocardiogram (ECG). Conduction through the AV node itself results in no waveform on the surface ECG. Conduction continues to each ventricle through large branches—the right and left bundle branches, respectively. Depolarization (or activation) of the ventricles results in ventricular contraction and is represented on the surface electrogram by the QRS wave. The right bundle branch is superficially located just beneath the RV endocardium and can "shut off" if bumped by a catheter during heart catheterization. When this occurs, a pattern referred to as a "right bundle branch block" can be seen. Recall that the right bundle travels in the moderator band that crosses the RV apex. The left bundle divides into two branches—a thin anterior and a large posterior branch. Between the AV node and the bundle branches lies an area wherein the fibers to each branch are identifiable and lined up in a packet known as the bundle of His. This area is not visible on the surface electrogram, but it can be identified by an electrical spike in the electrogram taken from within the heart (His spike). The recording of each of these areas of the conduction system can be readily accomplished using catheter electrodes. Chapter 14 covers the conduction system and electrophysiology studies in detail.

Normal Physiology

The cardiac cycle can be divided into two basic components. Ventricular systole describes the period during which ventricular contraction occurs. Ventricular diastole refers to the period during which the ventricles are filling with blood in preparation for the next systole. The right and left sides of the heart essentially work simultaneously to fill and then eject blood into the pulmonary and systemic arteries, respectively. The atria also have their systolic and diastolic periods. Atrial systole pushes atrial blood into the ventricle at the end of ventricular diastole (just before ventricular contraction). In that way, the atria push an extra boost of blood into the ventricles just prior to ventricular systole.

Figure 7–23 outlines the phases of the cardiac cycle, the LV motion and the position of the aortic and mitral valves during these phases. The RV motion and tricuspid and pulmonic valves follow a similar pattern. At the beginning of contraction, the pressure rises in the LV and closes the mitral valve. As contraction continues, a period occurs during which the mitral valve is closed but the pressure is not yet great enough to open the aortic valve. This brief period is referred to as the "isovolumic contraction period." Once the LV pressure rises higher than that in the aorta, the aortic valve opens and ventricular ejection begins. Ejection continues throughout systole and the LV empties. Following ejection, the LV begins to relax or go into its diastolic phase. As the LV relaxes, the pressure in the LV falls and the aortic valve closes. A period of brief isovolumic relaxation then occurs until the LV pressure falls below the LA pressure. When this happens, the mitral valve opens, and blood flows from the LA to the LV. The LV then rapidly fills with blood for about one-third of diastole, then it fills much more slowly until atrial systole kicks in, providing the last boost of blood just prior to the next ventricular systole. The whole process then repeats.

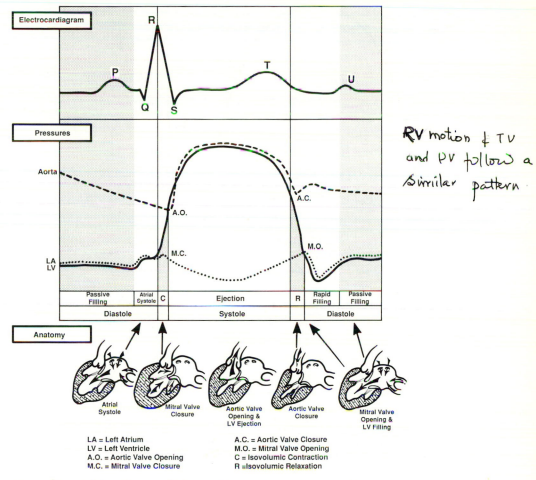

Figure 7–23. The phases of the cardiac cycle, and the position of the valves during those phases. Valve closure occurs at the pressure crossover points and result in the heart sounds being produced. Systole and diastole begin with isovolumic contraction and relaxation phases, respectively.

Normal Chamber Pressures

Figure 7–24 represents normal RA pressure and the position of the catheter in the RA from the right femoral vein. There are five waveforms identifiable. The A wave occurs during atrial contraction. The C wave occurs when the ventricle contracts and the tricuspid valve bulges into the RA. The X-descent is a fall in RA pressure that occurs when the atrium goes into diastole and the tricuspid ring is pulled into the RV (both enlarge the RA, and the pressure in the RA falls). The V wave occurs while the RA passively fills with blood from the venous system and peaks at the time the tricuspid valve opens and the RV goes into its diastole. The Y-descent reflects the fall in the RA pressure as the RA empties into the RV. The RA pressure thus rises with atrial systole (A wave), falls during ventricular

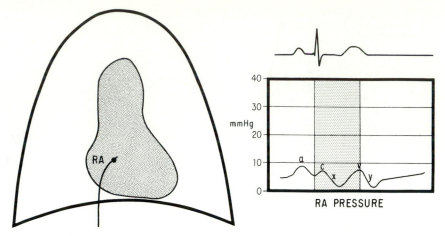

Figure 7–24. Normal right atrium (RA) pressure, and the position of the catheter in the RA (AP view). The shaded area represents electrical systole for timing of the pressure events with the ECG.

systole (X-descent), and falls during ventricular diastole (Y-descent). The filling of the RA occurs during the V wave. If the atrium is poorly compliant (stiff), the V wave will be higher than if it is not stiff.

The LA pressure is similar to RA pressure, with the exception that the LA is in a much more confined space and has a lower compliance (it is stiffer). Atrial contraction leads to a larger A wave, and atrial filling leads to a larger V wave. Left atrial pressure can be directly measured by transseptal puncture of the interatrial septum (Fig. 7–25) or indirectly by measuring the pressure from the pulmonary capillary wedge (Fig. 7–26). The pulmonary capillary wedge (PCW) can be used to record LA pressure because there are no valves between the LA and the PCW.

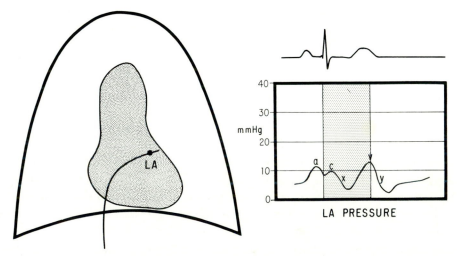

Figure 7–25. Normal left atrium (LA) pressure, and the position of the transseptal catheter in the LA (AP view).

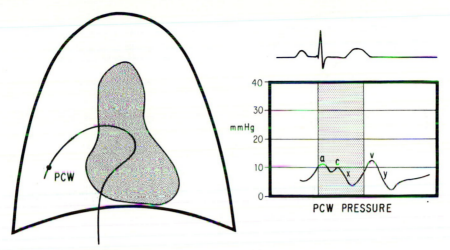

Figure 7–26. Pulmonary capillary wedge (PCW) pressure from the right lower lung. Catheter position and pressure tracing are shown. Note the pressure tracing is shifted in time from the LA pressure measured directly (Fig. 7–25).

    The RV pressure tracing is composed of an A wave due to atrial contraction, followed by the rise and fall of the ventricular systolic pressure. In early diastole, rapid filling occurs, and then slow filling (Fig. 7–27).

    Left ventricular pressure is similar to RV pressure, except that both the diastolic and systolic pressures are higher (Fig. 7–28). The LV or RV end-diastolic pressure is occasionally used as a rough measure of how stiff each ventricle is. The end-diastolic pressures are measured at the end of the A wave or with the peak of the electrocardiographic QRS wave if the A wave is difficult to see.

    Right ventricular ejection results in opening of the pulmonic valve and

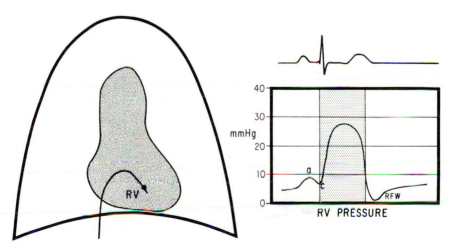

Figure 7–27. Right ventricular (RV) pressure. Catheter position and pressure tracing are shown. a = atrial contraction wave; c = initiation of contraction; RFW = rapid filling wave.

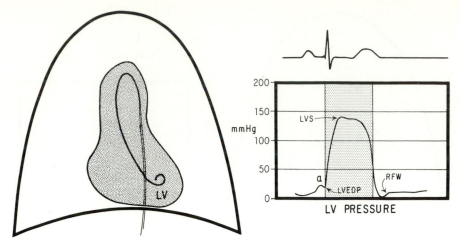

Figure 7–28. Left ventricular (LV) pressure. Catheter position and representative pressure are shown. a = atrial contraction component; LVEDP = LV end-diastolic pressure; LVS = peak LV systolic pressure; RFW = rapid filling wave.

pressure generation into the PA system. The pressure rises and then falls until the pulmonic valve closes. As the pressure wavefront returns from the pulmonary circuit back to the closed pulmonic valve, a small wave (the dicrotic wave) is usually observed (Fig 7–29).

The aortic pressure is made up of three components—the percussion wave, the tidal wave, and the dicrotic wave. The percussion wave corresponds to forward aortic flow, the tidal wave is a reflected wave from the upper extremity, and the dicrotic wave is a reflected wave from the lower extremity (Figs. 7–30 and 7–31). As one proceeds down the aorta, reflected waves move back into the

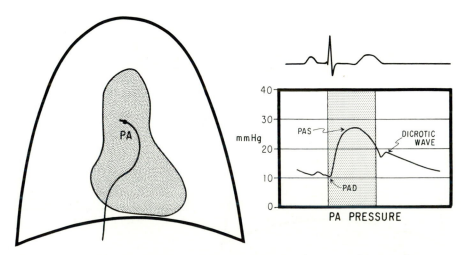

Figure 7–29. Pulmonary artery (PA) pressure. Catheter position and representative pressure are shown. PAD = pulmonary artery diastolic pressure; PAS = pulmonary artery systolic pressure.

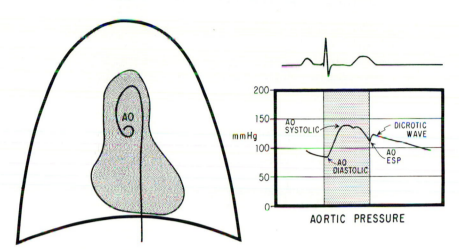

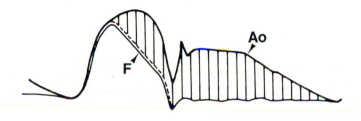

Figure 7–30. Aortic (AO) pressure. Catheter position from femoral artery shown with representative pressure. ESP = end-systolic pressure.

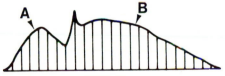

Figure 7–31. Components of the aortic (AO) pressure tracing. When the flow (F) curve is removed from the pressure curve, what remains is due to reflected waves. Reflected wave (A) likely arises from the upper extremity. This results in the tidal wave during ejection. Reflected wave (B) arises from the lower extremity. It results in the dicrotic wave during early diastole. (From O'Rourke MF. Arterial function in health and disease. New York: Churchill Livingstone, 1982:77; with permission.)

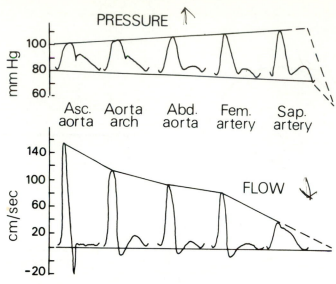

Figure 7–32. The *top* panel represents aortic pressure, and the *bottom,* aortic flow. Although forward flow is reduced as one goes from the ascending aorta to the periphery (*bottom*), the pulse pressure actually rises (*top*) owing to reflected waves. (From McDonald DA. Blood flow in arteries. Baltimore: Williams & Wilkins, 1974:358; with permission.)

pressure wavefront, becoming additive. Thus, the systolic pressure rises as one approaches the periphery (Fig. 7–32). Mean pressure is one-third of the way between systolic and diastolic pressure, because the waveform is roughly triangular in shape. There should be no difference between LV systolic pressure and aortic systolic pressure. However, peripheral systolic pressures are frequently higher than aortic, and this may become relevant when one is attempting to estimate a gradient across the aortic valve.

The Relationship Between Pressure, Volume, and Cardiac Output

As the heart fills in diastole, the pressure in the LV rises. The mean pressure in the LV during diastole can be approximated by the mean PCW pressure (mean LA pressure). The amount of blood the heart pumps out with each beat is referred to as the "stroke volume." The product of stroke volume times the heart rate provides the cardiac output. A fundamental relationship exists between filling pressures, how well the heart contracts (contractility), and cardiac output. This relationship can be best understood by analyses of the ventricular function curve (Sarnoff curve), shown in Figure 7–33.

At any given filling pressure (x-axis), the cardiac output produced is a function of the contractile state of the LV. If heart failure occurs, the normal function curve becomes flattened, and it takes a higher filling pressure to produce

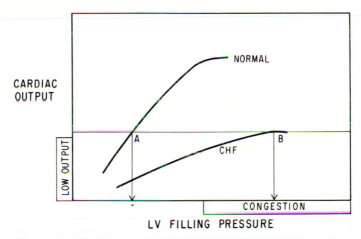

Figure 7–33. The ventricular function curve. A normal curve (NORMAL) is contrasted with a curve from a patient in heart failure (CHF). The relationship between cardiac output and filling pressure is nonlinear. In order to produce an adequate cardiac output in CHF, the filling pressure must be much greater than in normal. The same cardiac output is produced at a lower filling pressure in normals (A) than patients with CHF (B). To produce an adequate cardiac output leads to congestion. Conversely, simply reducing filling pressure leads to low output.

an adequate cardiac output. If the filling pressure rises too high, then pulmonary congestion may occur as the pressures "back up" into the lungs. If filling pressures are too low, then cardiac output is not adequate, and hypotension and low output (fatigue, and so forth) occur.

Under normal conditions, there is adequate cardiac output at an acceptable filling pressure. Under pathologic conditions, the curve may be altered. Therapy is then directed at optimizing filling pressure, contractile state, and the cardiac output. The cardiac performance is frequently described as being dependent on preload, afterload, and contractility. *Preload* is the amount of stretch of the heart muscle. Starlings' Law pointed out that the more the heart muscle was stretched, the stronger the muscle contracted. Preload can be estimated by using heart volume or the filling pressure. *Afterload* refers to the resistance against which the heart must work to contract. In the isolated heart muscle strip, it is simply the weight hung on the muscle as it contracts. In the intact heart, it is represented by the stress on the heart (or grossly represented by the systemic blood pressure). The less afterload, the more the heart can empty, and vice versa. *Contractility* represents the inherent ability of the heart muscle to contract and pump blood. It is referred to as its inotropic state. At the cellular level, contractile performance is dependent upon calcium moving to the actin-myosin apparatus within the heart cell.

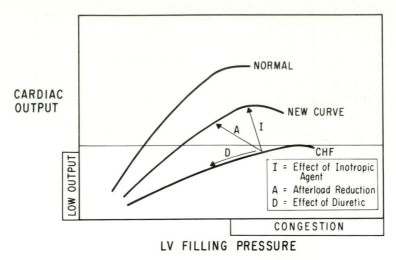

Figure 7–34. Effect of changes in preload, afterload, and contractility in the ventricular function curve. A diuretic reduces congestion by resulting in a lower filling pressure and lower output. Afterload reduction decreases filling pressure and raises cardiac output by shifting the ventricular function curve. An inotropic agent shifts the curve upward and results in improved cardiac output at about the same filling pressure. LV = left ventricle.

The ventricular function curve allows one to see how changes in preload, afterload, and contractility affect cardiac output (Fig. 7–34). A change in preload alone results in movement up and down the ventricular function curve. A change in contractility or afterload shifts the curve to a different level.

If someone is in heart failure, the curve is flatter than normal. This means that a higher filling pressure is required to achieve an adequate cardiac output. The price of having an adequate cardiac output is pulmonary congestion, however. Giving a diuretic alone will reduce the filling pressure and congestion, but results in a fall in cardiac output. To improve both cardiac output and the filling pressure, the afterload or contractility must also be improved. A reduction in afterload shifts the curve to the left and upward, so that an improved cardiac output can be produced at a lower filling pressure. Improvement in contractility shifts the curve upward alone, resulting in better cardiac output at each filling pressure.

Using this curve, one can predict how various drugs or devices (such as an intra-aortic balloon pump) affect the heart. Diuretics change the filling pressure and move one along any individual curve. Afterload reduction (with drugs such as captopril, hydralazine, enalapril) shifts the curve upward and leftward. Inotropic agents (such as digoxin, dopamine, amrinone) shift the curve upward. The idea is to operate out of the range where pulmonary congestion occurs without being in the low-cardiac-output range. In this manner, differing combinations of drugs allow the heart to work at an acceptable filling pressure and an acceptable cardiac output at the same time.

S E L E C T E D   R E F E R E N C E S

Anthony CP, Thibodeau GA. Textbook of anatomy and physiology. 11th ed. St.Louis: CV Mosby, 1983.

Bashore TM, Davidson CJ. Cardiac catheterization, angioplasty, and balloon valvuloplasty. In: Sabiston DC, Spencer FL, eds. Gibbons' Surgery of the Chest. 4th ed. Philadelphia: WB Saunders, 1989.

Davies ML. Cardiac roentgenology: Shadows of the heart. Chicago: Year Book Medical Publishers, 1981.

Gensini GG, et al. Anatomy of the coronary circulation in living men: Coronary venography. Circulation 1965; 31:780.

Gorlin R. Coronary artery disease, vol. XI. Smith L H Jr., ed. Major problems in internal medicine. Philadelphia: WB Saunders, 1976.

Kalmanson D. The mitral valve: A pluridisciplinary approach. Acton, MA: Publishing Sciences Group, 1976.

McDonald DA. Blood flow in arteries. Baltimore: Williams & Wilkins, 1974.

O'Rourke MF. Arterial function in health and disease. New York: Churchill Livingstone, 1982.

Wenger NK, Hurst JW, McIntyre MC. Cardiology for nurses. New York: McGraw-Hill, 1980.

CHAPTER 8

Basic Catheter Techniques

Charles J. Davidson, MD, and J. Kevin Harrison, MD

Historical Perspective

Werner Forssmann is generally credited with performing the first human heart catheterization. While receiving training as a surgeon in Eberswade, Germany, he used fluoroscopic guidance to advance a urethral catheter through his own left antecubital vein into the right atrium. In an attempt to develop a technique for direct delivery of drugs into the heart, he catheterized himself on several occasions. Because of intense criticism, however, he eventually abandoned this pursuit and undertook a career as a urologist.

In 1950, Zimmerman and coworkers performed the first left-heart catheterization. This technique was greatly facilitated by Seldinger, who described a method of percutaneous needle puncture with catheter exchange over a guidewire. Early attempts at visualization of the coronary arteries in human beings were accomplished with nonselective injection of radiopaque contrast media into the ascending aorta. In 1958, F. Mason Sones performed the first selective injection of contrast media into the coronary arteries utilizing a cutdown for the isolation of the brachial artery. The percutaneous femoral technique as modified by Judkins and the brachial technique pioneered by Sones are the most widely employed today. Each method offers its own set of disadvantages and advantages. The brachial technique, for example, is particularly useful in patients with severe peripheral vascular disease involving the abdominal aorta, illiac, and femoral arteries, whereas the femoral approach offers the advantage of not requiring arteriotomy and arterial repair. An advance in catheter design for right-heart catheterization came in 1970, when Swan introduced balloon-tipped catheters that could be introduced without fluoroscopy.

The advent of interventional coronary catheterization techniques occurred in 1977, when Andreas Gruentzig developed percutaneous transluminal coronary angioplasty (PTCA). While working in Zurich, Switzerland, and later at Emory University, he introduced a therapeutic technique within coronary arteries that has revolutionized the treatment of coronary artery disease. This interventional modality has become the standard against which future catheter therapies of coronary artery stenoses, such as atherectomy, laser, and interluminal stents, will be measured. More recently, percutaneous balloon valvuloplasty has been employed as a viable alternative for treatment of aortic, mitral, and pulmonic stenosis.

This chapter discusses the techniques of right- and left-heart catheterization and coronary arteriography. In addition, the technique of endomyocardial biopsy is reviewed. Discussion of the interventional procedures themselves is found in Chapter 9.

Internal Jugular Venous Cannulation

Anatomy (Fig. 8–1)

The internal jugular vein arises from the base of the skull and courses posterior and lateral to the internal and common carotid artery. It terminates lateral and anterior to the common carotid artery.

In relation to the sternomastoid muscle, the upper part of the vein runs medial to the muscle, whereas the middle segment courses posterior to the muscle in the triangle between the two inferior heads of the sternomastoid muscle. The

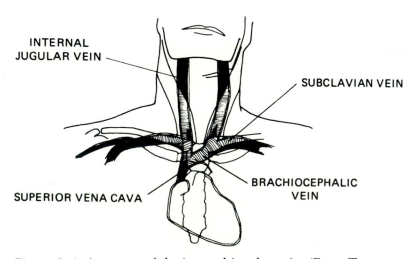

Figure 8–1. Anatomy of the internal jugular vein. (From Text-book of advanced cardiac life support. American Heart Association, 1987:147. Reproduced with permission of the American Heart Association.)

lower portion of the internal jugular vein runs behind the anterior part of the clavicular head. Finally, it joins with the subclavian vein at the medial end of the clavicle.

Indications

The indications for internal jugular venous access and for other central venous cannulation are summarized in Table 8–1.

Equipment

The equipment necessary for central venous cannulation using the Seldinger technique is shown in Figure 8–2 and is described in Table 8–2. It is possible to access the internal jugular vein by the over-the-needle technique or through-the-needle catheter devices (Angiocath, Intracath, Desert, and Jelco).

Technique

For all methods of internal jugular venous access, certain general principles apply. The patient is placed head down 15 to 30 degrees in the Trendelenburg position, and the patient's head is rotated in the opposite direction of the venipuncture. The entire side of the neck is prepared in a sterile fashion, then draped. The three approaches for cannulation of the internal jugular vein (central, anterior, and posterior) are described in Table 8–3.

Seldinger Technique

The Seldinger, or over-the-wire, technique is the most popular method for placement of a central venous or central arterial catheter. Although minor variations exist, this method as it is generally performed is described in Table 8–4.

TABLE 8–1
Indications for Central Venous Access

1. Emergent intravenous access.
2. Central venous pressure measurement and monitoring.
3. Rapid administration of large volumes of fluid.
4. Vasopressor or hyperalimentation administration.
5. Endomyocardial biopsy.
6. Right-heart catheterization, including measurement of pulmonary artery and capillary wedge pressure.
7. Insertion of a transvenous pacemaker.

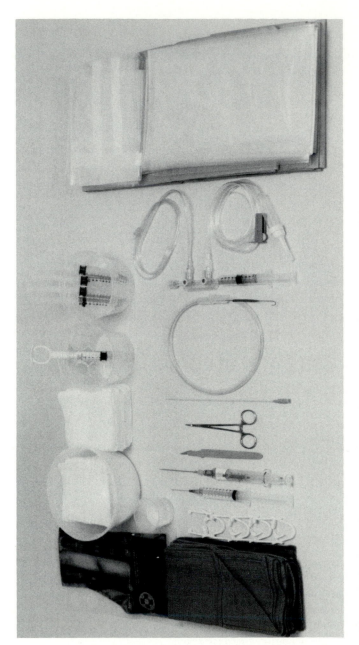

Figure 8–2. Example of equipment utilized for central venous or arterial access with the Seldinger technique.

TABLE 8–2
Equipment for Central Venous Cannulation Using the Seldinger Technique

Skin prep
Sterile prep
Gloves
Drapes
Suture
Antibiotic ointment
Dressing
Adhesive tape
Local anesthesia
   Lidocaine 1%
   22-gauge needle with plastic syringe
Cannulation equipment:
   Plastic syringe
   16- or 18-gauge 6-cm length thin-wall needle
   0.035-inch J-tipped guidewire
   Venous sheath

TABLE 8–3
Technique for Internal Jugular Venous Approach to Catheter Insertion

Central Approach
1. Palpate the triangle formed by the clavicle and the sternal and clavicular heads of the sternomastoid muscle.
2. Palpate the carotid pulse and retract it medially.
3. Infiltrate with local anesthesia by raising a skin wheal 3 to 4 cm above the clavicle.
4. While aspirating negative pressure, introduce the needle and syringe at the apex of the triangle formed by the two heads of the sternomastoid muscle.
5. Direct the needle laterally and caudad toward the ipsilateral nipple parallel to medial border of the clavicular (lateral) head of the sternomastoid muscle.
6. If the vein is not entered at a depth of 3 to 5 cm, slowly withdraw while maintaining negative aspiration pressure.
7. If the vein is still not cannulated, then direct the needle 5 to 10 degrees more laterally.

Anterior Approach
1. Retract the carotid artery medially with the left hand.
2. After anesthetizing the skin with a smaller needle, enter the skin at the midpoint of the medial aspect of the sternomastoid muscle.
3. Direct the needle at an angle of 30 to 45 degrees with the frontal plane caudad to the ipsilateral nipple.

Posterior Approach
1. After anesthetizing the skin, enter the skin at the lateral edge of the sternomastoid muscle one-third of the way between the clavicle and mastoid process (just above the site where the external jugular vein crosses the sternomastoid muscle).
2. Direct the needle caudally and medially under the lateral border of the sternomastoid muscle toward the midpoint of the sternal notch until blood is aspirated.
3. The vein should be cannulated at a depth of 5 to 7 cm.

TABLE 8–4
The Seldinger (Over-the-Wire) Technique

1. After entry into the jugular or subclavian vein, the plastic syringe is removed and the hub of the needle is covered by a finger to prevent entrance of air.
2. A 0.035-inch J-tipped guidewire is inserted through the thin-wall needle for a distance of 20 to 30 cm. The wire should pass freely through the vein.
3. The needle is removed, and a venous sheath and dilator assembly is advanced over the wire into the vein.
4. The dilator and guidewire are removed, leaving the sheath in place.
5. The side arm of the sheath is aspirated to insure free flow of blood, and is then flushed with saline.
6. The sheath is sutured into place.

Over-the-Needle and Through-the-Needle Techniques

After entry into the vein, these techniques require that the catheter is either advanced as the needle is withdrawn (over-the-needle technique), or the catheter is threaded through the larger gauge needle (through-the-needle technique).

Complications

The most common complications of the internal jugular venous cannulation are inadvertent puncture of the carotid artery and minor hematomas at the puncture site. Other potential complications are shown in Table 8–5.

Advantages of the Internal Jugular Venous Technique versus the Subclavian Venous Approach

There is a lower risk of pleural puncture and pneumothorax using the internal jugular venous approach compared with subclavian venous cannulation. Furthermore, if a hematoma occurs from accidental puncture of the carotid artery, compression of the area may be maintained by hand. If a pulmonary artery catheter is to be placed, then passage of a balloon-tipped catheter may be facilitated owing to the straight anatomic course to the right atrium.

TABLE 8–5
Complications Associated with Central Venous Access in the Internal Jugular Vein

Pneumothorax	Air embolism
Hemothorax	Catheter embolism
Hydrothorax	Neurologic: brachial plexus injury, phrenic and recurrent laryngeal nerve injury
Hydromediastinum	Carotid artery puncture
Hydropericardium	Hematoma at puncture site, if severe, may cause tracheal compression

Subclavian Venous Cannulation

Anatomy (Fig. 8–3)

The subclavian vein arises as a continuation of the axillary vein at the outer edge of the first rib and courses anterior to the scalene muscles. It joins the internal jugular vein to become the innominate, or brachiocephalic, vein. The subclavian vein lies anterior and inferior to the subclavian artery, whereas the anterior scalene muscle separates the subclavian vein and artery. The phrenic nerve runs immediately behind the junction of the subclavian and internal jugular veins. The apex of the pleura extends to the neck of the first rib near the origin of the innominate vein.

Indications and Equipment

The indications for subclavian venous cannulation are the same as those previously described for the internal jugular vein (see Table 8–1). Likewise, the equipment for the two methods of access is similar (see Table 8–2 and Fig. 8–2).

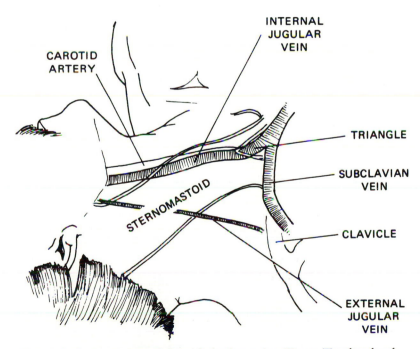

Figure 8–3. Anatomy of the subclavian vein. (From Textbook of advanced cardiac life support. American Heart Association, 1987: 147. Reproduced with permission of the American Heart Association.)

Techniques

The general principles for internal jugular venous cannulation apply to subclavian venous cannulation. Subclavian venipuncture is performed as outlined in Table 8–6.

Complications

The potential complications are similar to those for internal jugular venipuncture, except that subclavian artery puncture, rather than carotid artery puncture, may occur (see Table 8–5).

Advantages of Subclavian Venous Cannulation over the Internal Jugular Venous Technique

In comparison to the internal jugular vein, the subclavian vein may be more easy to locate, especially in patients with short, thick necks. Furthermore, if prolonged cannulation is necessary, the subclavian venous approach allows neck movement.

Femoral Venous Cannulation

Anatomy (Fig. 8–4)

The femoral vein lies medial to the femoral artery as it courses into the thigh below the inguinal ligament. The femoral artery may be palpated below the inguinal ligament, and the vein will lie immediately medial to it.

TABLE 8–6
Technique for Subclavian Venous Puncture

1. The right subclavian vein is usually cannulated to avoid the left-sided thoracic duct and because of the lower pleural dome on the right.
2. Raise a skin wheal at one finger's breadth below the inferior border of the midpoint of the clavicle with a small needle and syringe containing local anesthesia.
3. Place the index finger of the opposite hand in the suprasternal notch as a target.
4. With the syringe and needle assembly parallel to the frontal plane, point the needle medially and slightly toward the head.
5. Advance toward the suprasternal notch and under the clavicle. (Advancing the needle posteriorly or inferiorly results in the greatest likelihood of complication such as pneumo- or hemothorax.)
6. After the needle passes under the clavicle, aspirate gently until free return of venous blood occurs.
7. Detach the syringe, and immediately cover the hub of the needle.
8. Follow the same procedure as described for the over-the-wire, over-the-needle or through-the needle technique.

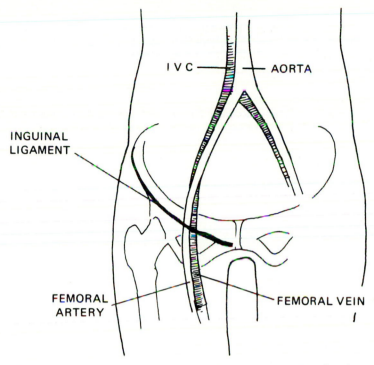

Figure 8–4. Anatomy of the femoral vein. (From Textbook of advanced cardiac life support. American Heart Association, 1987:146. Reproduced with permission of the American Heart Association.)

Indications

The indications for femoral venous cannulation include those described for the internal jugular venous technique. It may allow more rapid access of a central vein during cardiac resuscitation, without interruption of CPR. Femoral venous access is the most commonly used approach for cardiac catheterization procedures that require right-heart catheterization.

Equipment

The equipment is the same as that described for the internal jugular venous approach.

Technique

The technique of femoral venous cannulation is generally performed by the Seldinger technique. Femoral venous access is obtained as outlined in Table 8–7.

TABLE 8–7
Technique for Femoral Venous Cannulation

1. Prepare and drape the femoral area in a sterile fashion.
2. Palpate the femoral pulse 1 to 2 finger breadths (2 to 4 cm) below the inguinal ligament.
3. With a small needle and syringe filled, infiltrate the skin with lidocaine. This 22-gauge "finder" needle may be advanced posteriorly until the vein is entered. It may be disconnected from the syringe and left in place as a guide for the larger Seldinger needle.
4. Using a thin-wall needle attached to a syringe, medial to the femoral pulse, advance at a 45-degree angle with the skin.
5. Maintain negative suction while advancing the needle.
6. If no blood is obtained, slowly withdraw the assembly while maintaining gentle aspiration.
7. Upon obtaining free flow of blood, detach the syringe and either insert a J-tipped guidewire (Seldinger technique) or advance a catheter into the vein.

Complications

The most common complication of femoral venous access is hematoma at the puncture site. This is often due to difficulty in locating the vein or to inadvertent puncture of the femoral artery. Other complications include thrombosis, phlebitis, femoral nerve damage, or formation of arteriovenous fistula.

Advantages of the Femoral Venous Technique over the Internal Jugular and Subclavian Venous Approaches

The major advantage of the femoral venous route of access is that it allows compression of the artery if inadvertent puncture should occur. This may be of special importance in patients who have received thrombolytic therapy or are receiving anticoagulants. Also, cannulation does not require interruption of CPR. Because most left-heart catheterizations are performed via the femoral route, both venous and arterial puncture may be obtained within the same sterile field.

Right-Heart Catheterization

Indications

Right-heart catheterization allows measurement of right-heart pressures, including right atrial, right ventricular, pulmonary artery, and pulmonary capillary wedge pressure, as well as measurement of cardiac output.

Equipment

The same equipment is required for right-heart catheterization as for internal jugular venous cannulation (see Table 8–2). In addition, a balloon-tipped flotation catheter or a curved end-hole catheter (e.g., Lehman Catheter, USCI Corp., Bellerica, MA) is employed (Fig. 8–5). An 8 French sheath may be utilized or, if percutaneous insertion without a sheath is performed, a 7 French dilator is required. A pressure recorder, pressure transducer, manifold, ECG monitor, and connecting tubing are necessary.

Technique

The technique of right-heart catheterization is outlined in Table 8–8.

Complications

The most common complications of right-heart catheterization are nonsustained atrial and ventricular arrhythmias, e.g., premature atrial contractions, and premature ventricular contractions. A list of other potential complications is shown in Table 8–9.

Left-Heart Catheterization

Prior to cardiac catheterization, the procedure and potential complications should be explained to the patient and written informed consent obtained. The patient is generally fasting for at least 4 hr, and is usually premedicated with antihistamines such as diphenhydramine (25 to 50 mg, given intravenously). Other sedatives such as intravenous or oral benzodiazepines may be given prior to the procedure. An intravenous line should be established prior to the procedure. The patient is brought to the catheterization laboratory, and prepped and draped in a sterile fashion.

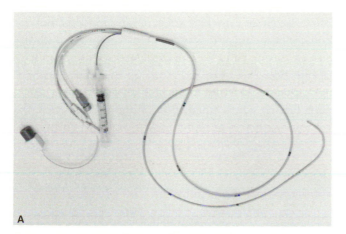
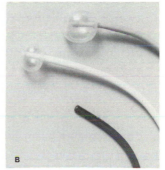

Figure 8–5. Example of two types of right-heart catheters: balloon-tipped and end-hole catheters.

TABLE 8–8
Technique for Right-Heart Catheterization

1. Balloon-tipped catheters should be test inflated.
2. End-hole catheters should have an additional curve made by wrapping the catheter around the index and middle fingers.
3. Obtain central venous access as previously described.
4. Utilizing the Seldinger technique, remove the needle over a guidewire.
5. Puncture the skin with a blade to provide a hole large enough for the introducer.
6. Either dilate the puncture site with a 7 French dilator or insert an 8 French sheath over the guidewire and remove the introducer.
7. Either insert the right-heart catheter percutaneously over the guidewire or insert the balloon-tipped catheter through the sheath.
8. Advance the catheter into the right atrium. (Remove the guidewire if not already done.)
9. Aspirate the catheter until all air is removed and blood is easily aspirated. Flush the catheter with saline. (If a balloon-tipped catheter is utilized, all ports should be aspirated and flushed.)
10. Connect the catheter or pulmonary artery distal port to the pressure manifold.
11. Record right atrial pressure.
12. If a balloon-tipped catheter is used, the balloon should be inflated at this time.
13. Advance the catheter into the right ventricle, pulmonary artery, and pulmonary capillary wedge positions while recording pressures.
14. Deflate the balloon. On end-hole systems, retract the catheter into the pulmonary artery position.

Percutaneous Femoral Arterial Technique (Judkins)

Equipment

Because of its relative ease, speed, reliability, and slightly lower rate of complications, the Judkins technique has become the most widely used method of coronary arteriography in this country. The preformed catheters used for the Judkins technique are shown in Figure 8–6. These catheters are generally made of polyurethane and polyethylene and contain either steel braid or nylon in the wall of the shaft, thus allowing improved torque control. The catheters are designed with a single end hole for contrast injection and a tapered blunt tip to reduce intimal trauma. Although the original catheters were usually 8 French, which were 2.7 mm in diameter (note that each French size is equal to 0.33 mm in diameter), the 6 (2.0 mm) and 7 French (2.3 mm) catheters are now most commonly utilized for

TABLE 8–9
Complications Associated with Right-Heart Catheterization

Arrhythmias	Catheter thrombus
Pulmonary infarction	Infection, including phlebitis
Pulmonary artery perforation	Balloon rupture
Catheter kinking or knotting	

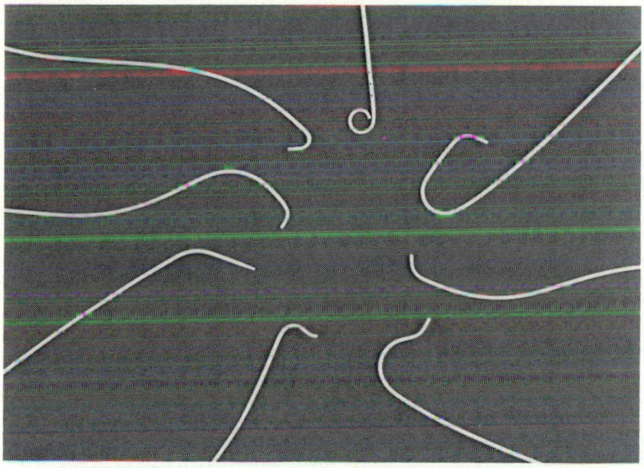

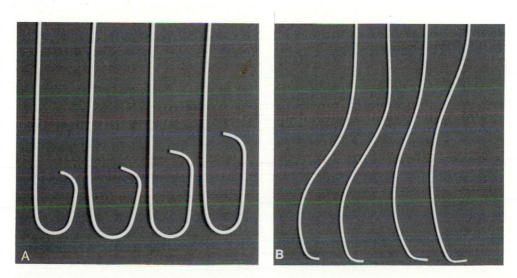

Figure 8–6. Various types of catheters utilized in cardiac catheterization with the percutaneous femoral technique. *A,* Beginning clockwise from top: the pigtail catheter, the left and right Judkins catheters, the left and right Amplatz catheters, a multipurpose catheter, a bypass graft catheter, and an internal mammary artery catheter. *B.*

adult coronary arteriography. All catheters have a primary, secondary, and tertiary curve. The Judkins left and right coronary catheters are available in four sizes that are commonly referred to as JL3.5, JL4, JL5, JL6, and JR3.5, JR4, JR5, and JR6. The numbers describe the length in centimeters of the secondary arm of the catheters (Fig. 8–7). The JL4 catheter is most commonly employed in patients

Figure 8–7. Judkins left and right coronary catheters. *A,* From left to right: Judkins left 3.5, 4, 5, 6. *B,* From left to right: Judkins right 3.5, 4, 5, 6.

with normal-sized aortic roots, whereas the JL5 and JL6 catheters are used in patients with progressively elongated or dilated aortic roots. The secondary bend represents the major difference in the left and right coronary catheters. The secondary bend of the left coronary catheter approaches 180 degrees, whereas the bend of the right coronary catheter is approximately 30 degrees.

Technique

After local anesthesia with a 1 percent lidocaine, percutaneous entry of the femoral artery is achieved by puncturing the vessel 1 to 3 cm below the inguinal ligament. The inguinal ligament, which can be palpated as it runs across a line from the anterior superior iliac spine to the superior pubic ramus, should be the landmark utilized rather than the often misleading inguinal crease. A transverse skin incision with a scapel is made over the femoral artery. An 18-gauge thin-wall needle is inserted at a 30- to 45-degree angle into the femoral artery and a J-tipped Teflon-coated guidewire with a 0.035-inch diameter is advanced into the needle. The guidewire should pass freely up the aorta. Fluoroscopy should be used to follow the course of the catheter. While applying firm pressure over the femoral artery, the needle is removed and a dilator, equal in size to the catheters to be used, is introduced over the guidewire. With the guidewire within the aorta, the coronary catheter is then passed over the guidewire to the ascending aorta. After the guidewire is removed, 3 to 4 cc of blood is aspirated from the catheter to remove thrombus or fibrin, and the catheter is then flushed with heparinized saline. The catheter is attached to a catheter-syringe manifold assembly, thus allowing both pressure monitoring and contrast injection. Systemic heparinization is generally recommended after arterial access is obtained.

The left coronary catheter is advanced near, but not into, the orifice of the left main coronary artery. With the image intensifier in a shallow left anterior oblique (LAO) projection, a flush injection of contrast is made to visualize the left main ostium prior to entry of the catheter. Following this and each subsequent injection, arterial pressure should be noted. If there is damping (fall in catheter-tip pressure) or ventricularization (normal systolic pressure, but low diastolic pressure), it may indicate a significant stenosis of the left main coronary artery and imply that the catheter tip has created total or near total obstruction of the vessel (Fig. 8–8). Alternatively, if there is damping of both systolic and diastolic pressure, it suggests an adverse position of the end hole of the catheter against the wall of the artery. In either case, the catheter should be removed immediately from the ostium, and the angiographer should reevaluate the possibilty of high-grade proximal coronary stenosis with further flush injections of the artery in multiple views. If ostial stenosis is present, further injections must be done rapidly and followed by immediate withdrawal of the catheter while contrast remains in the vessel. Prolonged injections in this situation may result in severe myocardial ischemia.

After arteriography of the left coronary artery is performed in multiple views with satisfactory visualization of any abnormalities (see section on coronary

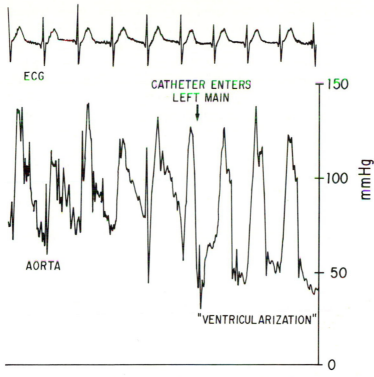

Figure 8–8. Pressure tracing demonstrating damping of distal catheter-tip pressure during occlusion of coronary orifice secondary to severe ostial stenosis.

arteriography), the left coronary catheter is withdrawn to the level of the diaphragm. The guidewire is reintroduced, and the left coronary catheter is replaced with the Judkins right catheter. The catheter is advanced to the ascending aorta about 3 cm above the right sinus of Valsalva. Whereas the Judkins left catheter almost automatically seeks out the ostium, the Judkins right catheter may require considerable manipulation to intubate the right coronary ostium. The tip of the right coronary catheter is slowly rotated (anteriorly) with steady withdrawal until it enters the orifice of the artery. The withdrawal is necessary because the catheter tends to descend within the aortic root as it is torqued anteriorly. Coronary catheters other than the Judkins catheter have been designed that require different manipulative techniques (i.e., the Noto, Amplatz, Schoonmaker, and so on).

Unlike the left coronary artery, damping and ventricularization of the right coronary artery is often due to spasm induced by the catheter tip. Other potential causes include a small-caliber artery, superselective cannulation of the conus artery, or severe proximal stenosis. The cause can usually be determined by nonselective test injections (flush shots) or administration of nitroglycerin. Once again, when damping or ventricularization is present, cautious injections with rapid withdrawal of the catheter should be accomplished to avoid ischemic complications.

Selective injection of aortocoronary bypass grafts via the percutaneous femoral approach can be accomplished with a right Judkins catheter, a right Amplatz catheter, or a specifically designed bypass graft catheter. To engage posterior or medial grafts, a specifically designed Judkins bypass catheter, which is similar to a right coronary catheter but modified such that the tip has a smooth, downward terminal curve, may be employed (see Fig. 8–6). Performing arteriography of aortocoronary bypass grafts is greatly facilitated if rings or metal clips have been placed at the origin of the graft at the time of coronary artery bypass surgery.

Arteriography of internal mammary artery grafts can be performed with a Judkins right coronary catheter or a specifically designed internal mammary catheter (see Fig. 8–6). Injection of these grafts with contrast often causes varying degrees of pain in the patient's extremities.

After coronary arteriography has been performed, the catheters are removed and firm pressure is applied to the femoral area for about 10 to 15 min either by hand or by a mechanical clamp. The patient should be instructed to lie in bed for several hours with the leg remaining straight to prevent hematoma formation. The time required for the patient to lie in bed is related to the size of the catheter or sheath that was utilized for the procedure.

The main advantage of the Judkins technique is the speed and ease of selective catheterization. However, these attributes should not preclude gaining extensive operator experience to assure quality studies with an acceptable degree of safety. The main disadvantage of this technique is its use in patients with ileofemoral atherosclerotic disease, which may prevent retrograde passage of catheters through areas of extreme narrowing or tortuosity.

Brachial Artery Technique

In 1959, F. Mason Sones introduced the first technique for coronary artery catheterization via a brachial artery cutdown. The Sones technique still retains popularity in many centers, although the percutaneous brachial technique is now more popular than brachial artery cutdown.

Equipment

The Sones catheter is available as a thin-walled woven Dacron or polyurethane design. It is 100 cm in length and 7 or 8 French in diameter, tapering to 5.5 French at the tip. It has an end hole and two to four side holes near the catheter tip. After direct exposure of the brachial artery (usually the right), an arteriotomy is made. The catheter is connected to a manifold and advanced through the subclavian artery and innominate artery to the ascending aorta using fluoroscopy and pressure guidance. If a tortuous innominate or subclavian artery is encountered, a guidewire may be useful. Patient maneuvers such as shrugging the shoulders, turning the head to the left, extension of the arm, or the taking of a deep breath may also be attempted in these situations. Pressure monitoring and safety precautions for the brachial artery technique are similar to those outlined with the Judkins techniques.

After advancement of the catheter into the central aorta, heparin is administered. In the Sones technique, the same catheter is used for both right and left coronary injections. After a flush injection has been made of the left main coronary artery, selective left and right coronary arteriography may be performed. With the patient in the LAO projection, the catheter is advanced to the left sinus of Valsalva and a J-loop is made. The catheter is then advanced and withdrawn until the left ostium is engaged.

To cannulate the right coronary artery, the catheter is withdrawn from the left coronary artery while maintaining a gentle loop and applying clockwise rotation. Damping due to spasm, selective catheterization of the conus artery, or wedging within a stenosis may occur with the Sones technique and should be carefully anticipated by noting pressure changes and the results of flush injections. The side holes may not allow the similar pressure changes observed with the end-hole catheters of the Judkins variety.

When the catheter is removed from the brachial artery, proximal and distal bleeding are permitted to remove potential small thrombi. A small probe may be placed gently into the distal artery if distal flow is inadequate. A Fogarty thrombectomy catheter may need to be utilized for this purpose when occlusion is obvious. The arteriotomy site is usually closed with a purse-string suture. After the skin is closed, a light pressure dressing is placed over the area.

Disadvantages of the Sones technique are that it is more difficult to develop expertise with this technique and the left coronary artery may be extremely difficult to cannulate. Furthermore, catheter seating may be less stable than with the Judkins technique, and biplane ventriculography or aortography may be difficult because the patient is being studied from the arm. Operator exposure to x-rays is usually higher than with the femoral approach. Left internal mammary grafts may also require the use of a left brachial approach. Advantages of the Sones technique are that the entire case, including bypass grafts, may be performed with a single catheter. The technique is especially useful in patients with severe iliofemoral vascular disease. In addition, the patient can ambulate quickly following the procedure.

Percutaneous Brachial Technique

A modification of the Sones technique is the percutaneous brachial technique with preformed Judkins catheters. Briefly, this technique employs the Seldinger method of percutaneous brachial artery entry. One commonly used method employs a 6 French sheath placed into the brachial artery; 5,000 units of heparin are then infused into the side port. A guidewire is then advanced to the ascending aorta under fluoroscopic control, and 5 French Judkins left, right, and pigtail catheters are then passed over the guidewire for routine arteriography and ventriculography. Occasionally, the guidewire may be necessary to direct the left coronary catheter into the left sinus of Valsalva and the ostium of the left main coronary artery. The right coronary catheter technique requires similar manipulation as the femoral technique. The main advantage of the percutaneous brachial technique is the avoidance of a brachial artery cutdown and repair. Sones catheters may also be used after percutaneous insertion.

Transseptal Left-Heart Catheterization

Transseptal left-heart catheterization is now used infrequently in many cardiac catheterization laboratories. However, with the growing popularity of the use of certain prosthetic valves in the aortic position (i.e., the disc valves and the St. Jude) that cannot be crossed retrograde during catheterization, and with the emerging technologic advances that allow balloon mitral valvuloplasty to be performed, a revival in the transseptal technique has occurred. Other indications for transseptal puncture include the inability to perform retrograde left-heart catheterization due to peripheral vascular disease or aortic stenosis, or the necessity to directly measure left atrial pressure. While the LA pressure and pulmonary capillary wedge pressure generally correlates well, discrepancies do occur (especially in patients with prosthetic mitral valves in place).

Technique

The transseptal procedure can only be performed via the right femoral vein. The transseptal catheter is a short, curved catheter with tapered tip and side holes (Fig. 8–9). It is placed in the right atrium over a 70-cm curved Brockenbrough needle that is inserted through the catheter until just inside the catheter tip. The exact technique varies, but generally the catheter-needle combination is manipulated into the fossa ovalis while continuously recording atrial pressure. Often mere advancement of the catheter system against the fossa ovalis results in entry of the catheter-needle apparatus into the left atrium. If this does not occur, a portion of the tip of the needle is abruptly advanced from the catheter into the left atrium. It is important to appreciate the relationship between the aortic root and left atrium. With the catheter in the left atrium, further manipulations are then used to advance the catheter into the left ventricle, and left ventricular pressures and angiography are obtained.

Although the risk of this procedure is low if it is performed by an experienced operator, complications, when they occur, tend to be serious. The major risk of transseptal catheterization is inadvertent puncture of right atrial structures, such as the free wall or coronary sinus, or entry into the aortic root.

Endomyocardial Biopsy

Endomyocardial biopsy has become popular since 1972, following the development of a bioptome at Stanford University that made the procedure relatively

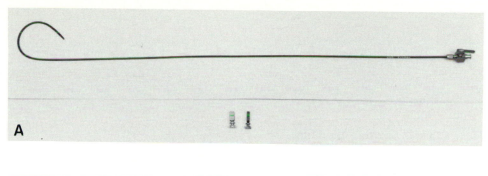

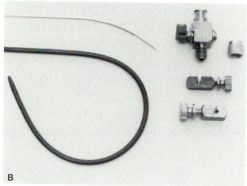
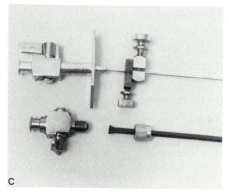

Figure 8–9. A, Transseptal catheterization equipment with the Brockenbrough system. Needle and catheter are shown (*B*), along with stopcock valve (*C*).

safe. Endomyocardial biopsy is used to monitor tissue rejection in heart-transplant recipients, allowing adjustment of immunosuppressive therapy. It is also used as a diagnostic tool for investigating patients with unexplained cardiomyopathy looking for inflammatory (myocarditis) or infiltrative (amyloidosis, hemochromatosis) disease processes that are potentially treatable.

Because of the relative ease of access and safety, the right ventricular septum is usually the area sampled. Although the left ventricle can be biopsied, control is more difficult, and the procedure is slightly more hazardous.

There are two general approaches for obtaining endomyocardial biopsies—one via the right internal jugular vein, and the other via the femoral vein. With the approach from the neck, access to the right internal jugular vein is achieved using the Seldinger technique. A 9 French transducer sheath is inserted that contains a side arm port for heparinized saline and a self-sealing diaphragm to prevent air emboli.

The bioptome (Fig. 8–10) is prepared by bending it at a 45-degree angle about 7 cm from the tip (see Fig. 8–10). The bioptome is inserted into the sheath by pointing the tip laterally towards the patient's right. The bioptome is advanced to the lateral right atrium under fluoroscopy, ensuring that the bioptome does not enter the right subclavian vein. With the bioptome in the mid atrium, the handle is rotated in a counterclockwise manner. This will rotate the tip anteriorly and

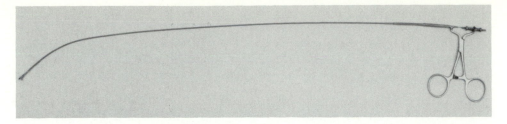

Figuure 8–10. Stanford bioptome.

then medially, and the bioptome can then be advanced across the tricuspid valve into the right ventricle. Once across the tricuspid valve, the bioptome is rotated further counterclockwise in order to point the tip posteriorly toward the right ventricular septum. This position can be verified using fluoroscopy or by use of a simultaneous recording of the intracardiac electrogram. The instrument is then gently advanced until it meets resistance or until premature ventricular contractions (PVCs) are induced. The tip will now be in the area of the right ventricular apex pointing toward the septum. The bioptome is withdrawn 1 to 2 cm, and the jaws are opened. The bioptome is then gently advanced until resistance is felt or PVCs are induced. The jaws of the bioptome are then closed, and the bioptome is withdrawn. Initially, resistance will be felt, and then there may be a sudden release of tension. The bioptome is withdrawn by rotating the handle anteriorly in a clockwise direction, and the instrument is pulled back through the sheath. The jaws of the bioptome are opened, and the biopsy is carefully removed with a 25-gauge needle, taking care to avoid crush artifact. The sample is placed in fixative such as glutaraldehyde or formalin. Numerous biopsies can be obtained by repeating the process.

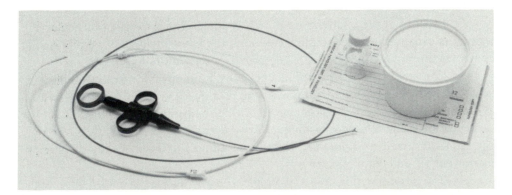

Figure 8–11. The long sheath with hemostatic valve for positioning of the flexible biopsy forceps is shown along with a 7 French multipurpose catheter used as an introducer, flexible biopsy forceps, and containers used to transport biopsy specimens.

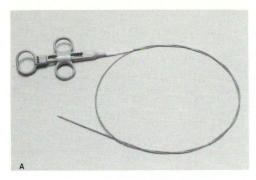
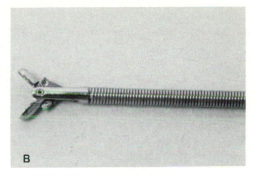

Figure 8–12. A, Flexible bioptome. *B,* Magnified view of biopsy forceps.

Biopsies via internal jugular vein can also be obtained using a flexible bioptome. This method uses a long sheath with a curve that directs the flexible bioptome toward the right ventricular septum (Figs. 8–11 and 8–12). The difference in this technique is that the guiding sheath remains in position in the right ventricle while the bioptome is advanced and withdrawn with each biopsy. At the end of the procedure, the entire apparatus (sheath and bioptome) is removed. The disadvantage of this approach is that the long, thin sheath provides less precise control over the ability to position the bioptome.

An alternative approach utilizes the femoral vein and employs the flexible bioptome. The bioptome is positioned on the right ventricular septum using the long, curved, radiopaque introducer sheath. Sterile access to the femoral vein is gained using the Seldinger technique. A J-wire is advanced to the level of the right atrium. A multipurpose catheter acts as an introducer and is inserted into the guiding sheath. This unit is then advanced over the wire into the right atrium, and the multipurpose catheter is withdrawn, leaving the sheath. The sheath has a self-sealing diaphragm and a side port. The side-port tubing is connected to a pressure transducer.

The sheath is advanced across the tricuspid valve into the right ventricle, and its position is confirmed by the right ventricular pressure tracing and fluoroscopy. Position of the sheath tip against the ventricular septum is essential to avoid biopsy of the right ventricular free wall or apex. The sheath position against the septum is confirmed by fluoroscopy and may be further verified by hand injections of radiocontrast through the sheath. Once the sheath is properly positioned, the bioptome is carefully introduced until the tip has just exited the sheath. It is imperative that the jaws of the bioptome be opened as soon as the tip of the bioptome has exited the sheath. With the jaws open, the instrument is gently advanced until resistance is felt or PVCs are induced. The jaws of the bioptome are closed. The bioptome is then removed from the sheath, the jaws are opened, and the specimen is carefully removed as previously described.

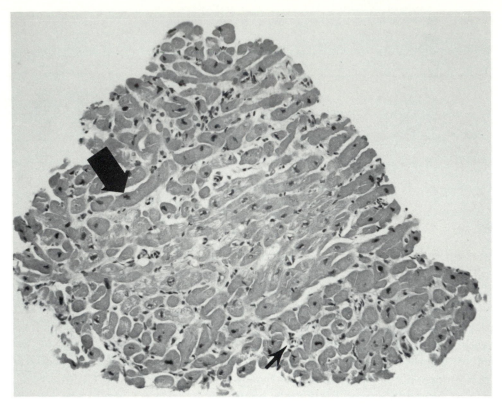

Figure 8–13. Hematoxylin and eosin stain of normal myocardium seen at low power. Normal cardiac myocyte and nucleus (*large arrow*) and capillary (*small arrow*). (Courtesy of Charles Steenburgen, M.D., Ph.D., Duke University Medical Center, Durham, N.C.)

The key to prevention of complications is that the bioptome should never be advanced without the jaws being open. The open jaws present a blunt surface rather than the "bullet-shaped" profile of the closed instrument (see Fig. 8–12). The jaws themselves are not sharp, and a "tearing action" results in the obtaining of the biopsy material.

A biopsy of normal myocardium as seen under low power is shown in Figure 8–13. An example of contraction artifact due to improper specimen handling is shown in Figure 8–14. Figure 8–15 illustrates findings seen in myocarditis. Samples can also be examined using electron microscopy (Fig. 8–16). Specific types of cells can be seen with special immunoperoxidase techniques (Fig. 8–17), allowing identification of the type of infiltrative cell present. Table 8–10 lists the potential uses for endomyocardial biopsy and the expected results.

The complication rate from this procedure has been low. The most serious risk is perforation of a cardiac chamber. Other potential complications include arrhythmias, air emboli, pneumothorax, infection, coronary artery to right

Text continues on page 134

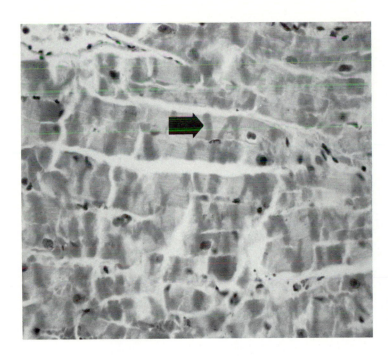

Figure 8–14. Contraction band artifact (*arrow*) (H & E, 40×). (Courtesy of Charles Steenburgen, M.D., Ph.D.)

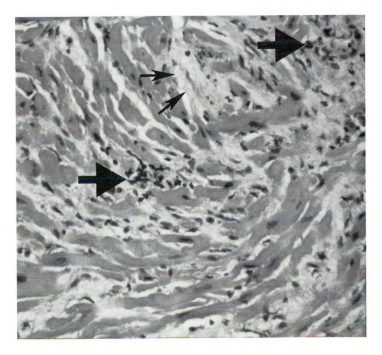

Figure 8–15. Hematoxylin and eosin stain of a myocardial biopsy in a patient with myocarditis showing extensive intercellular mononuclear cell infiltrate and intercellular proteinaceous debris. Intercellular mononuclear cell infiltrate (*large arrow*) and proteinaceous debris (*small arrow*). (Courtesy of Charles Steenburgen, M.D., Ph.D.)

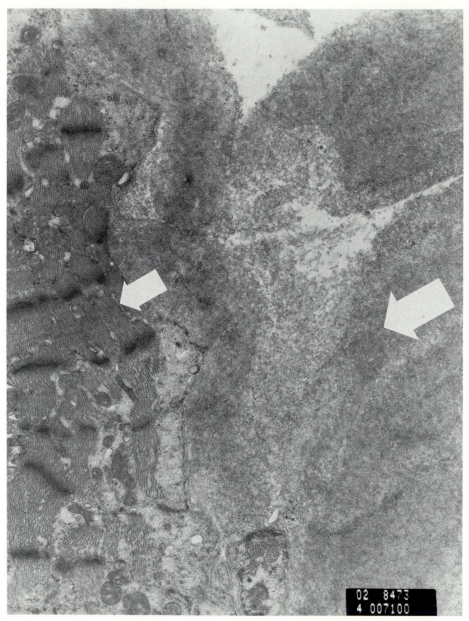

Figure 8–16. Myocardial biopsy viewed by electron microscopy. A normal myo-cyte is seen to the left, and the fibrillar proteinaceous debris characteristic of amyloidosis is seen to the right. Cardiac myocyte contractile elements (*small arrow*) and amyloid protein (*large arrow*). (Courtesy of Charles Steenburgen, M.D., Ph.D.)

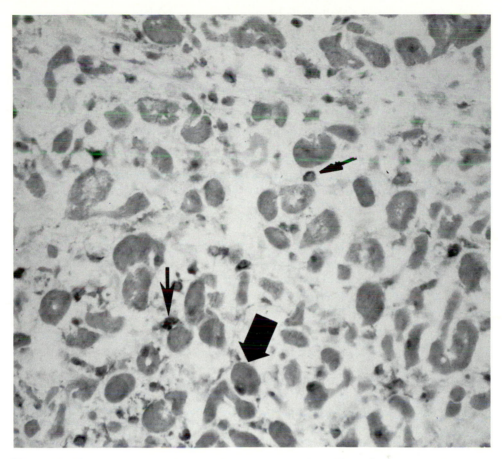

Figure 8–17. Immunoperoxidase stain identifying T-cell lymphocytes. Cardiac myocyte and nucleus (*large arrow*) and T lymphocyte stained with immunoperoxidase (*small arrow*). (Courtesy of Charles Steenburgen, M.D., Ph.D.)

TABLE 8–10
Representative Findings on Endomyocardial Biopsy

Disease	Histologic Findings
Myocarditis	Inflammatory cells, myocyte necrosis
Transplant rejection	Inflammatory cells, myocyte necrosis
Amyloidosis	Amorphous protein staining with Congo red stain
Hemochromatosis	Iron deposits
Sarcoidosis	Inflammatory cells, granulomas, multinucleated giant cells
Adriamycin toxicity	Myofiber degeneration, vacuoles within myocytes
Eosinophilic endomyocardial fibroelastosis	Eosinophils, endomyocardial fibrosis
Gaucher's/Pompe's disease	Storage vacuoles
Neoplasm	Neoplastic cells specific for the type of tumor

ventricular fistula, and right bundle branch block or complete heart block. As with other right-heart procedures, a temporary pacemaker should be immediately available in patients with underlying left bundle branch block.

SELECTED REFERENCES

Braunwald E, Swan HJC. Cooperative study on cardiac catheterization. Circulation 1968; 37 (Suppl III):1.

Brockenbrough EC, Braunwald E. A new technique for left ventricular angiocardiography and transseptal left heart catheterization. Am J Cardiol 1960; 6:1062.

DeFalque RJ. Percutaneous catheterization of the internal jugular vein. Anesth Analg 1974; 53:116.

Fenoglio JT. Endomyocardial biopsy technique and application. Boca Raton, FL: CRC Press, 1982.

Heupler F. Coronary arteriography and left ventriculography: Sones technique. In: King SB, Douglas JJ, eds. Coronary arteriography and angioplasty. New York: McGraw-Hill, 1985:137.

Intravenous techniques. In: Textbook of advanced cardiac life support. American Heart Association, 1987:141.

Judkins MP. Selective coronary arteriography. Part 1. A percutaneous transfemoral technique. Radiology 1967; 89:815.

Mason TW. Techniques for right and left ventricular endomyocardial biopsy. Am J Cardiol 1978; 41(2):887.

Phillips SJ. Technique of percutaneous subclavian catheterization. Surg Gynecol Obstet 1968; 127:1079.

Seldinger SI. Catheter replacement of the needle in percutaneous arteriography: A new technique. Acta Radiol 1953; 39:368.

Swan HJC, Ganz W, Forrester JJ, et al. Catheterization of the heart in man with the use of a flow-directed balloon-tipped catheter. N Engl J Med 1976; 283:447.

Wyte SR, Barker WJ. Central venous catheterization: Internal jugular approach and alternatives. In: Roberts JR, Hedges JR, eds. Clinical procedures in emergency medicine. Philadelphia: WB Saunders, 1985:321.

CHAPTER 9

Therapeutic Techniques

J. Kevin Harrison, MD, and Charles J. Davidson, MD

Therapeutic procedures have gained an increasingly important place in the catheterization laboratory. Pericardiocentesis, a potentially life-saving procedure for patients with cardiac tamponade, has been done for many years. Intra-aortic balloon pumps have proved useful for stabilizing patients with hemodynamic embarrassment. Balloon-catheter procedures are now being employed to treat a variety of diseases, including coronary artery disease, valvular stenosis, and congenital heart disease. Percutaneous transluminal angioplasty (PTCA) has become an alternative to coronary artery bypass surgery for many patients with coronary artery disease. In addition, percutaneous balloon valvuloplasty is being employed to treat selected patients with valvular heart disease. These techniques, as well as some new procedures under development, are discussed.

Percutaneous Transluminal Coronary Angioplasty

The first PTCA was performed on September 16, 1977 by Andreas Gruentzig in Zurich. The use of this technique has increased dramatically over the past 11 years; approximately 60,000 procedures were performed in 1984, and 200,000 procedures were performed in 1987. Postulated mechanisms of successful PTCA include plaque compression, plaque remodeling, intimal splitting, plaque disruption, local aneurysm formation, and smooth-muscle injury with loss of the elastic recoil of the outer layers of the artery.

135

Equipment

The catheter assembly for PTCA consists of two catheters: a guiding catheter and a balloon dilatation catheter. The guiding catheter is introduced through a sheath in the femoral artery or directly into the brachial artery. The catheters are pre-shaped similar to diagnostic catheters to allow positioning at the orifice of the left or right coronary arteries or bypass grafts. Guiding catheters are not tapered at the tip, however, thus allowing passage of the balloon dilatation catheter through the lumen. The primary function of the guiding catheter is to provide adequate support for the dilatation catheter as it is advanced over the area of stenosis. The guiding catheter is positioned at the orifice of the coronary artery or bypass graft without obstructing the orifice.

The dilatation catheter is advanced to the stenotic arterial branch. The original dilatation catheter by Gruentzig was a two-lumen catheter with the balloon at the distal end and a short, soft wire fixed to the distal end of the balloon. The wire allowed for direction of the catheter without injury to the artery. Other systems, including an over-the-wire steerable catheter system, are now utilized. Most coronary dilatation catheters are 135 cm in length, have an external diameter of 2.3 to 4.5 French, and contain two or three lumens. The central lumen is utilized for pressure measurements, contrast injection, or passage of a steerable guidewire. The second eccentric lumen is employed for balloon inflation and deflation. The third lumen is generally reserved for a venting wire to permit removal of air from the balloon during its preparation. Recent advances in balloon-catheter technology have included lower profile over-the-wire balloon catheters, a balloon attached to a 0.018-inch guidewire, and an autoperfusion balloon catheter that allows myocardial perfusion during balloon inflation. Representative examples of PTCA balloon catheters are shown in Figure 9–1.

The balloons are manufactured from polyvinylchloride, polyethylene, or irradiated polyolefin, and are 20 to 25 mm in length. Radiopaque markers are present in the center of the balloon, and balloons are filled with contrast and saline mixtures to allow visualization during fluoroscopy. Inflation and deflation of the balloon are controlled by a calibrated pressure pump that delivers up to 14 atm of pressure. It is important that inflation can be accomplished to a precise diameter to permit adequate distending forces to the stenotic area without over-distending the normal segment.

In the steerable catheter systems, the thin guidewire passes through the central lumen of the balloon catheter and out its tip. These guidewires are soft, radiopaque, and have excellent torque control. They can be advanced through tortuous and stenotic segments. Following placement of the guidewire across the lesion, the wire is utilized as a rail to allow advancement of the balloon catheter without risk of entering side branches or creating false lumens. Standard guidewire length is 175 cm; however, 300-cm wires are available for exchange of balloon catheters without disengaging the lesion. Guidewires are also available that allow docking of an extension wire to the distal end of standard-length guidewires, thus creating an exchange-length guidewire. The most popular outer-shaft

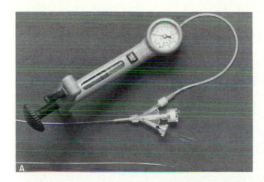
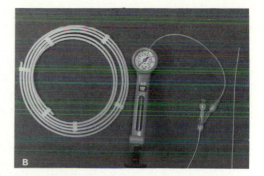

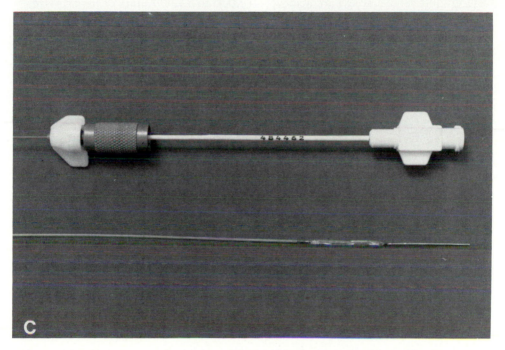

Figure 9–1. Representative examples of PTCA balloon catheters. *A,* A 2.5-mm Harzler LPS 1.0-cm fixed-tip wire (ACS; Mountain View, CA). USCI (Bellerica, MA) indeflator attached to balloon port. *B,* A 2.5-mm Simpson ultra-low profile II (SULP II) with 0.014-inch exchangeable guidewire (ACS). USCI indeflator attached to balloon port. *C,* A 2.5-mm probe (balloon on a wire) (USCI).

diameters are 0.014 and 0.018 inch. Guidewires also differ in the flexibility and steerability of the distal tips.

Procedure

In preparing the patient for coronary angioplasty, the benefits, risks, potential complications, and alternatives should be fully explained. In addition, the patient should consent to undergo cardiac surgery if the need arises during the procedure. It is therefore important that cardiac surgical support, as well as anesthesia support, be readily available.

Premedication with antiplatelet agents (including aspirin) and calcium antagonists is begun at least 24 hr prior to the procedure to prevent vessel spasm and platelet deposition on the disrupted endothelium at the PTCA site. The PTCA procedure may be performed via the femoral or brachial route. The femoral approach will be discussed in greatest detail.

Following local anesthesia, a temporary bipolar pacemaker is inserted through a femoral venous sheath and positioned in the inferior vena cava. After arterial and venous access are achieved, 10,000 to 15,000 units of heparin are administered intravenously. Baseline angiograms are obtained using a standard diagnostic catheter or guiding catheter.

The balloon is selected to closely approximate the diameter of the artery to be dilated, which is usually between 1.5 and 4.0 mm. The balloon is prepared by removing all air from the balloon and inflating with either full-strength contrast media or a mixture of contrast and saline. Balloon catheters vary in their method of removing air bubbles.

In over-the-wire systems, the guidewire is loaded into the balloon catheter, and a bend is made on the wire's distal tip. The guidewire is then withdrawn so that it lies just proximal to the tip of the balloon shaft.

The balloon catheter and guidewire assembly is advanced through a Y-connector that is attached to the guide catheter. The side port of the Y-connector is attached to a manifold to permit both flushing of the guide catheter and contrast injections. With the guide catheter positioned in the coronary ostium, the assembly is moved forward to the tip of the guide catheter.

Using images acquired during coronary arteriography as a roadmap, the guidewire is advanced across the stenosis to a distal position in the artery. Care is taken to assure that there is no kinking of the guidewire or entrance into small side branches. The balloon catheter is then moved over the guidewire and positioned over the lesion. In a fixed-wire system (see Fig. 9–1), a floppy tipped wire is attached to the balloon catheter. The catheter is advanced across as the tip is rotated. Care is taken to avoid buckling of the wire as the catheter is maneuvered to the proper location. The fixed-wire system and balloon on a wire system generally provide a lower profile than the over-the-wire system. This allows for improved visualization, especially in distal stenosis, and also permits the crossing of the most severely stenotic segments of artery.

As the balloon is inflated, a dumbbell-shaped "waist" is usually seen to disappear when adequate inflation pressure is attained. The total inflation time and maximal atmospheres of inflation pressure vary depending on patient tolerance, electrocardiographic (ECG) changes, arrhythmias, and operator preference. Inflation times may range from 30 sec to 15 min (usually 2 to 5 min), and inflation pressures range from 4 to 14 atm (usually 5 to 8 atm). After one to several inflations, the balloon catheter is withdrawn into the guide catheter while maintaining the guidewire across the lesion. If injection of contrast verifies that an adequate result has been achieved, the guidewire is removed and final cineangiograms or digital images of the artery are recorded.

The femoral sheaths are removed within 3 to 4 hr. Alternatively, the patient is maintained on a heparin infusion for 18 to 24 hr, and the sheaths are removed the following day. While there are many definitions of a successful result, the current criteria suggest that the residual stenosis should have less than a 50% diameter narrowing.

Complications

Major complications occur in 2 to 17 percent of patients. The risk is higher when multiple lesions are dilated at one setting. Death occurs in less than 1%. The most common major complications are myocardial infarction, side-branch occlusion, acute coronary occlusion (due to spasm, dissection, and plaque hemorrhage), and emergent coronary artery bypass surgery. Coronary artery rupture and coronary embolism are rare major complications associated with PTCA. A recent Task Force from the ACC/AHA has summarized lesion characteristics that are exceptionally complex and prone to complications (see Chapter 5).

Minor complications include those related to femoral artery and vein puncture (hematoma, arteriovenous fistula, or pseudoaneurysm), anticoagulant complications, and arrhythmias (ventricular tachycardia, ventricular fibrillation, or a new conduction disturbance). Chapter 6 summarizes a contemporary series from the Society of Cardiac Angiography regarding the risks of PTCA.

Atherectomy Catheters

Another approach being developed for the treatment of coronary artery disease is to cut away the atherosclerotic plaque, a process that is referred to as "atherectomy." The Auth and Kensey atherectomy catheters are rotational devices that are designed to grind or cut away the stenotic plaque (Fig. 9–2). These devices leave the debris in the arterial lumen. Other atherectomy devices, the Simpson and transluminal extraction catheters (TEC), are designed to remove this tissue once it is cut.

The Simpson atherectomy catheter has a cutting slot on the side of a metal capsule of the catheter. This slot is positioned over the area of stenotic plaque (Fig. 9–3). The plaque is then "shaved off" by advancing a rotary cutting blade across the slot in the catheter capsule. Plaque is collected in the distal capsule. The tissue is then removed by withdrawing the catheter and emptying the capsule. The process is repeated until the desired result is obtained.

Another atherectomy catheter, the transluminal extraction catheter, consists of a conical array of spinning blades mounted on the end of a catheter (Fig. 9–4 *A* and *B*). As the cutter moves through the atherosclerotic plaque, the tissue fragments are removed using a vacuum system. A series of passes are made through the lesion with a small-diameter cutter that may then be exchanged for

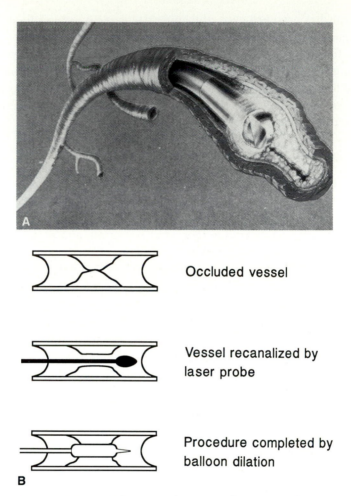

Occluded vessel

Vessel recanalized by
laser probe

Procedure completed by
balloon dilation

Figure 9–2. A, Schematic drawing of Kensey atherectomy catheter. *B,* Schematic drawing of method of combined laser and balloon angioplasty. (From the Society for Vascular Surgery and North American Chapter, International Society for Cardiovascular Surgery, with permission.)

progressively larger sizes (e.g., 6 French cutter followed by a 7 French cutter). Preliminary results with the Simpson and transluminal extraction catheters in obstructed leg and coronary arteries appear promising. The devices may be particularly useful for recanalization of totally occluded vessels. Restenosis rates in peripheral arteries have been variable, and it has been postulated, but not proven, that restenosis rates in coronary arteries might be lower than with conventional balloon PTCA. Ongoing trials should clarify the role of these devices in affecting restenosis rates.

Concerns with these devices are related to the wide exposure of the subendothelial tissues, which are potentially thrombogenic, the loss of endothelium, and the acute risk of coronary artery perforation.

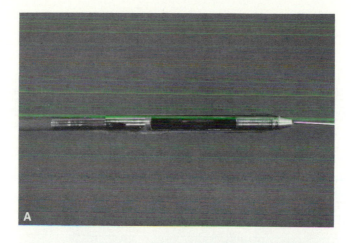

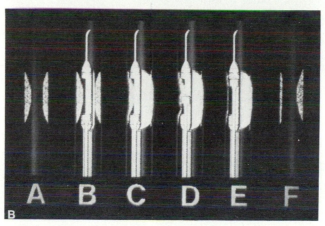

Figure 9–3. A, Magnified view of the cutting capsule on the Simpson atherectomy catheter. *B,* Schematic drawing of Simpson atherectomy catheter and various stages (A through F) of removal of atherosclerotic plaque.

Laser Angioplasty Catheters

Another recent area of investigation has been the use of laser ablation of atherosclerotic plaque. In these systems, fiberoptics are included in the catheter to carry the high-energy light. The high-energy laser is emitted directly (e.g., via a sapphire tip) to ablate plaque or is used to heat up a metal tip to thermally evaporate tissue. The challenge of this technology is to develop the ability to direct the laser energy at plaque while avoiding damage to the normal endothelium. There is the grave risk of vessel perforation with laser energy.

There are also catheters that combine technologies—catheters with both angioplasty balloons and lasers. The laser energy, via a hot-tip metal probe, is

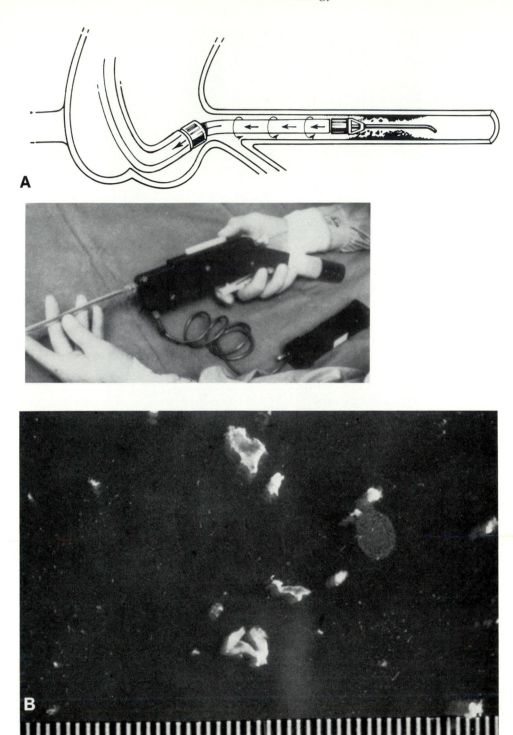

Figure 9–4. *A*, Schematic representation of transluminal extraction catheter (TEC) cutting device in operation. Below the schematic representation is the TEC controller, which includes a motor and suction. The thumb is located on the advancement control, and the index finger is located on trigger to activate the motor. (From Stack RS, Califf RM, Phillips HR, et al. New interventional technology. Am J Cardiol 1988; 62 (Suppl 11):12F; with permission.) *B*, Tissue fragments removed by the suction system.

used to initially open the occluded artery. The angioplasty balloon is then used as a second stage to further dilate the lumen (Fig. *9–2B*).

Other Catheter Devices Under Investigation

Catheters designed to improve qualitative and quantitative measures of the severity and character of coronary stenoses are under development. The hope is that these techniques might better guide and monitor the newer therapeutic techniques such as atherectomy and laser angioplasty.

Angioscopy is one such technique. In angioscopy, fiberoptics are included in the catheter to directly visualize the arterial endothelium (Fig. *9–5*). This requires the occlusion of the proximal portion of the artery by a balloon on the catheter so that the distal artery can be flushed with saline and visualized. In addition to the limitation imposed by the necessity to transiently occlude the artery, the acquired images give information only on the inner topography of the arterial endothelium and lumen.

Intravascular ultrasound utilizes ultrasound crystals mounted on a catheter. This technique yields two-dimensional images from which the degree of ste-

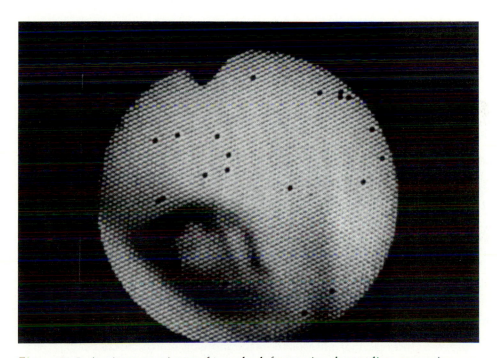

Figure 9–5. Angioscope picture from the left anterior descending artery in a patient with endothelial ulceration. (From Forrester J, et al. Cardiac angioscopy in acute ischemic syndromes. Am J Cardiac Imag 1988; 2 (3):180, Fig. 4; with permission.)

nosis, eccentricity, depth, and composition of atherosclerotic plaque might be defined (Fig. 9–6).

Catheters employing low-energy laser energy are also under development in the hope of acquiring information about the arterial endothelium. With this technique, a low-energy laser is emitted against the tissue. The fluorescent and reflected light energy that returns via the fiberoptics in the catheter is analyzed using spectral analysis. The spectral analysis returning from atherosclerotic plaque differs from that returning from normal endothelium, making it theoretically possible the catheter laser energy at atherosclerotic plaque rather than normal endothelium.

In addition to these newer catheter techniques for investigating and treating disease in the coronary arteries, there are also new catheter techniques for augmenting cardiac output. In patients with cardiogenic shock, percutaneous bypass procedures have been developed in order to stabilize a patient prior to performing a definitive intervention. Catheters can be quickly inserted into the femoral vessels and a pump oxygenator connected. The blood is removed from the femoral vein, and a pulsatile pump oxygenator returns it to the femoral artery with oxygen added. This external "heart-lung" machine can be used to provide external support to a failing heart. Another investigational device involves a catheter inserted via the femoral artery into the left ventricle. This catheter has a high-speed rotor that creates a vacuum, causing blood to be suctioned from the left ventricle and to exit through the catheter in the thoracic aorta, thus augmenting cardiac output. And finally, there are catheter devices under investigation that may be able to monitor blood pH, pCO_2, pO_2, glucose, potassium, or even blood urea nitrogen (BUN).

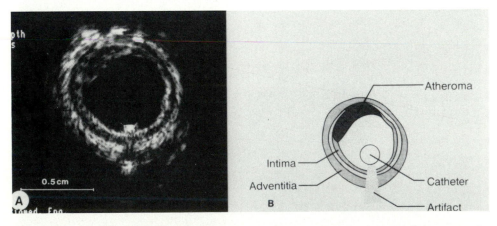

Figure 9–6. Intravascular ultrasound image showing lumen, layers of the arterial wall, and atherosclerotic plaque. *B*, Schematic diagram of structures seen in part *A*. (From Yock P, et al. Intravascular ultrasound: Development and clinical potential. Am J Cardiac Imag 1988; 2:190, Fig. 7; with permission.)

Balloon Valvuloplasty

Percutaneous Aortic Valvuloplasty

Indications

In 1986, Cribier and colleagues were the first to report successful dilatation of calcific aortic stenosis in the elderly utilizing percutaneous balloon valvuloplasty. Several studies have indicated that hemodynamic and symptomatic improvement occur immediately following balloon aortic valvuloplasty. The high early restenosis rate for aortic stenosis, however, makes the precise role of the procedure difficult to define. At 6 months, a high percentage of patients have evidence of restenosis, but many of these will continue to have sustained symptomatic improvement. At present, the indications for balloon aortic valvuloplasty in the elderly should be limited to the following patients: (1) patient at high risk for aortic valve replacement (i.e., advanced age of 70 years or older, or with serious coexisting medical illness; (2) patients who refuse surgery; (3) critically ill patients, as a "bridge" to aortic valve replacement; (4) patients who require noncardiac surgical procedures urgently. The mechanisms involved in the reduction in transaortic gradient includes tearing of commissural scar, fracture of valvular calcium and stretching of the aortic anulus.

Equipment and Technique

All patients should undergo routine right- and left-heart catheterization. A 7 French balloon-tipped catheter is inserted into the right femoral vein and utilized for recording right-heart pressures before and after valvuloplasty. Subsequently, a 5 French bipolar pacing electrode is percutaneously inserted through a 6 French sheath or, alternatively, through a pacing port that is available with balloon flotation catheters. The pacemaker should then be positioned within the right atrium or right ventricle.

Following percutaneous insertion of a 7 French pigtail catheter, supravalvular aortography is usually obtained immediately before and after balloon dilatation in order to determine any changes in the severity of aortic regurgitation. Cardiac output is measured before and after the procedure by either Fick or thermodilution methods, and the transvalvular gradient is obtained by simultaneous measurement of aortic or peripheral pressure with left ventricular pressure.

A 10, 12, or 14 French sheath is then percutaneously inserted in the femoral artery. Alternatively, a brachial approach may be used. The aortic valve is then crossed in a number of ways. A 7 French, 4-cm curved right coronary artery catheter and a 0.035-inch diameter straight-tipped guidewire are often used to initially enter the left ventricle. The right coronary catheter is then exchanged for a pigtail catheter using a 260-cm J-tipped guidewire. Left ventriculography is then performed before and after the balloon aortic valvuloplasty procedure.

The pigtail catheter is then exchanged over a 260-cm 0.035-inch or

0.038-inch J-tipped guidewire for a 20-mm valvuloplasty balloon catheter that is advanced across the aortic valve (Fig. 9–7). Dilatations are performed by hand injection of a mixture of contrast and saline to approximately 6 atm of pressure. A "waist" is usually seen to disappear in the balloon upon full inflation. The transvalvular aortic gradient and cardiac outputs are then remeasured and, if significant stenosis persists, either a larger balloon with a diameter of 23 mm or two valvuloplasty balloons may be utilized. Double-balloon valvuloplasty requires that a second sheath be placed in the opposite femoral artery, and the aortic valve recrossed.

Successful dilatation results in an immediate decrease in aortic transvalvular gradient and an increase in aortic-valve area (Fig. 9–8). Table 9–1 outlines results that can be expected.

Complications

The complications associated with aortic valvuloplasty are significant (15–20% overall), but must be understood in light of the high-risk profile of the patient population to whom it is applied. Systemic embolization occurs uncommonly (1–5%), and aortic regurgitation is generally unchanged. Peripheral vascular trauma

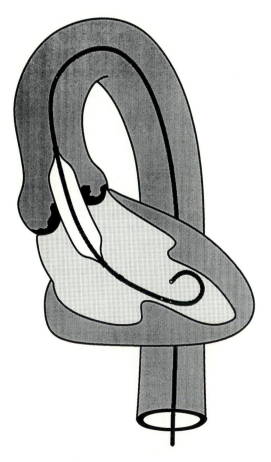

Figure 9–7. The single-balloon technique of aortic valvuloplasty is shown with the inflated balloon retrograde across the aortic valve.

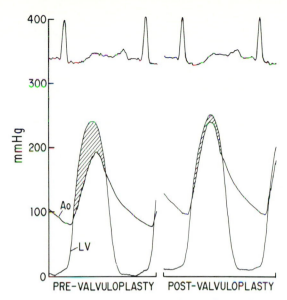

Figure 9–8. A representative hemodynamic result following successful percutaneous balloon aortic valvuloplasty. Note the reduction in aortic transvalvular gradient (*shaded area*).

related to the large catheters or sheaths used occurs in about 7–8 percent of patients and represent the most common complication. Death occurs in 1 to 2 percent of patients owing to failure of the procedure to relieve obstruction or to acute aortic regurgitation, anular rupture, myocardial ischemia or infarction, cardiac tamponade, ventricular arrhythmias, or stroke.

Percutaneous Mitral Valvuloplasty

Indications

In 1984, Inoue reported percutaneous balloon valvuloplasty as a treatment for mitral stenosis. In 1986, McKay and colleagues reported its application in adult patients. The mechanism responsible for the improvement in the mitral gradient and the effective orifice area appears primarily to be commissural splitting. Thus, it would appear that appropriate candidates for excellent long-term results from percutaneous mitral valvuloplasty would be similar to those in whom surgical commissurotomy would have been effective. As opposed to aortic valvuloplasty, restenosis appears to be uncommon when an adequate dilatation has been achieved. Younger patients appear to have better procedural results than elderly patients.

Equipment and Techniques

Routine diagnostic right- and left-heart catheterization are performed via the femoral route. Transseptal catheterization is performed with an 8.5 French Brocken-

TABLE 9–1
Typical Acute Hemodynamic Results Following Percutaneous Balloon Valvuloplasty

Aortic Valvuloplasty					
Mean Aortic Valve Gradient (mm Hg)		*Aortic Valve Area (cm²)*		*Cardiac Index (L/min/m²)*	
Before	*After*	*Before*	*After*	*Before*	*After*
75	35	0.6	0.9	2.0	2.1

Mitral Valvuloplasty					
Mean Mitral Valve Gradient (mm Hg)		*Mitral Valve Area (cm²)*		*Cardiac Index (L/min/m²)*	
Before	*After*	*Before*	*After*	*Before*	*After*
17	7	1.0	2.2	2.5	3.0

Pulmonic Valvuloplasty					
Peak RV Pressure (mm Hg)		*Peak Gradient (mm Hg)*		*Cardiac Index (L/min/m²)*	
Before	*After*	*Before*	*After*	*Before*	*After*
100	50	80	30	3.0	3.0

brough catheter positioned in the foramen ovale and then advanced into the left atrium. Hemodynamic measurements are obtained through the Brockenbrough catheter and a simultaneous left ventricular pigtail catheter. Left atrial and left ventricular pressure are compared for determination of mitral valve gradient. Cardiac output is determined by Fick or thermodilution methods, and the mitral valve area is calculated.

An 8 French Mullins sheath is then placed into the left atrium, through which a 7 French balloon flotation catheter is advanced into the left ventricle. A 0.038-inch diameter 260-cm guidewire with a coiled tip is then placed through the balloon flotation catheter into the left ventricle. The balloon catheter is removed and a double-lumen sheath is used to place a second coiled guidewire across the valve. The interatrial septum is then dilated with an 8-mm balloon to allow passage of either one or preferably two balloon dilatation catheters that are 15 to 20 mm in diameter. The balloons are positioned across the mitral valve and inflated by hand with a mixture of contrast and saline (Fig. 9–9).

Another technique of balloon mitral valvuloplasty involves retrograde cannulation of the mitral valve. This is accomplished by placing a transseptal sheath through the mitral and aortic valves. A guidewire (or guidewires) is inserted through this sheath, and is snared by a retrieval catheter from the femoral artery (or arteries) and exteriorized. The transseptal sheath is withdrawn into the left atrium, and the balloon catheters are inserted from the femoral arteries retrograde over the guidewires. The advantage of this approach is that the large balloon catheters are not advanced across the atrial septum; thus, problems with

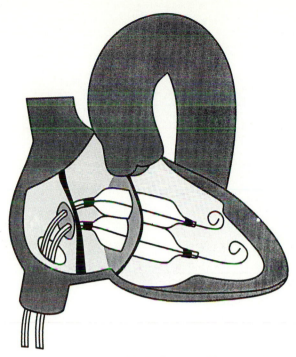

Figure 9–9. The double-balloon technique of balloon mitral valvuloplasty is shown schematically. The balloon catheters traverse the interatrial septum and are positioned over guidewires that are placed in the left ventricle.

balloon-created atrial septal defects or with pushing of the balloons across the septum are avoided.

Results

As in aortic valvuloplasty, mitral transvalvular gradient is decreased and mitral valve area is increased immediately following successful dilatation (Fig. 9–10 and Table 9–1). Preliminary long term results appear good in properly selected patients, and this procedure rivals operative commissurotomy for these patients.

Complications

In-hospital mortality appears to be almost 2 percent of patients undergoing balloon mitral valvuloplasty. Stroke from dislodged thrombus or calcium occurs in 2 to 7 percent of patients. To possibly reduce the risk of this complication, patients should be placed on warfarin 4 to 6 weeks prior to the procedure. Other reported complications include residual atrial septal defect (usually of small size, but in up to 20% of patients), cardiac perforation and tamponade, arrhythmias, and blood loss. In addition, perforated or torn mitral cusps may produce severe mitral regurgitation.

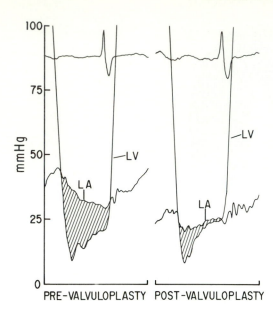

Figure 9–10. A representative hemody-namic result following successful balloon mitral valvuloplasty. The mean mitral valve gradient is dramatically reduced (*shaded area*).

Percutaneous Pulmonic Valvuloplasty

Indications

In 1979, Semb and coworkers were the first to successfully perform balloon dilation of the pulmonic valve in a patient with pulmonic stenosis. The procedure involved pulling an inflated balloon catheter back through the pulmonic valve. In 1982, Kan described static inflation of the balloon across the pulmonic valve.

The technique has now been applied to neonates, children, and adults, and is generally considered to be the treatment of choice for congenital pulmonic stenosis.

Although indications for pulmonic valvuloplasty are not well defined, several guidelines exist. Balloon pulmonic valvuloplasty should be considered in all patients with a transvalvular gradient of 50 mm Hg or greater. Previous surgical valvuloplasty or pulmonic valve dysplasia does not preclude success with percutaneous balloon valvuloplasty. The mechanism of improvement in the valve gradient generally involves disruption of the pulmonic leaflets, tearing of commissural scar and stretching of the pulmonic anulus.

Equipment and Technique

Pulmonic valvuloplasty is performed via the percutaneous right femoral venous approach. A pulmonary artery catheter is replaced by a guidewire, and the balloon catheter is then advanced over this wire and across the pulmonic valve.

The balloon size (6 to 25 mm in diameter), length (20 to 40 mm) and number of balloons vary. In general, balloons are chosen that are 1.2 to 1.5 times the pulmonary anulus diameter as assessed by echocardiography or angiography. A double-balloon technique is used when the pulmonic valve anulus exceeds the available single-balloon size. Balloon inflation time is approximately 5 to 10 sec at 3 to 5 atm of pressure.

Results

Balloon pulmonic valvuloplasty results in an immediate reduction in transvalvular gradient (Fig. 9–11). "Typical" results that have been described are summarized in Table 9–1. Acute changes may be affected by transient right ventricular dysfunction that would underestimate the final pulmonic valve gradient. Alternatively, the final transvalvular gradient would be overestimated if subpulmonic obstruction transiently worsened. If significant subpulmonic obstruction occurs acutely ("suicide ventricle"), it generally responds well to beta-blocker therapy.

Although balloon dilatation of pulmonic valve dysplasia may be less effective, larger balloon diameters may provide satisfactory results.

The true incidence of pulmonic regurgitation following balloon pulmonic valvuloplasty ranges from 0 to 74 percent depending on the methods employed to assess the regurgitation. Doppler evidence of pulmonic regurgitation of at least a mild degree is a frequent consequence of the procedure.

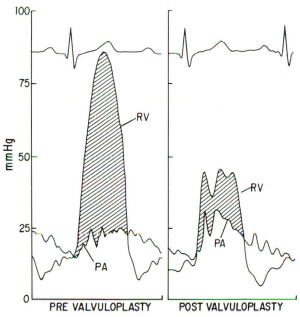

Figure 9–11. A typical result from successful balloon pulmonic valvuloplasty with dramatic reduction in transvalvular gradient (*shaded area*).

Complications

Procedural complications are uncommon (<5%) and include transient systemic hypotension, blood loss requiring transfusion, premature ventricular contractions, transient Q-T prolongation, and bradycardia.

Femoral venous occlusion occurs in 10 to 30 percent of patients and is most common in infants. Because the right ventricle is structured to handle a volume load rather than pressure, the long-term adverse effects of mild increases in pulmonic regurgitation may not be severe.

Interventional Catheter Techniques in Pediatric Patients

Therapeutic procedures in the cardiac catheterization laboratory have also been developed to treat patients with other forms of congenital heart disease. Balloon atrioseptostomy, known as the Rashkind procedure, is primarily used to palliate infants with D-type transposition of the great vessels. A sheath is inserted into the right femoral vein, and a balloon-tipped catheter is passed through the sheath into the right atrium. The catheter, with the balloon deflated, is directed across the foramen ovale and is advanced into the left atrium. The balloon is then inflated with about 2 ml of a saline-contrast mixture, which distends it to about 15 mm in diameter. The inflated balloon is then vigorously withdrawn through the atrial septum, creating a defect (Fig. 9–12). This defect allows improved mixing of the systemic and venous circulations. The balloon is then deflated while in the right atrium, and the catheter is removed.

Catheter-based devices for closing atrial and ventricular septal defects are being tested. The prosthesis consists of a spring-loaded wire skeleton with hooks for anchoring the device. The prosthesis is covered with polyurethane foam (Fig. 9–13A). The device is connected to a catheter-delivery system that allows it to be pulled back and compressed into a 12 to 14 French metal capsule. In the capsule, a spring-loaded conical wire array acts to center the prosthesis. The position and size of the septal defect are first determined by placing a balloon catheter through the septal defect and inflating the balloon. The catheter is then pulled back until the balloon occludes the defect. The balloon is slowly deflated, maintaining gentle traction on the catheter, until it just passes through the defect. The residual volume in the balloon is measured, and the catheter is withdrawn. The balloon is reinflated using the measured volume, and the balloon diameter is measured, thus allowing determination of the size of the septal defect. The position of the defect can also be clarified by cineangiograms that are taken when the balloon catheter is across the septal defect.

When the position of the defect has been determined and the proper prosthesis size has been selected, the catheter delivery system (with the prosthesis encased in the metal pod) is inserted into the venous system. Systemic heparinization is begun. The catheter is manipulated across the septal defect. The prosthesis is then extended from the pod, allowing it and the centering device to spring

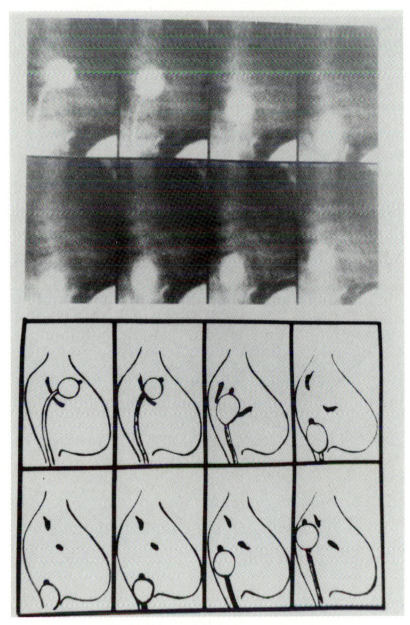

Figure 9–12. Fluoroscopic images (*above*) and diagramatic representation (*below*) of atrioseptostomy. (From Rashkind W. Interventional cardiac catherization in congenital heart disease. Cardiovasc Clin 1985; 15 (1):305, Fig. 1; with permission.)

open (Fig. 9–13*B*). The prosthesis is then slowly retracted into the defect, allowing the wire cone to funnel the prosthesis into the center of the defect. When the hooks have become firmly embedded into the septum, the prosthesis is released by withdrawing the locking wire. The catheter delivery system is then removed. Systemic heparinization is usually continued for about 48 hr.

A similar method for occlusion of a patent ductus arteriosus (PDA) is being developed. The occlusion prosthesis is a spring-loaded device that consists of three metal hooks that are filled with a cone of polyurethane foam. It is withdrawn into a metal pod on the end of the catheter, causing it to collapse and be encased within the metal capsule (Fig. 9–14*A*). The catheter is introduced into the femoral artery and advanced retrograde to the thoracic aorta. The capsule on the catheter tip is manipulated into the ductus arteriosus. The prosthesis is then extruded from the catheter and allowed to expand in the ductus. Gentle, but firm,

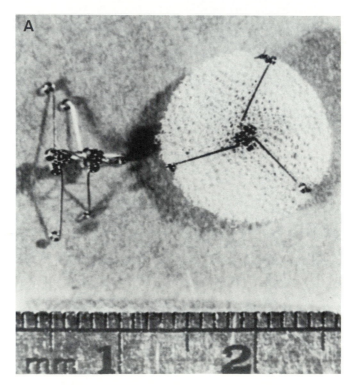

Figure 9–13. *A*, Magnified view of wire skeleton covered with polyurethane foam used for closure of atrial septal defects. (From Rashkind W. Interventional cardiac catheterization in congenital heart disease. Cardiovasc Clin 1985; 15(1):312, Fig. 7; with permission.) *B*, Schematic diagram of method of placing atrial septal defect closure device. (From Rashkind W. Interventional cardiac catheterization in congenital heart disease. Cardiovasc Clin 1985; 15 (1):309, Fig. 4; with permission.)

traction is put on the carrying device to firmly seat the hooks into the wall of the ductus. The transporting catheter is then detached from the prosthesis, and the catheter is removed from the femoral artery. Systemic heparinization is continued for about 48 hours.

An alternative PDA prosthesis being tested is a nonhooked, double-disc device (Fig. 9–14B). This device is passed via the pulmonary artery into the aorta. The distal disc is then extended and pulled back until it bends upon itself, forming a funnel shape in the ductus. The proximal disc is then anchored on the pulmonary artery side of the ductus, securing it in place.

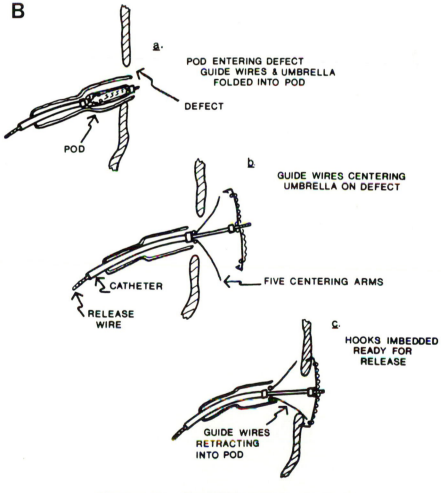

Umbrella Emplacement Sequence

Figure 9–13B.

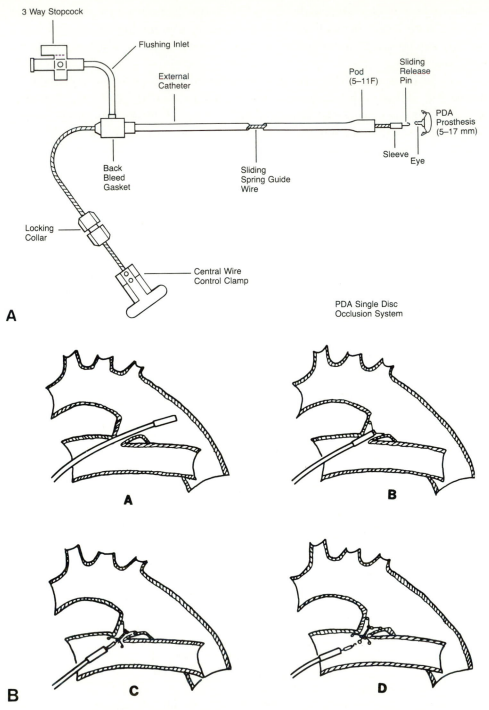

Figure 9–14. A, Diagram of the delivery catheter used to place the PDA occlusion prosthesis. (From Rashkind W. Interventional cardiac catheterization in congenital heart disease. Cardiovasc Clin 1985; 15 (1):311, Fig. 6; with permission.) *B,* Schematic drawing of the placement of the double-disc PDA occlusion prosthesis. (From Rashkind W. Interventional cardiac catheterization in congenital heart disease. Cardiovas Clin 1985; 15 (1):313, Fig. 8; with permission.)

Catheter-Retrieval Devices

Various catheter-based instruments for removal of intravascular foreign bodies have been devised. Some of the retrieval devices are shown in Figure 9–15. The majority of the foreign bodies are central venous pressure catheters which are inserted via through-the-needle technique. These catheters can be sheared off if the catheter is retracted with the needle still in place. These catheter fragments usually lodge in the superior vena cava, right atrium, or pulmonary artery.

The loop-snare type devices are the most frequently employed. The loop at the end of the catheter is manipulated around the foreign body. The loop is then tightened around the object by withdrawing the wire in the external end of the catheter. With the foreign body secured, the catheter is withdrawn.

Endoscopic grasping forceps or myocardial biopsy forceps can also be used to grasp and remove intravascular foreign bodies.

A catheter with a ureteral stone catcher on the distal end can also be used to snare intravascular foreign bodies. Once the wire basket is manipulated around the foreign body, the basket is closed by retracting the wire at the proximal end of the catheter.

These different catheter-retrieval instruments seem to be equally effective at successfully removing intravascular foreign bodies. Foreign bodies that are lodged in the distal branches of the pulmonary artery can be difficult to retrieve because of inability to direct the catheter system into the particular branch of the pulmonary artery required.

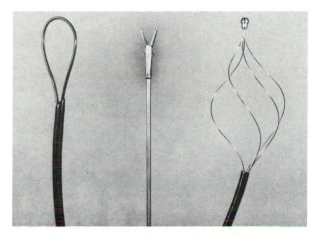

Figure 9–15. Various catheter-retrieval devices. From left: adjustable loop snare, bronchoscopic grasping forceps, and device similar to urologic basket stone catcher. (From Bloomfield D. The nonsurgical retrieval of intracardiac foreign bodies: An international survey. Cathet Cardiovasc Diagn 1978; 4:5; with permission.)

Pericardiocentesis

Pericardiocentesis is used as a therapeutic maneuver to relieve pericardial tamponade. The fluid obtained may also be used diagnostically to help define the etiology of the pericardial effusion.

The pericardial space usually contains a small amount of fluid (< 50 cc), which acts as a lubricating layer to facilitate the normal motion of the heart. Pathologic increases in the amount of pericardial fluid are caused by various disease processes (e.g., infection, tumor, inflammation, etc.). When large amounts of fluid accumulate in the relatively fixed pericardial space, diastolic filling of the cardiac chambers is impaired and cardiac output and systemic blood pressure fall. As seen in Figure 9–16, in the presence of large effusions, further small increments in the volume of fluid cause large increases in pericardial pressure. This

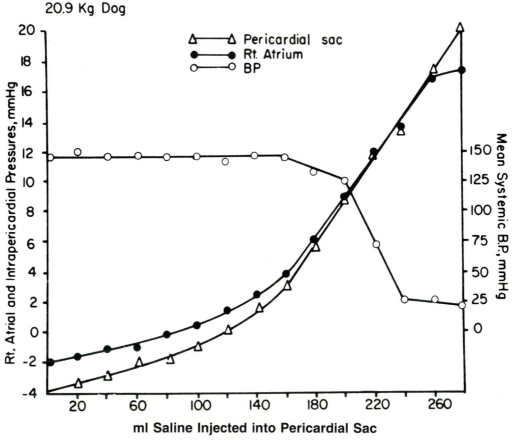

Figure 9–16. Gradual installation of volume into canine pericardial space demonstrating exponential nature of rise in pericardial pressure. Note fall in systemic blood pressure when critical volume is reached. (From Fowler NO. Cardiac diagnosis and treatment. No. 4. Hagerstown, MD: Harper & Row, 1980:982, Fig. 48.3; with permission.)

increase in pressure can rapidly embarrass cardiac output. Conversely, removal of small amounts of pericardial fluid in the setting of pericardial tamponade causes a significant fall in pericardial pressure. This allows for rapid improvement in diastolic filling and cardiac output and often dramatic clinical improvement in the patient.

The diagnosis of pericardial tamponade is a clinical one. Beck's classic triad (elevated jugular venous pressure, low systemic blood pressure, and a small, quiet heart) is helpful when present. Other common clinical features include chest pain, dyspnea, anxiety, and resting tachycardia. The classic standard laboratory features of the chest radiograph showing cardiomegaly with a "water-bottle" configuration or the ECG showing low voltage or electrical alternans may be absent. Echocardiography has replaced these as the confirmatory test when pericardial effusion is suspected; it has become the "gold standard" for defining pericardial effusions. In addition to confirming the presence of an effusion, it can often be helpful in defining the optimal area for needle insertion. This can be especially important in effusions that are difficult to reach, such as those that are loculated posteriorly.

Ideally, pericardiocentesis should be done in a controlled, monitored environment after echocardiographic confirmation of the effusion. An exception to this is the patient with cardiac arrest and electromechanical dissocation in whom pericardial tamponade is suspected. In the presence of pericardial tamponade, there is equalization and elevation (> 15 mm Hg) of the right atrial, right ventricular end-diastolic, pulmonary capillary wedge, left ventricular end-diastolic, and pericardial pressures. These pressures can be demonstrated by performing a right-heart catheterization at the time of pericardiocentesis (Fig. 9–17A and B). The pericardial pressure can be recorded in conjunction with these measurements. After pericardial fluid has been removed, these measurements can be repeated to confirm reduction of the filling pressures with an increase in systemic pressure and cardiac output.

The technique of pericardiocentesis involves sterile insertion of a needle into the pericardial space via the subxiphoid approach (Fig. 9–18 and Table 9–2 for details of procedure). An ECG lead is connected to the needle in order to detect injury current when the needle encounters myocardium. Injury current is demonstrated as S-T elevation on the ECG. As soon as possible, a wire is passed through the needle and the needle removed. A pigtail catheter is then inserted over the wire into the pericardial space. Prompt exchange of the pericardial needle is important in order to prevent perforation of a cardiac chamber (most commonly the right ventricle as the pericardial space diminishes). This can occur as the amount of pericardial fluid decreases, right-sided filling improves, and the right atrium and right ventricle re-expand. The pigtail catheter can be left in place for continued removal of fluid, but it is recommended that it be removed within 24 hr in order to diminish the risk of infection. The fluid that is removed is sent for diagnostic studies, including cell counts, culture, and cytology.

The most serious potential complication of pericardiocentesis is perforation of a cardiac chamber or a coronary artery. Other potential risks include hemothorax, pneumothorax, and infection of the pericardial space.

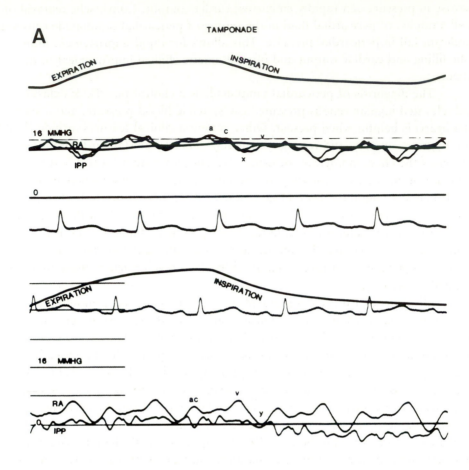

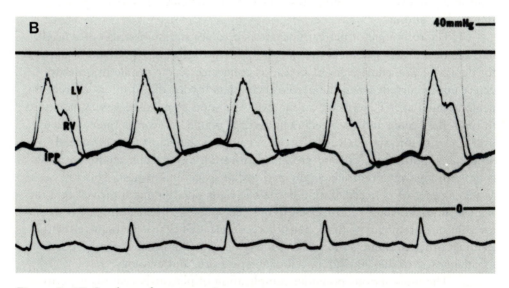

Figure 9–17. See legend on opposite page.

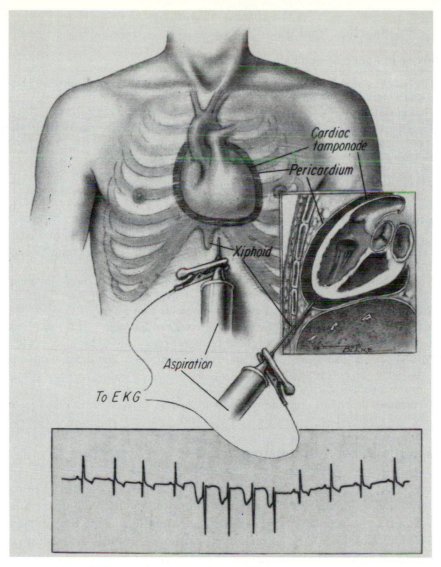

Figure 9–18. Schematic representation of the technique of pericardiocentesis. Note S-T elevation ("injury current") when the needle touches the myocardium. (From Sabiston D Jr. Gibbon's surgery of the chest. Philadelphia: WB Saunders, 1983:996, Fig. 31–1; with permission.)

Figure 9–17. A, Upper panel: right atrial, right atrial mean, and intrapericardial pressure contours in a patient with tamponade. Right atrial and intrapericardial pressures are elevated to 15 mm Hg and are equal. The X-descent is present, but note the absence of the Y-descent. Lower panel: Same patient following pericardiocentesis. Both pressures have fallen. Intrapericardial pressure is less than right atrial pressure, and the Y-descent is now present. (From Reddy PS. Hemodynamics of cardiac tamponade in man. In: Reddy PS, ed. Pericardial disease. New York: Raven Press, 1982:163; with permission.) *B,* Simultaneous right ventricular, left ventricular, and intrapericardial pressures in a patient with tamponade. Note the absence of an early diastolic "dip" in the ventricular pressures. (From Reddy PS. Hemodynamics of cardiac tamponade in man. In: Reddy PS, ed. Pericardial Disease. New York: Raven Press, 1982:175; with permission.)

TABLE 9–2
Technique of Pericardiocentesis

1. The patient is positioned sitting at a 30- to 45-degree angle to allow fluid to layer inferiorly.
2. The subxiphoid area is prepped with Betadine.
3. A syringe with lidocaine and three-way stopcock is connected to the 18-gauge thin-wall blunt-end needle.
4. The ECG V lead is connected to the needle with an alligator clip.
5. The pressure-monitor tubing is connected to the side arm of the stopcock.
6. The subxiphoid region is anesthetized with lidocaine, and a skin nick is made.
7. The needle is inserted and slowly advanced posterolaterally with continuous suction from the syringe and ECG monitoring.
8. The needle is advanced until the pericardium is entered with the return of fluid.
9. The needle should be withdrawn slightly if the ECG shows ST elevation ("injury current"), indicating the needle has encountered myocardium.
10. Needle position can be confirmed by echocardiography or fluoroscopy with contrast injection.
11. A wire is inserted through the needle, and the needle is removed.
12. A 6 French or 7 French pigtail catheter is inserted for drainage.
13. Pericardial and right-heart pressures can be measured.
14. Pressures can be remeasured once fluid has been removed to confirm resolution of the hemodynamic embarrassment.
15. Pericardial fluid is sent for cell counts, cultures, and cytology.
16. To diminish the risk of introducing infection, the pericardial catheter should be removed within 24 hr.

Intra-aortic Balloon Counterpulsation

The use of the intra-aortic balloon pump (IABP) is based on the theory of counterpulsation. The intra-aortic balloon is positioned in the descending aorta just distal to the left subclavian artery. It is inflated in diastole at the time of aortic-valve closure, thus increasing coronary perfusion pressure. It is deflated in systole at the time of aortic-valve opening, thereby decreasing left ventricular afterload and decreasing left ventricular work (Fig. 9–19).

Insertion of an IABP should be considered in patients with medically refractory unstable angina or in patients suffering cardiogenic shock. The IABP is also particularly indicated in patients with acute mitral regurgitation or with a ventricular septal defect in which the decrease in afterload provided by the IABP can produce hemodynamic stability. The use of IABP counterpulsation should be considered primarily in patients in whom further intervention such as cardiac surgery or angioplasty is deemed feasible, because it is considered a temporary stabilizing device that, by itself, has not been shown to improve survival.

Insertion of an IABP may be inadvisable or technically unfeasible in patients with severe femoral, iliac, or aortic atherosclerotic disease. It is also contraindicated in patients with significant aortic valve insufficiency, as the IABP may worsen the degree of regurgitation. A patient with a left-to-right shunt (e.g., patent ductus arteriosus) may suffer worsening of the shunt with the use of IABP counterpulsation.

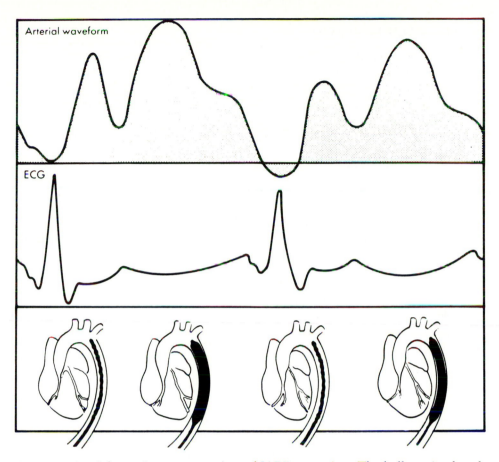

Figure 9–19. Schematic representation of IABP operation. The balloon is placed from the femoral artery and positioned just distal to the left subclavian artery. Two counterpulsation cycles are shown. The balloon is rapidly inflated at the beginning of diastole and is deflated just before the next systole. (From Quaal SJ. Comprehensive intra-aortic balloon pumping. St. Louis: CV Mosby, 1984:81; with permission.)

TABLE 9–3
Technique of IABP Insertion

1. The balloon is fully deflated by aspirating with a 50-cc syringe and stopcock.
2. Balloon is lubricated with sterile saline.
3. Inner stylet is removed.
4. An 8 French sheath is inserted into the femoral artery using Seldinger technique.
5. J-tipped 0.035-inch guidewire is advanced to the descending thoracic aorta.
6. The 8 French sheath is removed, and the IABP sheath and dilator are inserted over the wire.
7. Dilator is removed, leaving 1 inch of sheath above the skin so that bleeding can be controlled by pinching the sheath between the fingers and occluding the end with the thumb (Fig. 9–24A).
8. The IABP catheter is inserted over the J-wire through the sheath (rotating counter-clockwise to keep the balloon tightly wrapped).
9. The balloon is advanced under fluoroscopy until the tip is just distal to the left subclavian artery.
10. The J-wire is removed.
11. The central lumen is connected to the pressure monitor.
12. The balloon lumen is connected to the inflation compressor.
13. The IABP catheter and sheath are sutured to the skin.
14. Unless there is a specific contraindication, the patient is anticoagulated with heparin.

Detailed description of the technique of IABP insertion is found in Table 9–3. Once in proper position, the patient is usually systemically anticoagulated with heparin in order to try to prevent thromboembolic complications. Timing of the balloon inflation and deflation is essential in order to use the IABP safely and to maximize its effectiveness. The balloon should never be inflated during ventricular systole. The timing of inflation in diastole is important to maximize diastolic coronary perfusion pressure and to decrease presystolic left ventricular afterload.

The compressor is preprogrammed to deflate on the R wave. The device is begun at a 1:2 counterpulsation ratio, augmenting every other beat. The compressor has adjustment knobs for altering the timing of balloon inflation and deflation. These adjustments are made using the arterial pressure waveform as a guide to maximize the efficiency of the IABP. When balloon inflation is timed properly, the dicrotic notch assumes a V shape. Proper deflation has been achieved when the balloon-assisted aortic end-diastolic pressure (EDP) is lower than the native aortic EDP, and the balloon-assisted systolic pressure is lower than the native systolic pressure (Fig. 9–20).

The following are examples of improper IABP timing:

1. If early inflation occurs, the balloon is inflating during late systole and impedes left ventricular emptying. This problem is recognized by noting that the balloon inflation occurs prior to the dicrotic notch (Fig. 9–21).

2. With late balloon inflation, the pressure increase caused by balloon inflation occurs after the dicrotic notch (Fig. 9–22). This decreases balloon-pump effectiveness as it decreases the amount of time during which the diastolic coronary perfusion is augmented.
3. Early deflation decreases balloon-pump effectiveness as it fails to decrease the presystolic afterload. This type of timing error allows time in diastole for the diastolic pressure to re-equilibrate to baseline. This is recognized by a rise in diastolic pressure to baseline prior to the next systole and a lack of decrease in balloon-assisted peak systolic pressure (Fig. 9–23).
4. Late balloon deflation impedes early systolic emptying of the ventricle and prevents systemic runoff and the reduction in peripheral resistance that should occur. This problem is recognized by a lack of decrease in the balloon-assisted aortic EDP, as well as a decrease in the slope of the pressure rise (dp/dt) in the balloon-assisted systole (Fig. 9–24).

Once balloon inflation and deflation timing has been properly adjusted, the balloon counterpulsation assist ratio can be increased to 1:1 in order to augment every cardiac beat.

Cardiac catheterization can be performed in a patient with an IABP. This can be accomplished using the femoral artery technique, temporarily discontinuing counterpulsation while the catheter is being passed by the balloon. Once the catheter is in position in the aortic root, the balloon pump can be turned back on. Again, when the catheters are being withdrawn, the balloon is transiently turned off until the catheter tip has cleared the balloon.

Potential complications of intra-aortic balloon counterpulsation include vascular damage such as bleeding or thrombosis at the insertion site. Embolic events causing ischemia to the central nervous system, spinal column, kidneys, bowel, or limbs are other potential major complications. The risk of sepsis increases with the time the IABP is left in place. Hemolytic anemia, thrombocytopenia, and balloon rupture occur uncommonly.

Proper removal of the IABP deserves special attention. (Table 9–4 lists

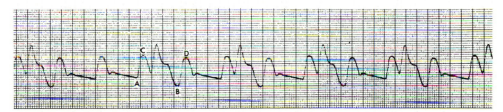

Figure 9–20. Pressure waveform demonstrating proper inflation-deflation timing. Balloon-assisted aortic end-diastolic pressure (B) should be lower than patient aortic end-diastolic pressure (A), and balloon-assisted systole (D) should be lower than nonassisted systole (C). (From Quaal SJ. Comprehensive intraaortic balloon pumping. St. Louis: CV Mosby, 1984:147; with permission.)

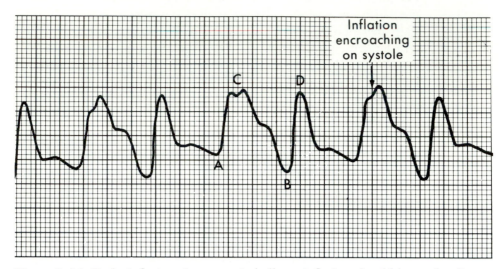

Figure 9–21. Early inflation. Intra-aortic balloon inflation should be at the dicrotic notch. Every other beat is augmented. Early inflation is occurring and encroaches on systole. The dicrotic notch is seen. A–C is the unassisted pressure. B–D is the assisted beat. (From Quaal SJ. Comprehensive intra-aortic balloon pumping. St. Louis: CV Mosby, 1984:163, with permission.)

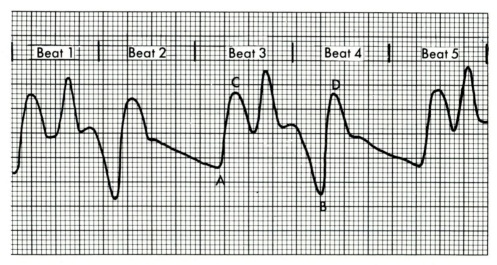

Figure 9–22. Late inflation. Every other beat is augmented. In beat 1, inflation occurs after the dicrotic notch. Inflation is close to the dicrotic notch in beat 3 and appropriately at the notch in beat 5. (From Quaal SJ. Comprehensive intra-aortic balloon pumping. St. Louis: CV Mosby, 1984:163, with permission.)

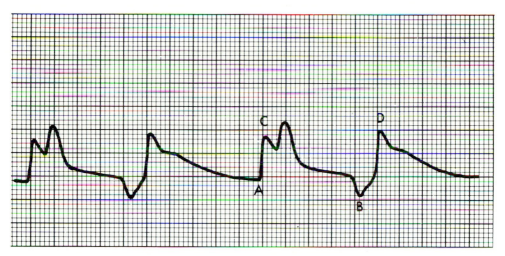

Figure 9–23. Early deflation. Every other beat is augmented. Note location of dicrotic notch on native beat. Balloon inflation occurs appropriately at dicrotic notch. Deflation occurs too early eliminating the fall in peripheral resistance seen with proper deflation timing. This results in balloon assisted systole (*D*) being greater than unassisted (*C*). (From Quaal SJ. Comprehensive intra-aortic balloon pumping. St. Louis: CV Mosby, 1984:163, with permission.)

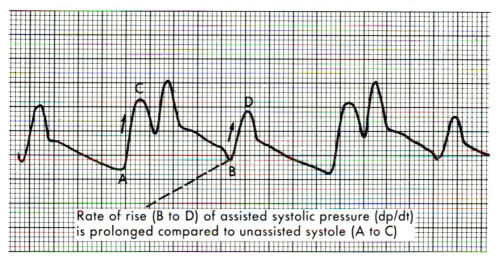

Rate of rise (B to D) of assisted systolic pressure (dp/dt) is prolonged compared to unassisted systole (A to C)

Figure 9–24. Late deflation. Every other beat is augmented. Late deflation prevents adequate peripheral runoff and the assisted beat begins at a higher end-diastolic pressure (*B*) then the unassisted beat (*A*). In addition, the rate of rise of the assisted beat (*B–D*) is slower than the unassisted (*A–C*). (From Quaal SJ. Comprehensive intra-aortic balloon pumping. St. Louis: CV Mosby, 1984:163, with permission.)

TABLE 9–4
Technique of IABP Removal

1. Discontinue anticoagulation.
2. Turn the compressor off.
3. Completely deflate the balloon by aspirating with a 50-cc syringe and stopcock.
4. Pull the balloon back until it is at the entrance of the sheath (do **not** withdraw the balloon through the sheath).
5. Remove the skin sutures to the sheath and balloon.
6. Apply pressure to the artery **distal** to the site of entrance of the catheter (Fig. 9–25).
7. The sheath and catheter are removed as a unit and a few seconds of bleeding are allowed to dispel any thrombus.
8. Pressure is then applied proximal to the entrance site and maintained until all bleeding has ceased.

the details of IABP removal.) When the IABP is no longer believed to be required, the augmentation ratio is usually "weaned down" from a 1:1 to a 1:4 counterpulsation ratio to ensure that the patient can clinically and hemodynamically tolerate removal. Anticoagulation is discontinued, and time is allowed for its effects to wear off. The balloon pump is turned off. The balloon is deflated, and a vacuum is created in the balloon by aspirating with a 50-cc syringe attached to the balloon lumen. The catheter is then pulled back to the entrance of the sheath. The balloon catheter is **not** withdrawn through the sheath in order to prevent the possibility of a portion of the balloon shearing off. The skin sutures to the sheath and balloon are removed. Pressure is then applied to the artery **distal** to the site of entrance to the balloon (Fig. 9–25). The sheath and catheter are then removed as a unit, and a few seconds of arterial bleeding is allowed. This allows any thrombus to be dispelled, and the distal pressure prevents a clot from being propagated distally in the femoral artery. Pressure is then applied proximal to the site of puncture to stop the bleeding. This pressure is maintained for approximately 30 min or until bleeding has ceased.

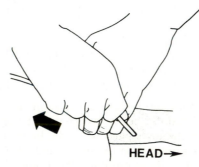

HEAD→

Figure 9–25. Removal of the intra-aortic balloon. Apply distal pressure to allow a few seconds of arterial bleeding to dispel any thrombus. (Courtesy of Datascope Corp.)

SELECTED REFERENCES

Al Zaibag M, Ribeirop AL, Kabsab SA, et al. Percutaneous double balloon mitral valvuloplasty for the rheumatic mitral valve stenosis. Lancet 1986; 1:757.

Block PC, Palacios IF, Jacomi ML, et al. Mechanism of percutaneous mitral valvotomy. Am J Cardiol 1987; 59:178.

Chokshi SK, Meyers S, Abi-Mansour P. Percutaneous transluminal coronary angioplasty: Ten years experience. Prog Cardiovasc Dis 1987; 30:147.

Cribier A, Saoudi N, Berland J, et al. Percutaneous transluminal valvuloplasty of acquired aortic stenosis in elderly patients: An alternative to valve replacement? Lancet 1986; 1:63.

Davidson CJ, Skelton TN, Kisslo K, et al. A comprehensive evaluation of the risk of systemic embolization associated with percutaneous balloon valvuloplasty in adults. Ann Intern Med 1988; 108:557.

Gruentzig AR, Sennsing A, Siegenthaler WE. Nonoperative dilation of coronary artery stenoses: Percutaneous transluminal coronary angioplasty. N Engl J Med 1979; 301:61.

Palacios I, Block PC, Brandi S, et al. Percutaneous balloon valvotomy for patients with severe mitral stenosis. Circulation 1987; 75:778.

Quaal SJ. Comprehensive intra-aortic balloon pumping. St. Louis: CV Mosby, 1984.

Rao PS. Balloon pulmonic valvuloplasty: A review. Clin Cardiol 1989; 12:55.

Rashkind, WJ. Interventional cardiac catheterization in congenital heart disease. Cardiovasc Clin 1985; 15(1):303.

Reddy PS. Hemodynamics of cardiac tamponade in man. In: Reddy PS, ed. Pericardial disease. New York: Raven Press, 1982:161.

Ryan TJ, Faxon DP, Gunnar RM, et al. Guidelines for Percutaneous Transluminal Coronary Angioplasty. Report of the ACC/AHA Task Force. J Am Coll Cardiology 1988; 12:529–45.

Safian RD, Berman AD, Diver DJ, et al. Balloon aortic valvotomy in 170 consecutive patients. N Engl J Med, 1988; 319:125.

Stack RS, Califf RM, Phillips HR, et al. New interventional technology. Am J Cardiol 1988; 62(Suppl II):12F.

Hemodynamic Principles

Thomas M. Bashore, MD, Laurence A. Spero, BSE, and Thad
Makachinas, BS

This chapter focuses on the "nitty gritty" of measuring pressure, oximetrics, cardiac output, and shunts in the catheterization laboratory. The theoretical basis of each topic is covered briefly, but emphasis is placed on the actual performance of each measurement in a practical manner. In many laboratories, these measurements are quite automated. Most are performed by technicians. This chapter is meant to provide a "cookbook" for the proper performance and interpretation of these studies using the equipment available in a representative laboratory.

Pressure Measurement

Background

In 1769, an English clergyman, Stephan Hales, first measured the arterial pressure in dogs and horses. He likened the pressure to a Windkessel, which is a large, inverted, air-filled dome with an input tube and an output tube that is used on fire engines. He envisioned the output strokes of the heart as intermittently filling the Windkessel from one side in a pulsatile manner with steady pressure emerging out the other side. The term "Windkessel" is still used to describe the cushioning function of the arteries. Arterial pressure is usually described in terms of a maximal systolic pressure and a minimal diastolic pressure, both fluctuating about the mean pressure. Most of the data in the cath lab represent pulsatile variables, and much of the information is influenced by physiologic variables, such as respiration, heart rate, LV-RV interaction, and so forth. It should not be disconcerting to appreciate that many measurements fluctuate normally.

Sources of Error in the Measurement of Pressure

One of the major goals of cardiac catheterization is the recording of the pressure waveforms and their magnitude from various vascular structures. Although this may appear to be readily obtainable, one should recognize certain errors inherent in the mesurement of these data in order to avoid overdependence on small variations in the values obtained.

It must be emphasized that any pressure data obtained from inside vascular organs reflect the influence of the pressures not only in the chamber being analyzed, but also in the contiguous structures that surround that chamber. For instance, because the heart resides in the pericardium and both structures are surrounded by the lungs, changes in either pulmonary or pericardial pressure will alter measurements of intracardiac pressure. Likewise, ventricular interaction results in the pressure of one ventricle affecting the pressure in the other. Physiologic variations such as simple respiration affect all of the pressure data. Thus, the "hard" numbers reported from cardiac catheterization data only reflect the average data at an arbitrary point in time. This does not imply that the data are incorrect, but rather that they represent an average value considering the expected physiologic variation seen normally. Certain pathologic states and conditions affect these values to a greater degree.

Sources of error in the measurement of pressures include the routine use of fluid-filled catheters and their poor response to pressure change; poor zeroing practices (wherein the transducer diaphragm is not placed at mid chest); air or other obstructions in the tubing between the catheter and the transducer diaphragm (resulting in damping of the pressure); and, perhaps most commonly, catheter whip artifact, which results from the fluid-filled catheter tip being thrown around inside the heart or great vessels. In addition, end-hole catheter pressure data may not be the same as side-hole catheter pressure data, particularly in areas of streaming or high velocity. In small vessels or valvular orifices, the catheters themselves also become obstructive and the resultant pressures altered.

Although micromanometer-tipped catheters (catheters with transducers built into them) greatly reduce many of these errors, their use has been too impractical in most clinical situations. It is imperative, therefore, that the interpretation of pressure data from fluid-filled systems be made with an appreciation of the pitfalls inherent in the actual data. When data do not fit the clinical situation, it is wise to re-examine the pressure data to insure that none of the artifacts mentioned are present.

Pressure and Resistance Measurements

The Arterial Pressure

In general terms, the arterial pulse pressure reflects both stroke volume and arterial cushioning (compliance), whereas mean pressure represents conduit function (peripheral resistance). With aging, both the pulse pressure and the mean arterial pressure rise owing to stiffening of the arteries.

The contour of the arterial pulse varies with the distance from the heart. As the pressure is transmitted down the aorta, the systolic wave progressively increases in size and becomes more triangular in shape (Fig. 10–1). A discrepancy thus occurs between the peak systolic pressure in the aorta and the peak systolic pressure in the peripheral vessels (brachial, femoral). This discrepancy is greatest in younger patients because there are more elastic fibers in the ascending aorta than in the peripheral vessels. As aging occurs, the elasticity of the ascending aorta declines, and the differences are reduced. When the peripheral or femoral pressure is used to assume ascending aortic pressure (such as when measuring an aortic valve gradient), the peripheral and aortic pressures should always be tracked together before entering the left ventricle in order to appreciate any discrepancy that may exist. If a difference exists, a "pullback" pressure (left ventricle then aortic pressure) should be used to determine the aortic gradient.

Vascular Resistance

Peripheral vascular resistance is generally determined by the smaller arteries (< 1,000 microns), the arterioles (20 to 200 microns), and the capillaries. An abrupt change in resistance occurs over a very short path between the arteries and veins. The upper-body vascular resistance is not quite the same as that of the lower body, and this difference is reflected in the resulting contour of the aortic pulse. Most physiologists believe that the contour of the systolic aortic pulse wave is the result of both flow and waveform reflection from the upper body whereas the diastolic (dicrotic) wave reflection arises from the lower body. In this concept, the percussion wave would represent the intrinsic flow wave, the tidal wave would be reflection from the upper body, and the dicrotic wave would be reflection from the lower body, as discussed in Chapter 7.

The fact that arterial reflections play a major role in the peripheral waveform is unquestioned. The high elastic content of the central aortic vessels results in little reflection (much like throwing a volleyball into a net), whereas the high resistance at the periphery can be likened to throwing a volleyball against a wall.

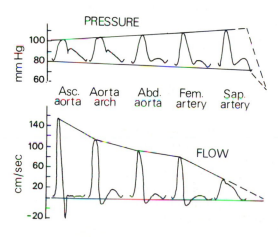

Figure 10–1. The systemic pressure from the ascending aorta to the periphery. The pressure rises despite a decrease in flow owing to reflected waves from the periphery. (From McDonald, DA. Blood flow in arteries. Baltimore: Williams & Wilkins, 1974:358; with permission.)

In the central aorta, much cushioning exists, whereas at the periphery, the high drop in pressure over a very short distance results in the "volleyball" bouncing back and summating with the incoming pressure pulse. The result is the amplification of the pulse pressure as the distance from the heart increases. Note in Figure 10–1 that the pulse pressure rises even though flow decreases as the periphery is approached.

In practical terms, peripheral resistance is measured by using an analog of Ohm's law. This is most easily represented by assuming a hollow tube where there is pressure at both ends. As shown in Figure 10–2, driving pressure through such a tube can be thought of similar to the cardiac output. The greater the pressure, the greater the flow. Conversely, the greater the resistance, the lower the flow.

In the cath lab, flow (cardiac output) can be measured by several methods, which are outlined below. Measuring the mean pressure on either end of the tube and knowing the cardiac output (CO) allows one to calculate vascular resistance.

For the pulmonary bed, the pulmonary vascular resistance (PVR) formula is

$$PVR = \frac{\text{mean PA - mean PCW}}{CO}.$$

The total pulmonary resistance (TPR) was originally used in children when pulmonary capillary wedge (PCW) pressure was not always available. It ignores the PCW pressure and is therefore defined as

$$TPR = \frac{\text{mean PA}}{CO}.$$

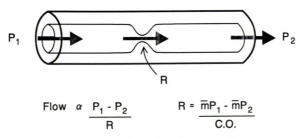

$$\text{Flow} \ \alpha \ \frac{P_1 - P_2}{R} \qquad R = \frac{\overline{m}P_1 - \overline{m}P_2}{C.O.}$$

Figure 10–2. Ohm's law for the vascular system. The flow through a tube increases with increased drop in pressure across the tube and decreases with the rise in resistance in the tube. Rearranging the equation allows one to calculate resistance if one knows the pressure on either end of the tube and the cardiac output.

Using this same concept, the systemic vascular resistance (SVR) is represented by

$$SVR = \frac{\text{mean AO - mean RA}}{CO}.$$

In practical terms, because the mean right atrial pressure is so small in comparison to the mean aortic pressure, the right atrial pressure is often ignored in the equation (the result is referred to as the "total systemic resistance").

When the mean pressure is expressed in mm Hg and the cardiac output in liters per minute, the resultant quotient represents the resistance in *Wood units* (or R units). One can convert these data to dynes $\times$ second $\times$ cm^{-5} by multiplying the quotient by a factor of 80. Table 10-1 lists the normal values.

A couple of practices common to pediatric cath data differ from those common to adult cath lab data. One is the use of the ratio of the PVR or TPR to the SVR. A ratio less than 0.5 (when PVR is used) and less than 0.7 (when TPR is used) implies operability. Ratios greater than those assume that pulmonary resistance is too high to operate. In addition, the conventional practice in pediatrics is to normalize vascular resistance for body surface area (BSA). It is not clear why this practice was never adopted in the adult cath labs, although it should have been. The way this is calculated in pediatrics is *not* to divide the resultant resistance by the BSA, but rather to substitute *cardiac index* (CO/BSA) for cardiac output in the resistance formulas (the results are different; try it).

The Balancing of the Hemodynamic Monitoring Systems

The importance of accurate pressure measurements during a cardiac catheterization procedure cannot be overemphasized. A monitoring system that has not been properly balanced or calibrated will not accurately reflect the patient's physiologic status and could potentially lead to a misdiagnosis. The following description outlines the steps to be used in a representative system.

Overview of the System

The entire system balance and calibration procedure should be performed at the beginning of each work day and checked prior to every catheterization. The fol-

TABLE 10–1
Normal Values for Resistance Measurements

	Absolute Units (dyne sec cm^{-5})	Wood Units (mm Hg $\cdot$ min $\cdot$ L^{-1}
Total pulmonary resistance	205 $\pm$ 51	2.5 $\pm$ 1.0
Pulmonary vascular resistance	67 $\pm$ 30	1 $\pm$ 0.5
Systemic vascular resistance	1170 $\pm$ 270	15 $\pm$ 3.5

lowing procedure is used in our own laboratories and can be modified depending on the manufacturer of the recording equipment.

A representative control room with its hemodynamic monitoring system is shown in Figure 10–3. Figure 10–4 schematically outlines the flow for the conversion of pressure in the heart to data on the monitor and paper printer. Figures 10–5 through 10–8 show actual component parts. Pressure within the heart is initially transmitted through the fluid-filled catheter to the *transducer* (Fig. 10–5). The transducer is basically an enclosed chamber with a diaphragm that is similar to a speaker or microphone. This diaphragm is deformd by pressure changes in the fluid-filled system. This deformation causes an electrical signal to be generated. The greater the pressure, the more the diaphragm moves and the greater the electrical signal that results.

The electrical signal produced, however, is very weak. It also has electrical "noise" in it that needs to be removed. The *conditioner* (Fig. 10–6) amplifies the signal and filters out the "noise" so that it is easier to interpret the waveforms. After the signal is processed, it is sent to *monitors* for display and to the *printer/recorder* (Fig. 10–7) so that a printout of the signal can be made available to the physician. The "traffic cop" that divides the signal and sends it to the monitor and the printer is the *system controller* (Fig. 10–8). To adjust the display on the monitor, a *display controller* is placed between the monitor and signal controller. The display controller controls the type of display that will show up on the monitor.

Each manufacturer has a different method for calibrating the system. The following outline is used with the Hewlett-Packard monitoring system. Although the basic concepts hold for all systems, certain steps will be quite different depending on individual monitoring equipment. In addition, much more automated systems may eliminate certain steps.

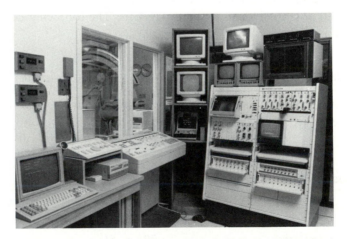

Figure 10–3. Typical control room. The hemodynamic recorder is on the right, and the x-ray console and other equipment are on the left.

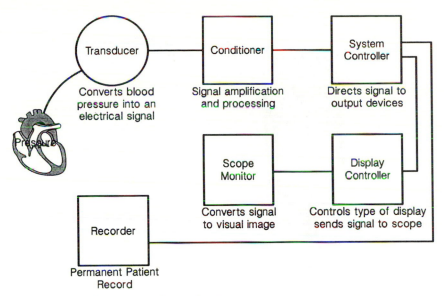

Figure 10–4. Outline of the methods that convert pressure in the heart to the waveforms seen on the monitor and printed on the recorder. The pressure is converted to an electrical signal in the *transducer*. This signal is amplified, and the "noise" is removed in the *conditioner*. A *system controller* then sends the signal to the *monitor* and to the *recorder*. It acts like a "traffic cop." The monitor is controlled by a *display controller*. In this fashion, pressure is simultaneously displayed on the monitor and printed on recorder paper.

The Transducer

If one uses a disposal dome system, the first step is to interface the disposal dome to the transducer. To achieve an air-free interface between the diaphragm and the plastic cover in the face of the quartz transducer, a small amount of saline solution is placed directly on the transducer. The disposable dome diaphragm is then interfaced to the transducer, making sure that no bubbles are present between the disposable diaphragm and the quartz face. If one is using a standard Statham fixed-dome system, similar care must be taken to insure that no air bubbles are present. Heparinized saline (5,000 units in a 1,000-ml bag of normal saline) can then be flushed through all of the lines and aseptically connected to the flushing port of the transducer cover (Fig. 10–9). This flush will purge the plastic dome in preparation for attaching the connecting tubing between the catheter and transducer.

Balancing the Recorder

Electrical signals from the signal conditioner result in fluctuations of a tiny beam of light in the cathode-ray tube at the back of the recorder. This cathode-ray tube can be observed if the thermal printer is simply removed from its cabinet (Fig. 10–10). Dots that appear on this cathode-ray tube will be recorded on paper as major and minor grid lines. The size of these grid lines will correlate with the size

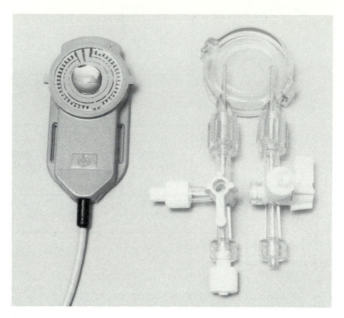

Figure 10–5. Example of a quartz transducer with disposable dome cover. A small bead of heparinized saline is placed in the middle of the transducer prior to placing the dome in place. This allows for an air-free seal between the base of the plastic dome and the transducer surface when the dome is attached to the transducer.

of the lighted dots. Three steps are necessary for the calibration of the system. Refer to Figures 10–4 and 10–10. First, the system controller to printer circuit is balanced. Then the conditioner to system controller is balanced. Finally the transducer to conditioner circuit is calibrated.

Figure 10–10 reviews the steps necessary to calibrate the system controller to the printer. The system-controller output box (see Fig. 10–8) has eight possible channels of output. The input to these channels can be selected from a total of 11 sources. Gain and position controls are located below each output channel. When the system control switch is placed at zero, the output should be aligned with the third major dot from the right on the cathode ray tube using the position button. From this zero point, an ELECTRICAL CALIBRATION needs to be added to the part of the system from the system controller to the recorder system. This is done by moving the *Zero/cal/use* switch to *Cal.* Using a screwdriver adjustment, the amount of deflection resulting from this electrical signal is adjusted until it lines up with the fifth major dot from the right on the cathode-ray tube. This tells the recorder that a certain amount of voltage change is represented by two large grid boxes. The system controller is then adjusted to align recorder and monitors. The system controller is switched to zero, and the posi-

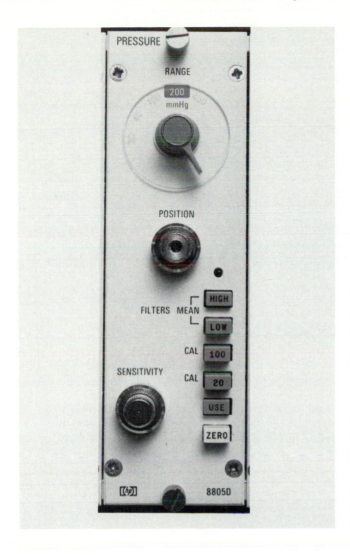

Figure 10–6. Front plate of signal conditioner. The range of pressures to be displayed is controlled by the range knob (*top*). The *Position* knob is used to move the tracing to an appropriate zero line. Within the *Position* knob is a *gain* control. The *Use/cal/zero* options are described in the text. The *Sensitivity* knob on the left is used to adjust the gain during mechanical balancing of the system. (See text for explanation.)

tion control is adjusted to center the dot between the third and fourth major dot from the right on the recorder and center of the screen on the monitor. The system controller is now set up to appropriately record data received from the signal conditioners. The monitors likewise need separate calibration, but this is generally performed by service individuals and not by cath-lab technicians. The monitors are normally calibrated to follow the recorder exactly.

Once this electrical calibration from the controller to the printer and monitors has been completed, then an electrical calibration of the system from the conditioners to the controller must be done. This is performed on the signal conditioner (Fig. 10–6) in a similar manner to that described above for the system controller. A zero is obtained by pressing the *Use* button out and adjusting the *Position* knob until the line on the monitor is at the 0 mm Hg point. Then the 100-CAL button is pressed in, and the gain is adjusted with a screwdriver so that

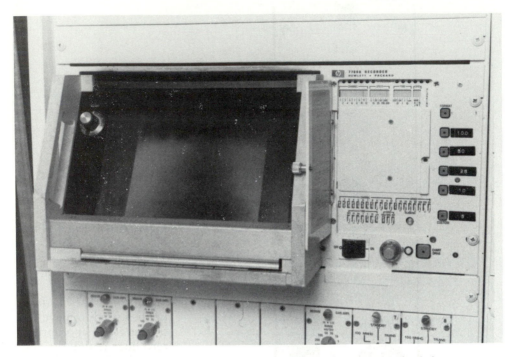

Figure 10–7. Thermal printer and its controls. When the unit on the left is removed, the cathode-ray tube described in Figure 10–10 is visible. The speed, grids, and channels to be recorded can be preselected by utilization of preset formats (shown on the right).

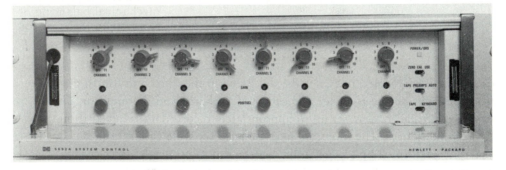

Figure 10–8. The system controller. A series of eight potential output channels is present (channels one through eight). The input to each of these channels can be selected from 1 of 11 sources by the top row of the control knobs. Below each channel output are gain and position controls. To the right are the switches described in the text. The *Zero* position is for determining a baseline zero, the *Cal* position is for calibrating using an electrical calibration signal, and the *Use* position connects the system controller to the transducer output through the signal conditioner.

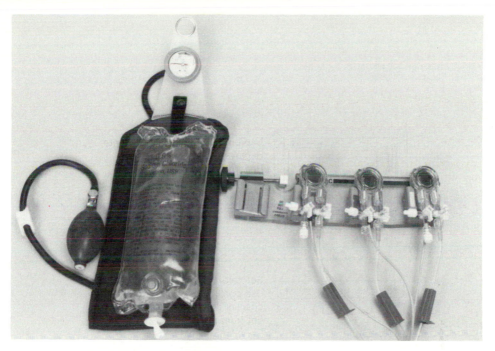

Figure 10–9. Connection between flush solution for transducers and the transducer system.

the monitor displays at a signal the 100 mm Hg point. Now only the transducer needs to be calibrated.

The final step is to add a *MECHANICAL CALIBRATION* signal to the transducer and make sure that what is mechanically added to the transducer is reflected on the monitor and printer. This is done by pushing the *Use* button on the conditioner and simultaneously measuring pressure with a mercury baumanometer (Fig. 10–11) or with a digital mechanical calibration device (Fig. 10–12). To adjust the mechanical pressure recorded, the *Sensitivity* knob on the conditioner is used. The transducer should then be leveled to the middle of the lateral chest wall by placing the open end of the tubing from the transducer at that level and pressing the *Zero* button on the conditioner. The transducer open to air should now reflect an appropriate zero point on both the screen and paper. The system has now undergone both electrical and mechanical calibration. The addition of mechanical pressure from the patients will now be accurately reflected on both the monitor and the printout.

Measurements of Cardiac Output

There is no truly accurate way to measure cardiac output in vivo. The best that can be done is to utilize rough estimates of cardiac output based on a variety of

Recorder

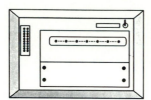

Use button **OUT** on conditioners.
Remove recorder transport.
Record with switch to **WIDE**.
MAJ and MIN grid switches **UP**.
Depress FORMAT (**6**).
Engage chart drive.

System Controller

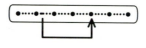

Set zero/cal/use switch to **ZERO**.
Use position control to line up all
channel dots on the **THIRD** major
dot from the right.

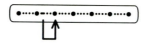

Set zero/cal/use switch to **CAL**.
Use gain control (screw driver
adjustment) to line up all channel
dots on the **FIFTH** major dot
from the right.

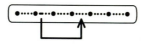

Set zero/cal/use switch to zero.
Use position control to line up all
channel dots **BETWEEN** the **THIRD**
and **FOURTH** major dots from the
right.

Figure 10–10. The recorder and its balancing sequence. At the top of the figure is a schematic of the cathode-ray tube that results in the imprinting of the pressure and grids on the printer paper. The printer shown in Figure 10–7 has been removed. To balance the data going to the printer, a zero is established, an electrical calibration signal is added and calibrated to the movement of two large grid lines (dots), and then the zero-voltage point is defined. This sequence is described in the right panels, and the corresponding diagrams on the left display the alignments. (See text for further explanation.)

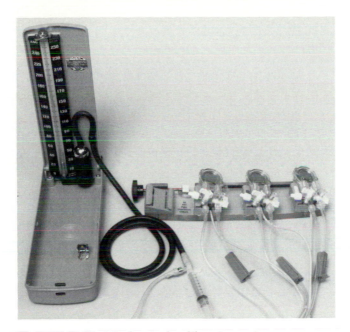

Figure 10–11. Mechanical calibration using a mercury Baumanometer. Pressure is added to the system using a syringe. Simultaneous pressure is produced on the transducer and in the manometer, and a stop-cock allows for the pressure to be held steady. The pressure in the mercury manometer and that produced by the recording system should be exactly equal.

assumptions. In general, the two major methods utilized for the measurement of cardiac output are the Fick method and the indicator-dilution method (of which thermodilution is most commonly used). Cardiac output is often normalized for patient size based on the BSA and expressed as cardiac index. This assumption, like many "facts" in medicine, is certainly open to question, but its use has generally been accepted clinically. Normal cardiac output is 5 to 7.5 L/min (2.5 to 4.5 L/min/m²) in adults.

Indicator Dilution Measures of the Cardiac Output

General Principles

The indicator dilution method has been used, with modifications, to measure cardiac output since its introduction in 1897. The basic equation, which is commonly referred to as the "Stewart-Hamilton equation," is as follows:

$$\text{cardiac output (L/min)} = \frac{\text{amount of indicator injected (mg)} \times 60 \text{ sec/min}}{\text{mean indicator concentration (mg/ml)} \times \text{curve duration}}.$$

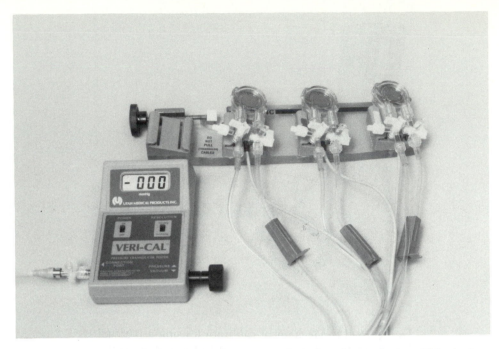

Figure 10–12. Mechanical calibration using a digital-pressure device. This device allows more precise pressure to be added to the system via the screw knob on the left than the mercury manometer system.

This is basically the law of conservation of mass and can be expressed as

$$\text{cardiac output} = \frac{\text{amount of indicator injected}}{\text{area under concentration-time curve}}.$$

One assumes that the injection of a certain amount of an indicator into the circulation will appear and then disappear from any downstream point in a manner commensurate with the cardiac output. A representative curve is shown in Figure 10–13. For instance, if the indicator appears at a given point downstream quickly and washes out quickly, then the assumption is that the cardiac output is high. Although variation may occur, the site of injection is usually a systemic vein on the right side of the heart, and site of sampling is generally a systemic artery. Most commonly, the pulmonary artery is the injection site and the systemic artery is the sampling site. If a right-heart catheterization has not been performed, the left ventricle can adequately serve as the injection site and a peripheral artery as a sampling site. The normal curve itself has an initial rapid upstroke that is followed by a slower downstroke and the eventual appearance of recirculation of the tracer. In reality, this recirculation creates some uncertainty at the end of the curve, and assumptions are made to correct for this distortion. Because the indicator concentration declines exponentially in the absence of recir-

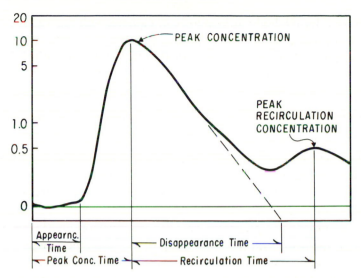

Figure 10–13. Indicator-dilution curve. The density of the dye is detected as a rapid early rise and a slower wash-out. After passing through the body, a second recirculation curve appears. Definitions and timing intervals are as shown.

culation, the initial data points from the descending limb are used to extrapolate the area under the ascending and descending limb by plotting the concentration on semilogarithmic paper. In this manner, the exponential fall is expressed linearly. The results, therefore, assume that the ascending and descending limbs form a triangular shape on the semilogarithmic plot. The base of this triangle then represents the total curve duration, and the mean area of the triangle can be assumed to be a function of the mean indicator concentration. Both of these can be used to determine the cardiac output using the Stewart-Hamilton equation. Small analog computers are now routinely used to measure the area under the curve and digitally display the results. These computers have replaced the time-consuming manual methods of replotting the curve on semilogarithmic paper.

There are several sources of error in this particular approach. When in-docyanine green dye is used, it should be prepared freshly because it is unstable over time and can be affected by light. The exact amount of dye injected is also critical to the performance of the study. It must be measured accurately, generally in a tuberculin syringe, and injected as a single bolus over a brief period. Once injected, the indicator must also mix well before reaching the sampling site, and the dilution curve must have an exponential downpoint that occurs over a long enough period so that extrapolation can occur. This latter problem is particularly significant if, for instance, there is severe valvular regurgitation or a low output state in which the washout decline of the indicator is so prolonged that recirculation begins well before there has been an adequate fall in the curve. For this reason, the green-dye method works poorly in patients with regurgitant lesions or low output. Intracardiac shunts may also greatly affect the shape of this curve. And finally, respiration and vascular obstruction may interfere with the result. Cardiac output is accurate to about ± 10 percent using this method.

Thermodilution Techniques

The more tedious and time-consuming nature of performing indicator-dilution techniques has been replaced in most catheterization laboratories by the use of the thermodilution techniques. The popularity of the Swan-Ganz catheter and its use have greatly expanded the ability to obtain thermodilution cardiac outputs in many clinical settings (Fig. 10–14).

The thermodilution procedure requires the injection of a bolus of cooled liquid (saline or dextrose) and the monitoring of the resultant change in the temperature during continuous sampling by a thermistor mounted downstream from the injection site. The change in temperature can be plotted in a manner similar to the dye-dilution method described previously. The cardiac output is then calculated by a rather complex equation that takes into account the temperature of the injectate and the temperature of the blood along with the volume and the specific gravity of the injectate. In addition, certain calibration factors are utilized. Remember, each manufacturer's catheter may require a different calibration factor for any given cardiac-output computer. Cardiac output is inversely related to the area under a thermodilution curve plotted as temperature versus time. If the tem-

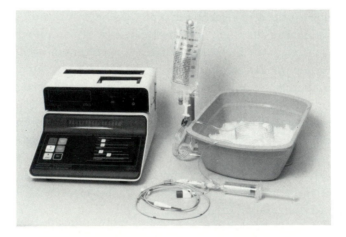

Figure 10–14. Thermodilution setup. The intravenous fluid is passed through plastic coils in a pan of ice. From this tubing, a calibrated syringe of iced fluid is drawn and injected into the proximal port of the catheter. The thermistor on the catheter is connected to the output computer shown on the left. (See text for details.)

perature-change curve is brief and ends rapidly, the cardiac output is obviously high. If the curve is lengthy and slow to fall, the output is low.

The thermodilution method has several advantages. Not only does it not require withdrawal of blood or arterial puncture, it is also less affected by recirculation. Perhaps its greatest advantage is that with the application of computers, it allows rapid display of results that are usable clinically. Most computers utilize the washout rate from the downslope of the curve to obtain a decay constant. This allows reconstruction of the complete triangle-shaped curve and the area under the curve.

Thermodilution cardiac outputs are susceptible to the same problems as indicator-dilution methods using green dye. Because the data represent only right-heart output, tricuspid regurgitation can be a problem due to disruption of the bolus of ice water. Thermodilution tends to over-estimate the cardiac output in low cardiac output states because of the loss of the cold temperature to the surrounding cardiac structures and the subsequent reduction in the total area under the curve. The method is also inaccurate at very high flow states (> 10 L per minute). Other problems include fluctuations in blood temperature during respiratory or cardiac cycles, irregular respiration, intracardiac shunts, and the warming of the injectate temperature prior to its injection into the cardiac chambers.

From a practical viewpoint, thermodilution cardiac outputs have become quite standard. Their range, however, can be relatively broad, so small changes should not be overinterpreted. It is estimated that, overall, cardiac output data can only be defined to $\pm$ 10 to 15 percent.

The Fick Principle

Overview

In many cath labs, the cardiac output and the amount of right-to-left or left-to-right shunting are determined by oximetric methods. It is important to be familiar with the equipment involved and the calculations used to obtain the desired results.

The Fick principle, first espoused by Adolph Fick in 1870, assumes that the rate at which oxygen is consumed is a function of the rate of blood flow $\times$ the rate of oxygen pickup by the red blood cells. The basic assumptions are shown schematically in Figure 10–15. In simple terms, it is assumed that the same number of red blood cells that enter the lung leave the lung. If one knows how many oxygen molecules were attached to the red blood cells entering the lung, how many oxygen molecules were added to the red blood cells as they leave the lung, and how much oxygen was consumed during their travels through the lung, then one can determine the rate of flow of these red cells as they pass through the lung (Fig. 10–15). This can be expressed in the following terms:

$$\text{Cardiac Output (L/min)} = \frac{O_2 \text{ consumption (ml/min)}}{AVO_2 \text{ difference (volume \%)} \times 10}$$

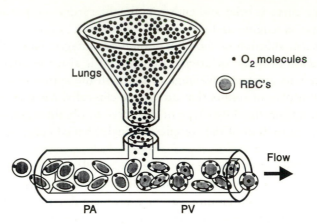

Figure 10–15. The Fick principle. Red blood cells
that enter the lungs contain less oxygen than
those leaving the lung. If the amount of oxygen
consumed is known, and the amount of oxygen
on the red cells determined, then the rate at which
the red cells travel through the lungs can be found
and flow (cardiac output) determined. (See text
for details.)

In practice, the arterial venous oxygen difference (AVO_2) is derived from
systemic (left ventricular, aortic, or femoral) oxygen content and the pulmonary
arterial oxygen content by drawing blood from these areas and directly measuring
the oxygen concentrations. In the strictest sense, the pulmonary arterial blood
and the pulmonary venous blood should be used, because this reflects blood flow
across the lung bed. Because the pulmonary venous blood is rarely sampled, the
assumption is made that left ventricular, aortic, or femoral arterial blood is similar to pulmonary venous blood. In actual fact, because of bronchial venous and
thebesian venous drainage, the oxygen content of systemic arterial blood may be
slightly lower than pulmonary venous blood. The difference is generally irrelevant, though. The variability in the Fick determined cardiac output is ± 5 to 10
percent.

The Measurement of Oxygen Consumption

Measurements must be performed in steady state. The patient must not be receiving supplemental oxygen. Automated methods can determine the oxygen content
within the blood samples; the more difficult measurement is that of oxygen consumption. Traditionally, the Van Slyke method has been used, wherein expiratory
gas samples are collected in a large bag (Douglas bag) over a set period of time.
Measuring the oxygen content in room air and within the bag and knowing how
much air is in the bag over a set period of time (i.e., 3 to 5 min) allow one to
determine the amount of oxygen that was consumed. When the volume of air is

measured and the time it takes to obtain this volume is measured, then oxygen consumption per minute can be derived. Newer devices now allow for measurement of oxygen consumption directly by using a polarographic method, wherein expired oxygen can be quantitated by noting the change in electrical current between a gold cathode and a silver anode imbedded in potassium chloride gel. These devices can be connected to the patient by use of a plastic hood (Fig. 10–16) or via a mouthpiece and tubing. This direct measurement of oxygen consumption is now the preferred method because of its simplicity.

The Fick method suffers primarily from the vagaries of obtaining accurate measurements of oxygen consumption and the inability to obtain a steady state under certain conditions. Age, sex, respiration, heart rate, BSA, lean body weight, and the basal status of the patient all affect oxygen consumption. It requires considerable time and effort on the part of the catheterization laboratory to obtain the appropriate data. The advantage of the direct Fick method is that it is most accurate in patients in whom there is low cardiac output; thus, it provides better data in these situations. It is also independent of the factors that affect curve shape using thermodilution or indicator-dilution methods. It is particularly important that automated devices for the measurement of oxygen consumption are well calibrated and allowed to remain at a constant room temperature for at least 15 to 20 min before using them. Some laboratories use an "assumed" Fick in which oxygen consumption is assumed based on the patient's age, sex, and BSA. The assumed Fick oxygen consumption can be estimated by using a value of

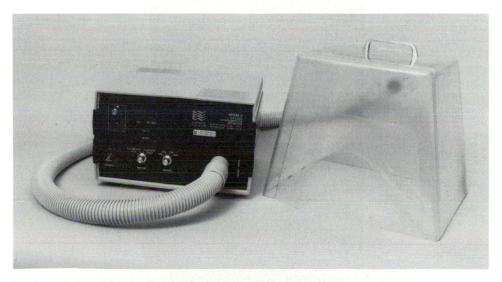

Figure 10–16. Measurement of oxygen consumption. An example of an online monitor that can be used to directly measure oxygen consumption. The hood acts as a mixing chamber, and air is withdrawn at a known rate from the hood. By measuring the oxygen present in the sample and subtracting that amount from what would have been expected if only room air had been sampled, the oxygen consumed can be determined.

125 ml per minute per m^2 for all patients. Improved methods for deriving the assumed Fick oxygen consumption have been published for both the pediatric age group (Saksena, 1983) and the adult population (Crocker et al, 1982). The assumed Fick oxygen consumption is reasonable to use only in patients hemodynamically normal.

The Measurement of the Oxygen Content of Blood

The blood samples in our laboratory are measured on a co-oximeter (Fig. 10–17). Briefly, the whole-blood sample is aspirated into the instrument, mixed with diluent, hemolyzed, and brought to a predefined temperature in a cuvette. Monochromatic light at four specific wavelengths is then passed through the cuvette to a photodetector that provides data regarding absorbances. A dedicated micro-

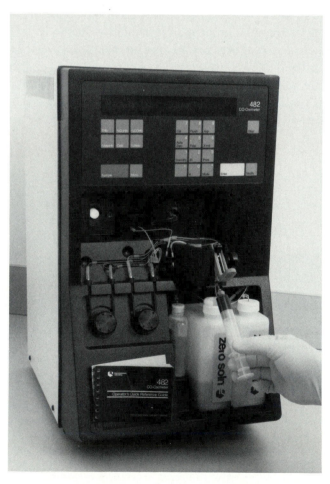

Figure 10–17. A representative co-oximeter. Used for measuring the oxygen content of the blood samples. (See text for details.)

computer calculates the total hemoglobin concentration (RHb), the percent oxygen O_2 hemoglobin (% O_2 Hb), the percent carbon monoxide hemoglobin (% CO Hb), and the percent methemoglobin (% met Hb). The reason for all these types of values is that one needs to know the total hemoglobin concentration that can accept oxygen. If the hemoglobin is tied up with other molecules, then it is not available to have oxygen attached to it. A smoker may have a considerable amount of hemoglobin tied up with carbon monoxide, for instance.

The oxygen capacity (THb) can thus be determined by subtracting hemoglobin attached to carbon monoxide and methemoglobin from the total hemoglobin (RHb). The measured oxygen content can then be expressed in terms of how much of the actual oxygen capacity has oxygen attached.

The oxygen content (volume % O_2) is derived from the following equation:

$$\text{volume \% } O_2 = 1.39 \times \text{THb} \times \frac{O_2 \text{ Hb}}{100},$$

where THb represents the total hemoglobin in the sample capable of carrying oxygen (the oxygen capacity) and O_2 Hb represents the amount of hemoglobin that was measured to have oxygen attached. Hemoglobin can carry 1.36 ml per gram of oxygen. It is assumed that about 0.03 mg per gram of oxygen is dissolved in the blood. The equation thus defines how much of the total capacity for carrying oxygen actually is used by oxygen in the blood sample. This is the volume content of oxygen. The difference between the oxygen content in the arterial system and that in the venous system is referred to as the "AVO_2 difference." The normal value for the AVO_2 difference is generally considered 4.0 ± 0.6 volume percent. When a patient has low cardiac output, more of the oxygen is removed from the blood, and the AVO_2 difference becomes greater.

Measurement of Shunts

Oximetric Measurements

A variety of techniques are available to assist in the determination of intracardiac shunts. In most cases, intracardiac shunting is suspected prior to catheterization. With fewer routine right-heart catheterizations being performed, the opportunity to detect small left-to-right shunts at catheterization has declined. The increased use of echocardiography, however, has clearly allowed the cardiac catheterization procedure to be more focused, and this has surely compensated for this loss. Radionuclide methods can likewise help define shunt presence and severity. In the invasive laboratory, left-to-right shunts are most commonly measured by noting a stepup in the oxygen saturation in venous chambers. The continuous registration of oxygen saturation is now possible using a fiberoptic catheter, and this can simplify the procedure.

Before the oxygen stepup can be utilized as an accurate measure of shunting, however, a review of the normal chamber saturations is of obvious importance. The oxygen content of the inferior vena cava is essentially always higher than the oxygen content of the superior vena cava. This is because the kidneys utilize substantially less oxygen relative to cardiac output than other organs. Renal-vein oxygen saturation is therefore high. As blood returns to the right atrium from the inferior vena cava, it is directed toward the intra-atrial septum by the Eustachian valve. This creates turbulence and nonuniform mixing in the right atrium. In addition, markedly unsaturated blood flows into the right atrium in small amounts from the coronary sinus. Thus, the right atrium receives three different sources of blood (from the superior vena cava, inferior vena cava, and coronary sinus) with differing saturations and in differing amounts. For this reason, a great deal of physiologic variability in oxygen saturation is seen in the right atrium. It is important to appreciate that random right atrial blood samples may vary considerably. More and more mixing of the blood occurs as it enters the right ventricle. In the pulmonary artery the blood is well mixed. Because of this, when there is no shunt, the mixed venous saturation is best measured by sampling blood from the pulmonary artery.

As expected from the physiologic variability noted, the maximal allowable stepup in oxygen content also varies considerably from one right-heart chamber to another. This variability makes it hard to detect a small shunt at the atrial level. In fact, assuming a systemic cardiac index of 3.0 L/minute per m^2, oximetry cannot accurately detect a left-to-right shunt ratio at the atrial level of less than 1.5:1. The shunt ratio is the quotient of the right heart cardiac output over the left heart cardiac output. This means that for each liter of blood the left heart pumps, the right heart must pump 1.5 L. The smallest detectable shunt at the ventricular or great-vessel level is 1.3:1.

To detect a shunt precisely, an oximetry run must be properly performed with an end-hole catheter. A complete run (rarely done) would include each pulmonary artery; the main pulmonary artery; the outflow, midflow, and inflow of the right ventricle; the high, mid, and low right atrium; the low and high superior vena cava; and the inferior vena cava above and below the renal veins. Seldom are all of those sites sampled in practice; therefore, several formulae have been devised to determine the mixed venous saturation using only samples from the superior and inferior vena cava. The most common formula used is

mixed venous O_2 content
$$= \frac{3 \, (\text{SVC } O_2 \text{ content}) + 1 \, (\text{IVC } O_2 \text{ content})}{4}.$$

It is important in obtaining samples to expel any heparin in the syringe prior to filling. Only 2 to 4 cc of blood is required for each sample. When these data are obtained, the presence or absence of a shunt can be defined as shown in Table 10–2. After a shunt has been found, the next step is to determine its magnitude.

TABLE 10–2
Minimum Variability in Oxygen Content and Saturation Among Right-Heart Structures In Order to Declare a Shunt is Present

Shunt	Sites	Minimal Change in Oxygen Content	Minimal Change in Oxygen Saturation Changes
PDA	RV to PA	0.5 vol. %	5%
VSD	RA to RV	0.9 vol. %	7%
ASD	MV to RA	1.9 vol. %	11%

To determine the size of a left-to-right shunt, both the pulmonary blood flow and the systemic blood flow must be determined. If a shunt is present, the pulmonary and systemic blood flow will obviously not be equal. The methods used are similar to those described for Fick cardiac outputs. In order to understand how this is done, a new term—the "effective pulmonary blood flow" (EPBF)—must be introduced. The EPBF is defined as the fraction of mixed venous return received by the lungs without contamination by shunt flow. In the absence of a shunt, the EPBF, the systemic blood flow (SBF), and the pulmonary blood flow (PBF) are all equal. As described previously, to determine the flow across any organ bed, one must measure the oxygen content at the inlet to the organ and the oxygen content at its outlet. The quotient of the oxygen consumption and this AVO$_2$ difference define flow across the organ bed. Pulmonary blood flow thus uses pulmonary artery (Pa) saturation and pulmonary venous (PV) saturation. Systemic blood flow uses the systemic arterial (Sa) and the mixed venous (MV) saturations. The equations for deriving the pulmonary blood flow and systemic blood flow are as follows:

$$\text{PBF (L/min)} = \frac{O_2 \text{ consumption (ml/min)}}{(PVO_2 - PaO_2) \times 10}$$

$$\text{SBF (L/min)} = \frac{O_2 \text{ consumption (ml/min)}}{(SaO_2 - MVO_2) \times 10}$$

If the PBF is equal to the SBF, no shunt is present. In that case, the Sa saturation can substitute for the PVO$_2$ and the PA saturation for the mixed venous saturation.

In the presence of a shunt, however, the effective PBF must be determined. The EPBF uses saturations from the site proximal to any chamber receiving shunt blood in the lungs (the mixed venous in the case of an atrial septal defect) and from the site following the addition of oxygen in the lungs (the pulmonary vein).

$$\text{EPBF (L/min)} = \frac{O_2 \text{ consumption (ml/min)}}{(PVO_2 - MVO_2) \times 10}$$

If the pulmonary vein is not entered, then use an assumed 98 percent saturation for the pulmonary venous oxygen.

For a Left-to-Right Shunt,

$$PBF = EPBF + \text{left-to-right shunt}$$

$$\text{Left-to-right shunt} = PBF - EPBF$$

The equation is as follows:

$$\text{left-to-right shunt} = \frac{O_2 \text{ consumption}}{(PVO_2 - PaO_2) \times 10} - \frac{O_2 \text{ consumption}}{(PVO_2 - MVO_2) \times 10}$$

Or, more simply, if there is no concurrent right-to-left shunt, one can substitute systemic saturation (Sa) for pulmonary venous saturation:

$$\text{left-to-right shunt} = \frac{O_2 \text{ consumption}}{(SaO_2 - PaO_2) \times 10} - \frac{O_2 \text{ consumption}}{(SaO_2 - MVO_2) \times 10}$$

The magnitude of a left-to-right shunt is thus defined as the PBF minus the effective PBF. As an example, the blood samples to be used for an atrial septal defect are shown diagramatically in Figure 10–18. Note that the appropriate saturations to be measured are those from the chamber or vascular structure just prior to the shunt origin and from either side of the shunt destination.

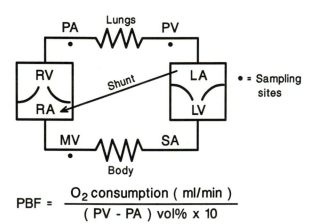

$$PBF = \frac{O_2 \text{ consumption (ml/min)}}{(\text{ PV - PA }) \text{ vol\% x 10}}$$

$$EPBF = \frac{O_2 \text{ consumption (ml/min)}}{(\text{ PV - MV }) \text{ vol\% x 10}}$$

L→R shunt = PBF - EPBF

Figure 10–18. The determination of a left-to-right shunt at the atrial level. The dots represent the key sampling sites (before the shunt and on either side of its destination). (See text for explanation.)

This works in a similar manner for right-to-left shunts. In a right-to-left shunt, the shunt flow is added to the effective PBF to obtain total systemic blood flow.

Rearranging the equation, we get the following:

$$\text{right-to-left shunt} = SBF - EPBF$$

$$\text{right-to-left shunt} = \frac{O_2 \text{ consumption}}{(SaO_2 - MVO_2) \times 10} - \frac{O_2 \text{ consumption}}{(PVO_2 - MVO_2) \times 10}$$

Or, more simply, if there is *no bidirectional shunt*, one can substitute the pulmonary artery (Pa) saturation for the mixed venous saturation:

$$\text{right-to-left shunt} = \frac{O_2 \text{ consumption}}{(SaO_2 - PaO_2) \times 10} - \frac{O_2 \text{ consumption}}{(PVO_2 - PaO_2) \times 10}$$

As in the previous example, a right-to left shunt at the atrial level requires measurement of oxygen saturation from the structure just prior to the shunt (the mixed venous saturation) and from the structures just before and after the shunt destination (the pulmonary venous and left ventricular saturations respectively). The method of calculating right-to-left shunt at the atrial level is shown in Figure 10–19. Using the same logic, shunts at any level (ventricular, great vessel) can be determined. These same equations are used to determine bidirectional shunts.

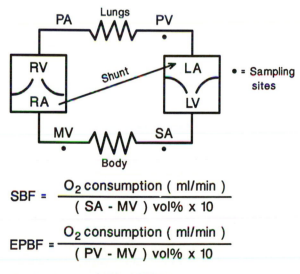

$$SBF = \frac{O_2 \text{ consumption (ml/min)}}{(SA - MV) \text{ vol\% } \times 10}$$

$$EPBF = \frac{O_2 \text{ consumption (ml/min)}}{(PV - MV) \text{ vol\% } \times 10}$$

R→L shunt = SBF - EPBF

Figure 10–19. The determination of a right-to-left shunt at the atrial level. (See text for explanation.)

A summary of these formulae follows:

1. **To calculate a shunt at the ventricular level:**

   LEFT-TO-RIGHT SHUNT (VSD)
   PBF   = EPBF + Shunt
   Shunt = PBF − EPBF
   $$\text{Shunt} = \frac{O_2 \text{ consumption}}{(PVO_2 - PaO_2) \times 10} - \frac{O_2 \text{ consumption}}{(PVO_2 - RaO_2) \times 10}$$

If no right-to-left shunt, one can substitute SaO_2 for PVO_2. Ra = right atrium.

   RIGHT-TO-LEFT SHUNT (VSD)
   SBF   = EPBF + Shunt
   Shunt = SBF − EPBF
   $$\text{Shunt} = \frac{O_2 \text{ consumption}}{(SaO_2 - RaO_2) \times 10} - \frac{O_2 \text{ consumption}}{(PVO_2 - RaO_2) \times 10}$$

If no left-to-right shunt, one can substitute PaO_2 for RaO_2.

2. **To calculate a shunt present at both the atrial and ventricular levels (ASD and VSD):**
   a. At atrial level (RABF = right atrial blood flow, RVO_2 = right ventricular oxygen content)

   RABF = SBF + Shunt
   Shunt = RABF − SBF
   $$\text{Shunt} = \frac{O_2 \text{ consumption}}{(RVO_2 - MVO_2) \times 10} - \frac{O_2 \text{ consumption}}{(SaO_2 - MVO_2) \times 10}$$

   b. At ventricular level (RVBF = right ventricular blood flow):

   RVBF = RABF + Shunt
   Shunt = RVBF − RABF
   $$\text{Shunt} = \frac{O_2 \text{ consumption}}{(PaO_2 - RaO_2) \times 10} - \frac{O_2 \text{ consumption}}{RVO_2 - MVO_2) \times 10}$$

The Indicator-Dilution Method

Shunt detection by indicator-dilution methods is more sensitive than shunt detection by oximetric methods, but it suffers from a variety of limitations. There is a growing trend away from the use of indicator-dilution methods in the catheterization laboratories, so lack of familiarity also presents some disadvantage. An indicator such as indocyanine green dye is injected into one chamber, and while sampling through a catheter from another chamber, the density of dye over time is detected in a densitometer and displayed on paper. Indicator-dilution methods are

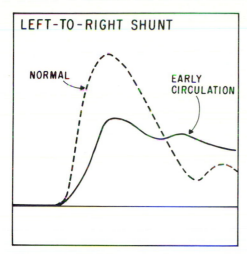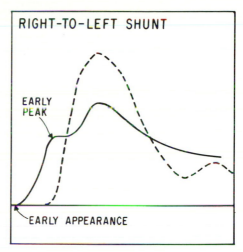

Figure 10–20. Representative shunt curves from an atrial septal defect. The *dotted line* represents the normal curve when the right atrium is the injection site and the brachial artery the sampling site. The left panel reveals the early recirculation peak from the left-to-right shunt. The right panel represents an early-appearance peak from a right-to-left shunt.

now used more for qualitative than quantitative detection of shunt presence, but both the diagnosis and quantitation of shunts can be obtained using these methods.

For instance, injecting dye into the pulmonary artery and sampling at the brachial artery results in the observation of a wavefront of dye, which rises, then declines. This is followed by a second smaller wavefront that appears after the sample has circulated throughout the body. If there is a *left-to-right intracardiac shunt*, say at the atrial level, some of the dye injected in the pulmonary artery will first pass quickly to the brachial artery, and some of the dye will pass to the left atrium, the right atrium, and then return to the pulmonary artery, left atrium, and the systemic artery. This second pass will create a second wavefront owing to the recirculation of dye through the shunt. This phenomenon is referred to as "early recirculation." If a *right-to-left shunt* is to be detected, one must inject dye into a right-heart chamber prior to the defect and sample anywhere downstream in the arterial system. A certain amount of dye will go through the shunt and appear prematurely in the arterial system. The location of any shunt can thus be found by varying injectate sites and sampling sites. Examples of left-to-right and right-to-left shunt at the atrial level are shown in Figure 10–20.

SELECTED REFERENCES

Crocker RH, et al. Determinants of total body oxygen consumption in adults undergoing cardiac catheterization. Cath Cardiovasc Diagn 1982; 8:363.
Saksena FB. Normogram to estimate the oxygen consumption index from the age, sex, and heart rate. Pediatr Cardiol 1983; 4:55.

CHAPTER 11

Angiographic Techniques and Data Analysis

Thomas N. Skelton, MD

The goal of invasive diagnostic techniques in cardiology is the acquisition of angiographic, hemodynamic, or electrophysiologic data for use in making patient-management decisions. This chapter focuses on technical aspects of acquisition and analysis of angiographic information in the cardiac catheterization lab. Compared to hemodynamic measurements, the analysis of ventricular performance, coronary artery stenosis, or valvular dysfunction is often rather subjective. In recent years, however, there has been a trend toward more objective description of angiographic data that has been aided, in many cases, by the application of computers to data analysis. Although there are numerous potential variations in the techniques of data acquisition and analysis, this chapter focuses on those considered to be "standard." It includes brief discussions about good angiographic technique as well as standard methods of data analysis.

Ventriculography: Technical Aspects of Imaging

Left ventriculography is most often accomplished by power injection of 40 to 50 ml of contrast through a pigtail or other multihole catheter that has been introduced retrograde across the aortic valve into the left ventricle. Ideal positioning of the catheter in the mitral inflow tract allows for good mixing of contrast with blood and avoids or minimizes the mechanical stimulation of ventricular ectopic beats during injection. Cineangiography frame rates of at least 30 frames per second are needed to assess ventricular-wall motion and to accurately identify end-diastolic and end-systolic images for ventricular-volume measurement.

In most laboratories where multimode image intensifiers are used, ventriculography is performed in a 9-inch (or similar large-field) mode. This usually allows for visualization of the left ventricular chamber, the surrounding myocardium and pericardium, the left atrium, and the proximal portion of the aortic root, all of which should be evaluated when reviewing the cineangiogram.

In general, the "standard" projections for biplane left ventriculography are the 30-degree right anterior oblique (RAO) and 60-degree left anterior oblique (LAO) views (Fig. 11–1). In a single-plane laboratory, the 30-degree RAO view is used, except in specific cases (such as ventricular septal defect) in which another projection may provide more useful information. Although the 30-degree RAO and 60-degree LAO specifications are generally useful, the optimal angulation may be somewhat different based on an individual patient's chest configuration.

In the RAO projection, the portion of the ventricular outline leftmost on the image will be the basilar part of the mitral valve; therefore, the left atrium (visualized only in the presence of mitral regurgitation during a left ventriculogram) will lie to the left (on the image) of the mitral valve. Optimal angulation in the RAO projection (Fig. 11–2A) will place the ventricle such that there is no overlap with the descending thoracic aorta, so that most of the left atrium will be located between the ventricle and the spine, and so that a portion of the aortic root is visible in the top portion of the image. When the ventricle overlaps the descending aorta, more RAO angulation is needed.

The LAO projection (Fig. 11–2B) should be set up so that the heart shadow on fluoroscopy is adjacent to, but does not overlap, the spine. In this view, the left atrium lies above and slightly to the right (on the image) of the ventricle. Some angiographers will modify the LAO view by adding cranial skew (Fig. 11–3). This modification often permits a better evaluation of the interventricular septum and should usually be used when evaluating ventricular septal

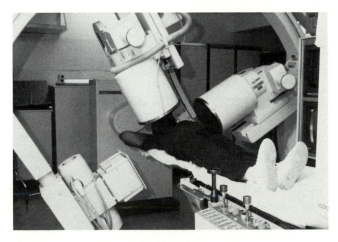

Figure 11–1. The cath-lab technician demonstrates camera positions for straight 30-degree RAO and 60-degree LAO ventriculography in a biplane laboratory.

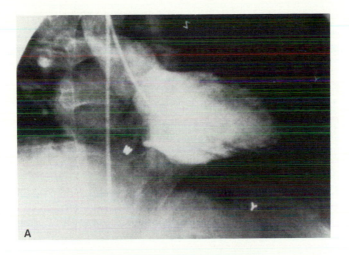

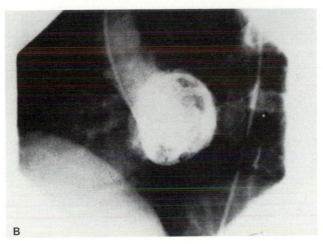

Figure 11–2. A and *B* are typical 30-degree RAO and 60-degree LAO views, respectively, of the left ventricle at end diastole.

defects. The addition of cranial skew has the disadvantage of causing the ventricle to partially overlap the diaphragm. The added density of the diaphragm may make adequate exposure difficult, depending on the size of the patient.

The final setup of camera angles and table position should be done during deep inspiration. This maneuver tends to move the heart inferiorly and anteriorly. In the RAO projection, the heart moves down on the image, and in the LAO view, the heart moves down and to the left on the image. If not set up with these changes in mind, the ventricle may be partially "cut off" on the film.

Measurement of Ventricular Volumes

Numerous disease states result in dilation of the left ventricle with or without reduction in systolic performance. Measurement of ventricular volume provides

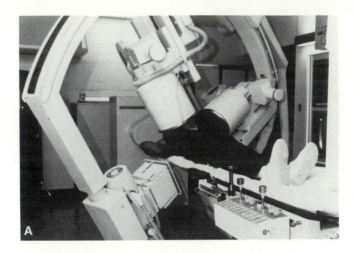

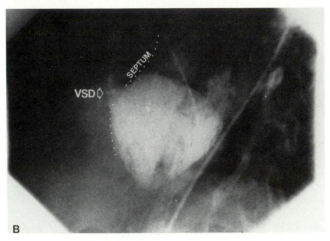

Figure 11–3. *A* illustrates modification of the LAO ventriculogram with cranial skew (compare with Figs. 1 and 2). *B,* A cinefilm frame of the LAO cranial view in a patient with a ventricular septal defect (VSD) shows the cranial modification enhancing the image of the interventricular septum (SEPTUM), although a portion of the ventricle is overlapped by the diaphragm.

an objective description of chamber size, and the comparison of end-diastolic volume and end-systolic volume provides additional information such as ejection fraction (defined below). Left ventricular ejection fraction is a powerful predictor of prognosis in patients with ischemic heart disease (O'Callaghan and Hinohara, 1988). Although there are other methods of estimating ventricular volumes and parameters derived from them, cineangiographic analysis is maintained as the "gold standard."

Definitions

End-diastolic volume (**EDV**) is the maximum left ventricular volume during the cardiac cycle and occurs immediately prior to the onset of systole. In patients in sinus rhythm, the EDV occurs immediately after atrial contraction. End-systolic volume (**ESV**) is defined as the minimum left ventricular volume during the cardiac cycle. Left ventricular stroke volume (**SV**), the amount of blood ejected with each beat, is the difference between **EDV** and **ESV**. Left ventricular ejection fraction (**EF**) is the percentage of the **EDV** that is ejected with each beat. Stroke volume and EF are expressed in the following equations:

$$SV = EDV - ESV$$

$$EF = \frac{SV}{EDV} = \frac{EDV - ESV}{EDV}$$

Technical Considerations for Imaging

Determination of ventricular volumes depends upon identifying cineangiogram frames corresponding to end diastole (ED) and end systole (ES), and upon being able to outline the dye-filled ventricular chamber. For accurate selection of the ED and ES images, a cinefilm frame rate of at least 30 frames per second is necessary. To obtain good definition of the ventricular outline, a contrast injection volume of 40 to 50 ml at a flow rate of 10 to 15 ml per second is generally used. In digital-imaging laboratories where subtraction techniques can be used to enhance image contrast, diagnostic studies can be obtained with as little as 5 ml of contrast diluted in saline.

Factors causing potentially nonanalyzable studies can usually be avoided by attention to detail during setup of the angiogram. The ventricular apex may be "cut off" the edge of the image owing to poor positioning during setup or to failure to allow for a normal amount of "overframing" on the cinefilm. The latter refers to the fact that the cinefilm image is often set up to record only the central portion of what is visible on the image intensifier. In the RAO view, there should be a relatively small amount of lung, which is highly radiolucent, adjacent to the anterior heart border. Inclusion of an excessive amount of lung in the image may alter the exposure parameters such that the anterior ventricular wall is not discernable adjacent to the very "bright" lung field. This anterior wall "burn-out" can also be minimized by inclusion of a radiodense shield over the lung field to partially or totally block the high transmission of x-rays in that area.

Ectopy during the ventriculogram is another cause of nonanalyzable studies. Even when a "quiet" catheter position is found during setup for the ventriculogram, however, the force of power injection or slight recoil of the catheter may mechanically stimulate ventricular ectopy. A modest reduction in the injection flow rate will sometimes reduce or eliminate the ectopy. In difficult cases, the catheter can be pulled back into the aortic root immediately following injection of most of the contrast. There is usually enough dye remaining in the ventricle to adequately define ventricular outlines for the subsequent beat or two.

Volume Measurement: The Area-Length Method

Although there are several valid methods for determining ventricular volumes, one of the most commonly used is the area-length method of Dodge and associates (Dodge, Sandler, Ballew, et al, 1960). Although originally applied to the anteroposterior (AP) and lateral projections, it has been widely used in single-plane and biplane oblique ventriculography. The area-length method begins with the assumption that the ventricle is shaped like an ellipsoid (Fig. 11–4). The volume of an ellipsoid is

$$V = \frac{4}{3} \pi \frac{L}{2} \frac{M}{2} \frac{m}{2},$$

where **V** is the volume of the ellipse, **L** is the long axis, and **M** and **m** are the minor axes. The long axis **L** is measured as the distance from the aortic valve plane to the apex for each of the two views. In the biplane calculation, **L** is the shorter value from the RAO and LAO views. The minor axes are not measured but are calculated from the area of the projected ventricular silhouette in each view, (hence the name "area-length") as follows:

$$M = \frac{4A_{RAO}}{\pi L_{RAO}} \qquad m = \frac{4A_{LAO}}{\pi L_{LAO}}$$

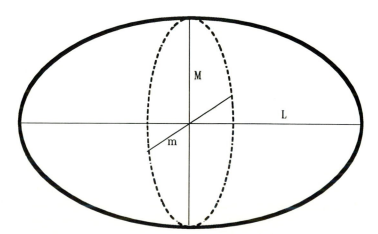

Figure 11–4. For volume determination, the shape of the left ventricle is approximated by a solid ellipsoid with a major diameter L and minor diameters M and m. (See text for discussion).

Substitution of the above for M and m, and 3.1416 for π in the equation for the volume of the ellipsoid results in the *biplane area-length formula*:

$$V = 0.849 \cdot \frac{A_{RAO}\, A_{LAO}}{L_{min}}$$

where L_{min} is the *shorter* of the long axes, L_{RAO} or L_{LAO}. In a single-plane analysis, the axes are assumed to be the same length in each view. Therefore, the *single-plane area-length formula* reduces to

$$V = \frac{8A^2}{3\pi L} \quad \text{or} \quad V = 0.849 \cdot \frac{A^2}{L}.$$

Correction Factors

Two major "correction factors" are involved in obtaining accurate volume determinations: magnification correction and regression parameter adjustment.

Magnification Correction

The image projected onto the image-intensifier screen is magnified as a result of the geometry of the divergent x-ray beam (Fig. 11–5). The degree of magnification is determined by the relative location of three points: the x-ray tube ("source"), the heart ("object"), and the image-intensifier screen ("image"). Relative magnification (M) is the ratio of the source-to-image distance (SID) to the source-to-object distance (SOD):

$$\text{magnification} = \frac{SID}{SOD}.$$

If a calibration object (such as two small lead dots mounted a known distance apart) is mounted on the faceplate of the image intensifier, the volume of the projected image can be determined by the area-length (or other) method and subsequently multiplied by a magnification correction factor to obtain the volume of the true object (the heart). Because the magnification M from the above equation applies to each linear dimension, a three-dimensional volume is magnified by a factor of M^3. The volume of the heart, V_{heart}, therefore, is related to the volume determined from the calibrated image, V_{image}, as follows:

$$V_{heart} = V_{image} \cdot \frac{1}{M^3} \quad \text{or} \quad,$$

$$V_{heart} = V_{image} \cdot MCF^3$$

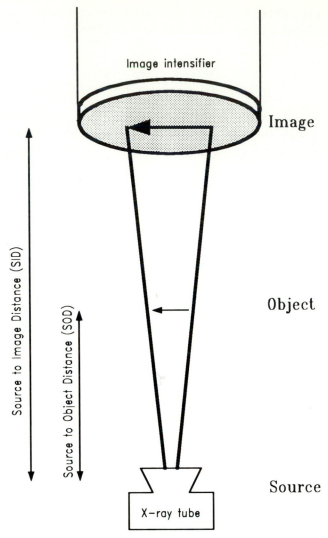

Figure 11–5. Schematic illustration of the magnification of an object caused by divergence of the x-ray beam. (See text for discussion).

where the magnification correction factor, **MCF** = $1/M$. In a biplane setting, **MCF**[3] will be a combination of RAO and LAO magnification factors.

An alternate means of deriving the size calibration is by use of the grid calibration technique. In this method, immediately following the ventriculogram, the patient is moved from under the image intensifier and a grid with lines spaced 1 cm apart (Fig. 11–6) is placed at the approximate location of the heart during the angiogram, and a short cinefilm run is recorded. Later, during volume measurement, this grid image is used as a direct size calibration for the heart. No magnification correction is needed, because the heart and grid are magnified to the same degree in the image.

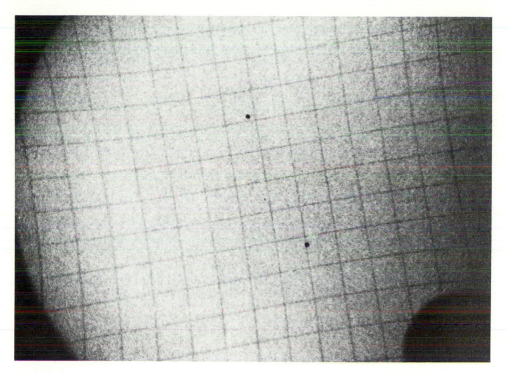

Figure 11–6. Radiographic image of a calibration grid with lines spaced 1-cm apart that form squares, each with area of 1 cm².

Regression Parameters

Because of the geometric assumptions made by the area-length method, the calculated ventricular volume (after application of any magnification correction), V_{calc}, is uniformly higher than the true volume, V_{true}. Thus, it is necessary to apply linear-regression parameters to obtain accurate data:

$$V_{true} = A \cdot V_{calc} + B ,$$

where **A** and **B** are regression parameters. Table 11–1 lists published regression parameters for adults. Ideally, each laboratory should determine its own regression parameters. This requires imaging phantoms of known volume, often radiopaque latex casts of dog or human autopsy ventricles (Fig. 11–7). The area-length method is applied to the images of these casts, but no regression parameters are used. Then, the calculated volume is compared with known true volume and linear regression analysis is applied to determine the equation of the line that best fits the data (Fig. 11–8). Regression parameters must be applied even for labs that use the direct-grid calibration method.

TABLE 11–1
Published Regression Parameters for Application to Calculated Left Ventricular Volumes

Angiographic Technique	Reference	Regression Parameters*	
		A	*B*
Biplane RAO/LAO	Wynne, *et al*[3]	0.989	− 8.1
Single plane RAO	Wynne, *et al*[3]	0.938	− 5.7
Single plane RAO	Kennedy, *et al*[4]	0.81	+ 1.9
Biplane AP/LAT	Sandler, *et al*[5]	0.928	− 3.8
Single plane AP	Sandler, *et al*[6]	0.951	− 3.0

*Parameters to the equation $V_{true} = A \cdot V_{calc} + B$.

Making the Measurements

The following list summarizes the basic steps for determination of ventricular volumes:

1. Selection of ED and ES images.
2. Tracing of ventricular outlines for ED/ES and RAO/LAO.
3. Size calibration (use of direct-grid measurement or calculated magnification-correction factors).
4. Calculation of volume using area-length formula.
5. Application of regression parameters.

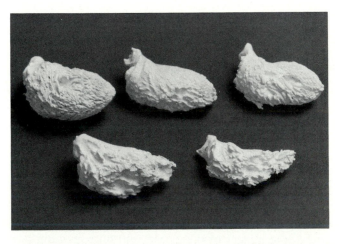

Figure 11–7. Photograph of latex casts of left ventricles of various sizes. These are imaged to determine regression parameters for an individual laboratory. (See text for discussion.)

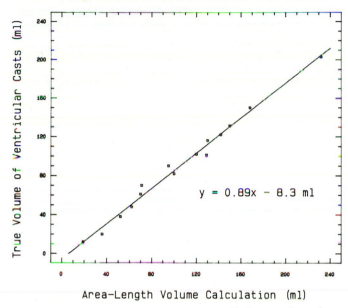

LV VOLUME CALIBRATION
Regression of TRUE vs CALCULATED Volume

$y = 0.89x - 8.3$ ml

Figure 11–8. Linear regression is applied to a plot of calculated volume versus known true volume of ventricular casts imaged in a newly constructed cath lab. The resulting equation is applied to all calculated volumes (x) from the same laboratory.

Step 1: Selecting ED and ES Images

The beat selected for analysis should be the earliest beat in the cineangiogram in which there is adequate contrast filling for delineating ventricular borders and that is not a premature ventricular contraction (PVC) or a post-PVC beat. By moving frame by frame within the selected beat, one can visually determine the largest (ED) and smallest (ES) ventricular silhouette for analysis. By observing the "negative contrast" (blood without contrast material) entering the left ventricle from the atrium, the last diastolic frame can usually be distinguished from the first systolic frame, which is recognized by initial closure of the mitral valve.

Step 2: Tracing the Ventricular Outline

To determine the projected area and length of the ventricle, its perimeter must be outlined. Using a film projector, the ventricle can be traced onto thin tracing paper or a plastic transparency for analysis. The tracing should be made at the outer margin of any visible contrast material. Therefore, trabeculations and papillary muscles are included *within* the ventricular outline (Fig. 11–9). The aortic

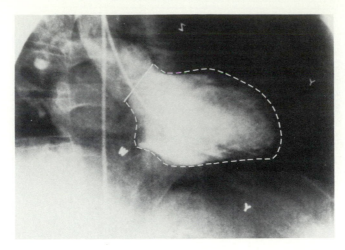

Figure 11–9. End-diastolic frame of the left ventricle in the RAO projection. The traced outline lies just outside all visible contrast and includes trabeculations and papillary muscles within it.

valve plane is drawn across the lower margins of the sinuses of Valsalva to complete the tracing. *Consistency* in tracing the ventricular outline is of utmost importance.

Step 3: Size Calibration

Three factors affect the size of the ventricle as seen on the film projector: (1) magnification of the object due to nonparallel x-rays (see Fig. 11–5), (2) minification of the image during image intensification and recording onto 35-mm film, and (3) remagnification of the film image when projected onto the projector's viewing screen. It is not practical to measure the magnitude of *each* of these factors, so, in practice, a size-calibration marker is filmed either at the level of the heart (direct-object calibration) or at the level of the image (markers mounted on the image-intensifier faceplate). The latter requires knowledge of the degree of magnification of the object (the heart), which is calculated based on the geometry of the individual catheterization laboratory (discussed below).

In the direct-object calibration method, a grid of uniformly spaced radiopaque lines or an object of known size is imaged at the level of the heart immediately following the ventriculogram. In a biplane lab, accurate placement of the grid is easier. To image the grid on the RAO camera, fluoroscopy with the LAO camera is used to position the grid in the center of the LAO image but perpendicular to it. This will assure that the grid is parallel to the face of the RAO image intensifier and that the grid is located in the isocenter of the imaging system. An analogous process is performed to image the grid on the LAO camera. Using this technique, both the heart and the grid are subjected to the same three factors that affect size of the projected image. If manual planimetry is to be done, the traced RAO-ED ventricular outline can be superimposed over the projected image of the grid. Alternatively, widely available computer-assisted methods allow planimetry using a graphics-input tablet to mark the grid points and to trace the ventricular outlines. The number of grid squares (each measuring 1 cm^2) included within the outline corresponds to the area (A_{RAO} in the area-length formula). The distance from the mid aortic valve plane to the apex is the long axis of the ellipsoid (L_{RAO}). For a biplane volume determination, A_{LAO} and L_{LAO} are analogously measured, and these data are applied in the area-length formula to obtain EDV.

If magnification-correction factors are to be used, radiopaque image-calibration markers a known distance apart (mounted on the face of the image intensifier during filming) should be present on the film image and should be marked along with the ventricular outlines when they are traced. Areas and long-axis lengths are determined based on the image calibration. Most often, computer-assisted methods are used to actually perform the planimetry and to calculate the magnification correction.

As discussed previously, magnification is determined by the ratio of the source-to-image distance (**SID**) to the source-to-object distance (**SOD**). The ease of determination of the **SID** and **SOD** for calculation of magnification correction depends on the geometry of the individual catheterization laboratory. In many modern biplane labs, when the heart is placed at the center of the image in both planes simultaneously (the "isocenter"), the **SOD**s are always the same, making magnification determination much simpler, because the remaining factor, **SID**, is available via digital readout. In a single-plane setting, the **SOD** may have to be estimated as the distance from the x-ray tube to the approximate location of the heart within the chest using a simple mechanical ruler.

Step 4: Calculation of Volume with the Area-Length Formula

For the volume calculation in a biplane lab, magnification must be determined for each plane independently and the magnification-correction factor, MCF, applied to each linear factor in the area-length formula. Thus, L_{LAO} is multiplied by MCF_{LAO}, A_{RAO} is multiplied by MCF_{RAO}^2, and so on. For example, in the usual case where L_{LAO} is shorter than L_{RAO},

$$V_{heart} = 0.849 \cdot \frac{A_{RAO}\,A_{LAO}}{L_{LAO}} \cdot \frac{MCF_{RAO}^2\,MCF_{LAO}^2}{MCF_{LAO}} \quad \text{or}$$

$$V_{heart} = 0.849 \cdot \frac{A_{RAO}\,A_{LAO}}{L_{LAO}} \cdot (MCF_{RAO}^2 \cdot MCF_{LAO}).$$

Step 5: Application of Regression Parameters

The final step in obtaining accurate ventricular volumes is the application of regression parameters, a step that adjusts for the area-length formula's assumption that the ventricle is perfectly ellipsoid in shape. Thus, the final volume $V = A \cdot V_{heart} + B$, where A and B are the regression slope and intercept, respectively, and V_{heart} is the volume corrected for magnification.

Application of Digital Imaging to Volume Measurements

A growing number of cath-lab installations are including digital-imaging capabilities. These systems offer the advantages of immediate review, enhancement, and analysis of the image. For example, with digital-subtraction techniques, diagnostic-quality ventriculography can be obtained with as little as 5 to 15 ml of contrast material. In general, the task of ventricular-volume measurement is performed in a manner exactly as described above, but the computer is used to assist in the tracing of the ventricular outlines and in making appropriate length and calibration measurements. There are technqiues currently under development that may allow the computer to automatically determine the ventricular borders ("automatic edge detection"), but it is likely that the computer operator will still have to review and perhaps edit the data to assure accuracy.

Regional Ventricular-Wall Motion Analysis

In patients with coronary artery disease, ischemic injury to the myocardium is seen as *regional* (as opposed to *global*) dysfunction. For example, a patient who has single-vessel disease with total occlusion of the right coronary artery that is causing an inferior myocardial infarction will have decreased motion of the inferior wall but may have normal or supernormal function of the anterior and lateral walls. Methods of objectively describing these *regional wall-motion abnormalities* are discussed in this section.

The interest in regional wall-motion analysis has been rekindled with the increasing use of thrombolytic therapy for acute myocardial infarction. In early clinical trials, when the effect of reperfusion on ventricular function was measured only by the ejection fraction (a measurment of *global* ventricular function), surprisingly little change was seen in patients who had excellent clinical results from thrombolysis. It was found that although the infarct region may be severely abnormal, the noninfarct regions of the ventricle may be supernormal in an effort to compensate for the loss of function in the infarct region. After reperfusion, a significant improvement in wall motion in the infarct region was often accompanied by a loss of the supernormal compensation in the other regions. The net effect may be one of little or no change in a global parameter such as ejection fraction, but a marked difference in wall motion of the infarct region (O'Callaghan and Hinohara, 1988). Therefore, regional wall-motion analysis may be a powerful tool for description of changes due to coronary disease and for objective measurement of the efficacy of therapeutic interventions.

Definitions

In the standard 30-degree RAO and 60-degree LAO projections, regions of the ventricular outline can be defined as shown in Figure 11–10. The following terms are used to denote the degree and direction of contraction abnormality from comparison of the end-diastolic ventricular outline to the end-systolic outline:

Hyperkinesis—Wall motion greater than normal.

Hypokinesis—Wall contraction is present, but it is less than normal.

Akinesis—No wall motion.

Dyskinesis—Wall bulges outward during systole.

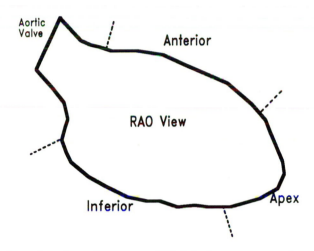

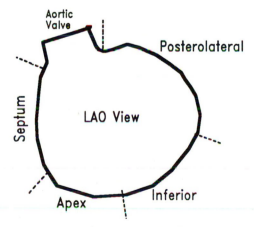

Figure 11–10. Outlines of the RAO (*top*) and LAO (*bottom*) projections of the left ventricle. Regional wall designations are shown.

Regional Wall Motion: Qualitative Visual Analysis

The severity and extent of regional dysfunction can usually be appreciated by visual inspection of the cineangiogram. One way of describing regional wall motion is by using the terms *"hypokinesis," "akinesis,"* and *"dyskinesis"* to describe the severity of contraction abnormality, and using the terms *"mild," "moderate,"* and *"severe"* to denote the extent of the region involved, referring to whether one-third or less, one-third to two-thirds, or more than two-thirds of the region is involved. For example, an inferior wall in which less than one-third of the wall is akinetic would be termed "mild inferior akinesis."

Visual inspection of the cineangiogram can also reveal subtle abnormalities in the *timing* of contraction called "tardokinesis," a milder form of regional dysfunction.

Regional Wall Motion: Quantitative Analysis

A variety of computer-assisted methods of analyzing regional wall motion are utilized. Two commonly used methods are the radial method and the centerline method. In each case, the ED and ES ventricular outlines as traced for volume determination are used for wall-motion analysis.

In the radial method (Fig. 11–11), the ED and ES outlines are first superimposed at a single point, usually the centroid, or geometric center, of the silhouette. Some variations superimpose the midpoints of the long-axis lines instead. Motion is measured along multiple "radii" extending out from the central point. The length of the radius extending to the ED contour, L_{ED}, is compared with the length of the radius extending to the ES contour, L_{ES}. These data are often expressed as fractional shortening, $FS = (L_{ED} - L_{ES})/L_{ED}$. Regional wall motion may be expressed as the average FS for all the radii within a region and compared with normal data.

The radial method has the advantage of being conceptually and computationally simple, and it remains in relatively widespread use today. It has disadvantages, however. The initial step of realigning the ED and ES contours so that their centroids are superimposed necessarily alters the spatial relationship between the two outlines and, therefore, may significantly alter distances between ED and ES points. The amount of movement needed for realignment will vary from patient to patient depending upon the shape of the ventricle and upon its contraction pattern.

The centerline method of regional wall-motion analysis overcomes some of the limitations of the radial method at the expense of a more complex algorithm that must be computer driven. This method, developed at the University of Washington (Bolson, Kliman, and Sheehan, 1980), does not alter the spatial relationship between the ED and ES contours. In this algorithm, a line, the "centerline," is constructed midway between the ED and ES contours. Wall motion is described as the lengths of 100 lines or "chords" equally spaced around the centerline and drawn perpendicular to it, intersecting the ED and ES borders. These

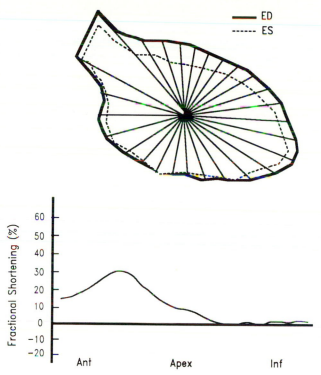

Figure 11–11. The radial method of wall-motion analysis describes motion as fractional shortening from end diastole (ED) to end systole (ES) along multiple radii extending from the superimposed centroid of the ED and ES outlines (RAO view).

chord lengths are then compared with those of a database of normal patients. To eliminate the effect of different heart sizes, the chord lengths are divided by the perimeter length of the ED contour. Data for each of the 100 chords are expressed as a percentage of normal chord length (with 100 percent representing normal wall motion), or as the number of standard deviations (SD) above or below normal motion (with 0 SD being normal).

Figure 11–12A graphically depicts chord-length data compared with a normal database of 100 patients for a patient suffering an acute anterior wall infarction. Figure 11–12B depicts wall motion 7 days following successful thrombolytic therapy that shows significant improvement in the anterior region. Figure 11–12C plots wall motion for this patient 6 months later, indicating return to normal.

In clinical trials of reperfusion therapy in acute infarction, the centerline method has been utilized to describe regional wall motion and its changes with intervention (Sheehan, Mathey, Schofer, et al, 1983, 1985). In addition, its developers have validated that the severity of regional wall-motion abnormality by the centerline method has a reasonably good correlation with a rough clinical mea-

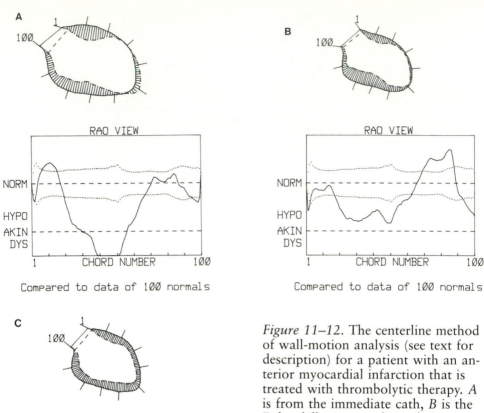

Figure 11–12. The centerline method of wall-motion analysis (see text for description) for a patient with an anterior myocardial infarction that is treated with thrombolytic therapy. *A* is from the immediate cath, *B* is the 7-day follow-up study, and *C* is a 6-month follow-up study. The anterior and apical walls, which are distinctly abnormal acutely, normalize with time. Motion for each of the 100 chords around the ventricle is graphically depicted in the plot beneath each set of ED/ES outlines. The area between the dotted lines on the graph is considered normal chord motion. NORM = normal. HYPO = hypokinesis. AKIN = akinesis. DYS = dyskinesis.

surement of infarct size by cardiac-enzyme determinations (Sheehan, Bolson, Dodge, et al, 1986).

Based on the centerline method, various methods of quantitating infarct-zone abnormalities and changes with therapy have been proposed. Figure 11–13, for example, shows an infarct zone determined as all the contiguous chords with motion worse than 1 SD below normal. The remaining chords are the "noninfarct zone." Data shown reflect the extent of the infarct zone, the severity of abnormality within it, and a "function index" that combines extent and severity data into a single parameter. Quantitative analysis methods such as those just

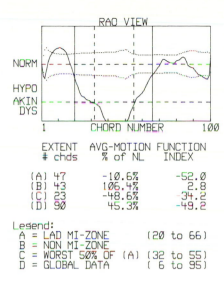

EXTENT # chds	AVG-MOTION % of NL	FUNCTION INDEX
(A) 47	-10.6%	-52.0
(B) 43	106.4%	2.8
(C) 23	-48.6%	-34.2
(D) 90	45.3%	-49.2

Legend:
A = LAD MI-ZONE   (20 to 66)
B = NON MI-ZONE
C = WORST 50% OF (A) (32 to 55)
D = GLOBAL DATA   (6 to 95)

Figure 11–13. Centerline analysis of the infarct region from Figure 12*A* defined as the set of contiguous chords with motion worse than −1 SD below normal (lower *dotted line*). Data are expressed as extent (number of chords involved) and severity (average motion as a percent of normal) of wall-motion abnormality, and as a "function index," which combines the two data. These data quantitatively describe infarct region dysfunction and can be used to follow changes in regional motion over time. LAD = left anterior descending.

described hold great promise as objective means of assessing the efficacy of therapy, and perhaps as means of estimating prognosis.

Analysis of Coronary Angiograms

Noninvasive tests that assess the coronary circulation provide *physiologic* data (information about cardiac function, metabolism, or coronary blood flow). These include exercise stress testing, thallium perfusion imaging, positron emission tomography, exercise echocardiography, and exercise radionuclide angiography. The unique capability of invasive coronary angiography is to provide *anatomic* detail of the coronary circulation.

In coronary atherosclerosis, coronary angiograms allow description of the severity of lumen stenosis and the number of vessels involved. In clinical practice, angiographers extrapolate the physiologic impact of coronary artery stenoses from the severity of luminal narrowing. In general, there is little impact on coronary blood flow until the diameter of the coronary lumen has been reduced to at least 50 to 75 percent of normal (Fig. 11–14).

Coronary angiography may disclose other information such as collateral circulation, coronary aneurysms, and acquired or congenital coronary anomalies.

Coronary Angiography: Technical Considerations

The accurate analysis of the coronary angiogram depends upon good technique of contrast injection, view selection, and panning. To avoid "streaming" of contrast material mixed with blood, the contrast injection rate should be sufficient to produce a small reflux of contrast out of the coronary orifice into the aortic root throughout the cardiac cycle. If the entire coronary artery will not fit within the

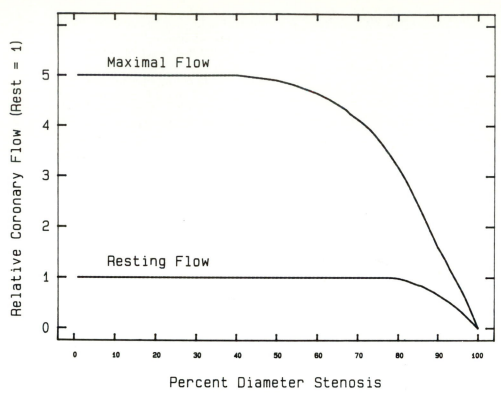

Figure 11–14. Theoretical plot of resting and maximal coronary blood flow as a function of percent diameter stenosis. There is little effect on maximal flow below 50 to 60 percent stenosis and little effect on resting flow below 75 to 85 percent stenosis.

image-intensifier field, the table may have to be moved, or "panned," so that the image moves from the proximal portion to the distal portion of the vessel during the angiogram. Selection of appropriate projections to clearly image all parts of the coronary tree is a very important part of good angiographic technique.

Commonly Used Views during Angiography

Selection of appropriate angulation for imaging the coronaries is usually based on a series of "standard" views for the beginning angiographer. The experienced angiographer, however, will recognize the need to slightly modify these views or to select a nonstandard angulation in order to confidently image all segments of the coronary circulation.

In cardiac catheterization labs, the x-rays emanate from a source beneath the table, pass through the patient, and strike the image intensifier located above the patient. In this context, the terms describing angulation refer the location of the image intensifier with respect to the patient. The terms "*right anterior oblique*" (RAO) and "*left anterior oblique*" (LAO) refer to rotation of the image intensifier to the patient's right or left, respectively, in the transverse plane (i.e., the camera moves side to side with no movement toward the patient's feet or head). The amount of rotation is expressed as degrees from the straight PA view where the image intensifier is directly above the patient's chest; for example, the "30-degree RAO view." *Cranial* skew refers to movement of the image intensifier toward the patient's head (along the patient's head-to-foot axis). The term "cranial" is actually a shortened form of "*caudocranial*" (meaning "tail to head"), which more fully describes the direction taken by the x-ray beam. *Caudal* (or *craniocaudal*) skew refers to movement of the image intensifier toward the patient's feet. In the following discussion, the term "*straight*" refers to the lack of any cranial or caudal skew.

Views of the Right Coronary Artery

Generally, two views of the right coronary artery (RCA) are sufficient—the straight RAO and LAO views. The LAO view (Fig. 11–15A) should be of sufficient angulation that the distal vessel does not project over the spine. This is usually accomplished with a 45-degree to 60-degree LAO projection. Ideally, the posterior descending branch, or other larger distal branches, should project in the "groove" made by the shadow of the diaphragm meeting the spine. A straight RAO view of approximately 30 degrees (Fig. 11–15B) places the proximal RCA just to the right (on the image) of the catheter ascending the thoracic aorta.

When an additional view of the distal RCA is needed, particularly to visualize the takeoff of the posterior descending branch, the straight RAO can be modified with cranial skew. In this case, the distal RCA may project over the diaphragm, making adequate exposure difficult; ideally, however, the branch requiring the special view can be placed in the groove between the diaphragm and spine.

Views of the Left Coronary Artery

There are eight commonly used views of the left coronary artery (LCA): three RAO (straight, cranial, and caudal), three LAO (straight, cranial, and caudal), straight PA, and straight left lateral. Each view tends to provide clear imaging of certain branches, but variations in heart configuration within the chest make view selection and modification of standard views of the left coronary artery particularly challenging.

Many angiographers will perform a "left main flush" shot before actually engaging the catheter tip into the left main coronary artery. This adds a margin of safety by early recognition of left main coronary artery stenosis. When left main coronary artery disease is found, the angiographer should watch even more carefully for damping of the pressure tracing, indicating occlusion of the left main artery by the catheter tip, and should manipulate the catheter with caution to avoid mechanical trauma to a plaque in the left main artery that could result in catastrophic dissection and occlusion of the artery. The left main flush is filmed

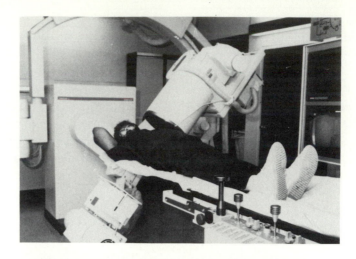

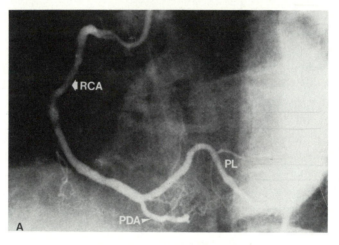

Figure 11–15. Camera angles (*top*) and cineangiograms (*bottom*) for standard views of the right coronary artery (RCA). *A,* Right coronary artery in the LAO view. Note that most of the distal vessel projects between the diaphragm and the spine, providing a clear view. A small coronary aneurysm is present. *B,* Right coronary artery in the RAO view. The vessel projects just to the right of the descending aorta. PDA = posterior descending artery. PL = posterolateral branch to the left ventricle.

with the coronary catheter in the left coronary sinus near, but not in, the orifice of the left main artery. Because the contrast is diluted in the aortic root, up to 10 ml may be required. The left main flush is filmed either in a straight PA view, in which the left main artery is often most perpendicular to the x-ray beam but overlies the spine, or in a shallow LAO angulation such that it lies just to the left (on the image) of the spine.

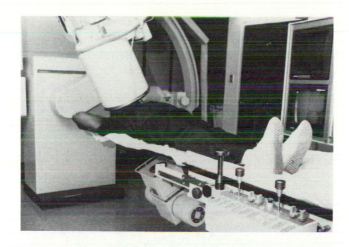

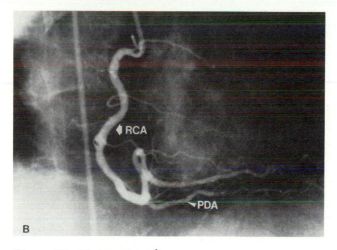

Figure 11–15 (continued)

RAO Views of the Left Coronary Artery

Figure 11–16A, B, and C illustrates typical images of the left coronary artery in the straight RAO, RAO cranial, and RAO caudal views, respectively.

The degree of straight RAO angulation should be approximately 30 degrees, or sufficient to place the left main and circumflex branch slightly to the right (on the image) of the ascending aorta (marked by the catheter within it if the femoral approach is being used). The straight RAO view gives a good overview of the LCA (see Fig. 11–16A), and often provides nonoverlapped images of the mid and distal anterior descending branch and of the mid and distal circumflex, with its marginal and posterolateral branches.

Addition of caudal skew to the same degree of RAO angulation provides a better view of the origin and proximal portion of the circumflex (see Fig. 11–16B). The mid circumflex and the obtuse marginals are seen well in this view. Although the RAO caudal is primarily a "circumflex view," it may give valuable

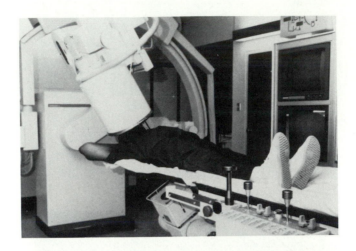

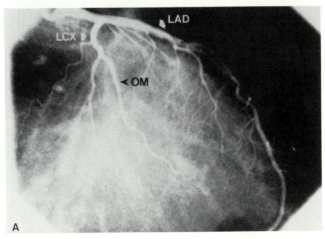

Figure 11–16. Camera angles (*top*) and cineangio-grams (*bottom*) for RAO views of the left coronary artery (LCA). *A,* Left coronary artery in the straight RAO view. This provides a good general overview of the LCA, but there is overlap of diagonal branches with the left anterior descending (LAD) artery, and the origin of the left circumflex (LCX) artery is not seen well. *B,* Left coronary artery in the RAO caudal view. The origin of the LCX and a small optional diagonal branch are seen well. *C,* Left coronary artery in the RAO cranial view. This "LAD view" shows the diagonal and septal perforator branches well in a sort of "fishbone" appearance. D# = diagonal. OM = obtuse marginal. Sp = septal perforator. (Fig. 11–16C appears on page 224.)

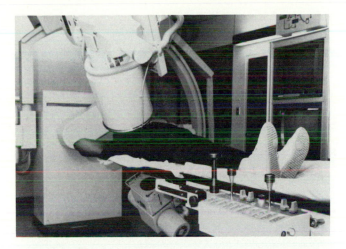

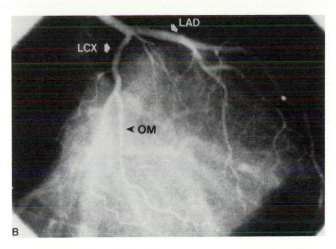

Figure 11–16 (continued)

information on segments of the left anterior descending (LAD) branch as well. In obese patients, caudal skew markedly increases the patient thickness through which x-ray beams must travel, making adequate exposure difficult. In these cases, a slight decrease in the caudal skew may significantly improve the image.

The RAO cranial view is designed as an "LAD view." With cranial skew (and often a little more RAO angulation), the circumflex branches are projected above or to the left (on the image) of the LAD. The diagonal, or anterolateral, branches of the LAD project upward on the image, and the septal perforators project downward in a sort of "fishbone" appearance (see Fig. 11–16C). This view ideally provides a clear view of the full length of the LAD (except perhaps its takeoff) and of the origins of the diagonal branches. There are a number of pitfalls to this view. Insufficient cranial skew or RAO rotation may cause many vessels to overlap on the image. The cranial skew will cause the LAD to lie in a narrow portion of the heart projecting between the lung and the diaphragm,

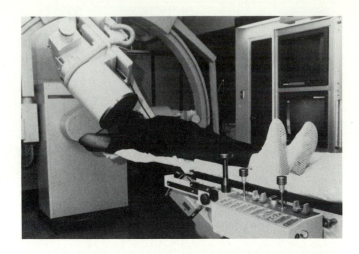

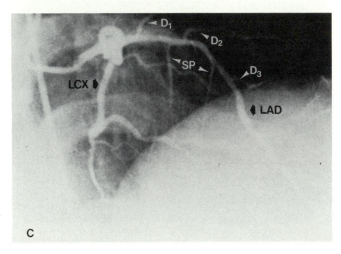

Figure 11–16 (continued)

making the heart's position within the image-intensifier field critical to obtaining optimum exposure. The final setup of the shot should be during deep inspiration. The commonest problem is "burnout" of the coronary artery due to inclusion of excess lung field in the image.

LAO Views of the Left Coronary Artery

Figure 11–17*A*, *B*, and *C* illustrates typical images in the straight LAO, LAO cranial, and LAO caudal views, respectively.

The straight LAO view is usually angulated approximately 60 degrees so that the circumflex branch does not overlap the spine (see Fig. 11–17*A*). This usually provides good images of the mid and distal circumflex (but not its marginal branches) and of the distal LAD. The proximal and mid LAD and its diagonal branches are usually foreshortened in this view, limiting its usefulness for the LAD. A steeper LAO or left lateral (see below) may provide a better view of the mid LAD.

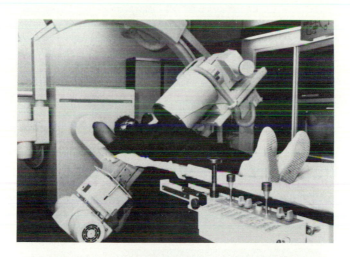

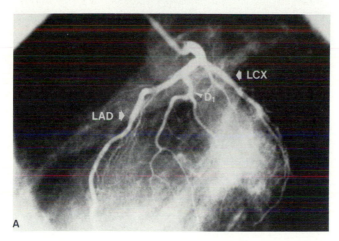

Figure 11–17. Camera angles (*top*) and cineangiograms (*bottom*) for LAO views of the left coronary artery (LCA). *A,* Left coronary artery in the straight LAO view. Angulation should be steep enough that the left circumplex (LCX) artery does not project over the spine. The proximal portions of the left anterior descending (LAD) artery and LCX artery are not seen well in this view. *B,* Left coronary artery in the LAO cranial view. This view is designed to image the proximal LAD and its diagonal branches well. The LAD projects just the left of the spine in the groove between it and the diaphragm. *C,* Left coronary artery in the LAO caudal view. Adequate exposure is often difficult, but the proximal portions of the major vessels may be seen well in this projection. D# = diagonal. OM = obtuse marginal. OD = optional diagonal. (Fig. 11–17B and C appear on the following pages.)

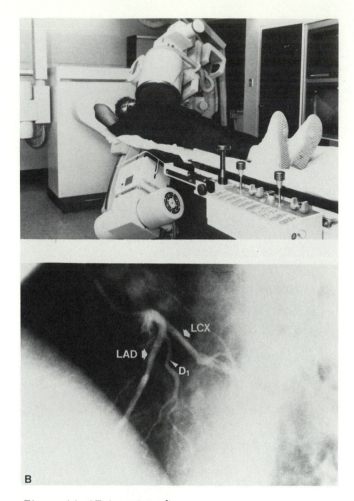

Figure 11–17 (continued)

The LAO cranial view is another "LAD view." With proper LAO angulation for this view (about 30 degrees rather than the 60-degree angle for the straight LAO), the LAD projects parallel to the spine and slightly to the left of it on the image (see Fig. 11–17*B*). Maximum cranial skew allowed by the geometry of the lab should generally be used. This places the proximal and mid portions of the LAD in the groove between the diaphragm and the spine on the image. In some patients with "vertical hearts," maximum cranial skew will place too much of the LAD below the diaphragm, and less cranial angulation may be optimal. Although a good LAO cranial view will be easily obtained in these patients, a good LAO caudal view will be difficult or impossible. In other patients with "horizontal hearts," even maximum cranial skew may still produce foreshortening of the proximal LAD, limiting the usefulness of the LAO cranial view in these patients, but the LAO caudal view may provide an excellent view of the proximal LAD.

The LAO caudal view (see Fig. 11–17*C*), often called a "spider" or

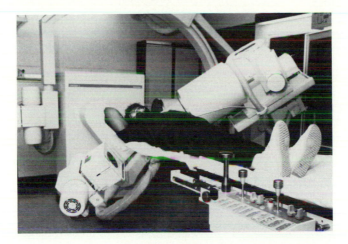

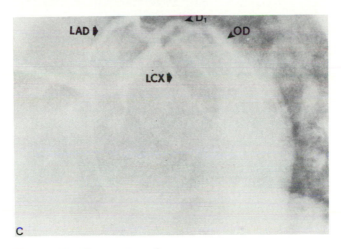

Figure 11–17 (continued)

"weeping willow" view because of the configuration of the branches on the image, is filmed with 45-degree to 60-degree LAO rotation and caudal skew. The amount of caudal skew is usually 15 degrees to 30 degrees, but should be limited as much as possible only by the ability of the x-ray to penetrate the thickness of the patient, often imaging through the diaphragm as well. This is usually a good view of the bifurcation of the left main artery, particularly of the origin of the circumflex, and ideally gives a good image of the proximal portions of both the circumflex and LAD.

Left Lateral View of the Left Coronary Artery
The lateral view of the LCA (Fig. 11–18A) should be considered a variation of the 60-degree LAO view in that similar portions of the coronary tree are seen well. Often the lateral view will show the mid LAD with less foreshortening than the 60-degree LAO view, however. With the image intensifier at the patient's left

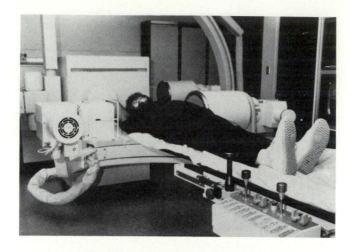

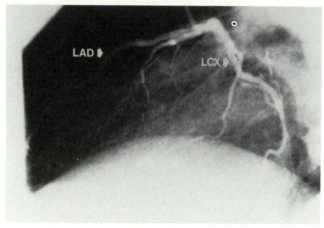

A

Figure 11–18. Camera angles (*top*) and cineangiograms (*bottom*) for lateral and PA views of the left
coronary artery (LCA). *A*, Left coronary artery in the
left lateral view. Often, the mid and distal parts of the
main vessels are seen well. *B*, Left coronary artery in
the PA view. The LCA partly overlaps the spine and
descending aorta in this view, but it often gives a good
image of the left main (L Main) coronary artery. LAD
= left anterior descending. LCX = left circumflex.

side, the coronary artery is centered within the image by raising or lowering the
table, rather than by horizontal motion of the table.

PA View of the Left Coronary Artery

With the image intensifier directly over the front of the patient's chest, the left
coronary artery usually projects partially over the spine (Fig. 11–18*B*). Despite
this limitation, the PA view may be an excellent view of the mid and distal circumflex and, particularly, the origin of the obtuse marginals, which will usually

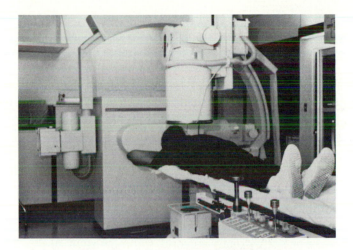

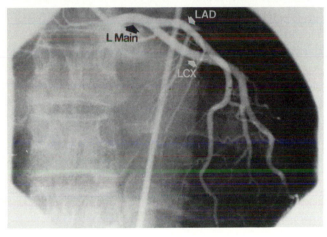

B

Figure 11–18 (continued)

project to the right (on the image) of the spine. This is also a good view of the left main coronary artery, although it usually projects partially over the spine.

Visual Analysis of the Coronary Angiogram

The goal of analysis of coronary stenosis is to determine the percent diameter narrowing and extrapolate the probable significance of the lesion to the coronary circulation. There are three important features of techniques of measuring coronary obstruction: (1) reproducibility, (2) accuracy, and (3) correlation with physiologic obstruction to blood flow as manifested by patient symptoms or by other truly physiologic means of assessing coronary flow.

Most often, angiographers visually estimate the percent reduction in luminal diameter and express the lesion on a scale of "minimal," 25 percent, 50 percent, 75 percent, 95 percent, 99 percent, or 100 percent stenosis, or on a scale of 10 percent, 20 percent, . . . , 90 percent, 100 percent. A substantial degree of variability between different angiographers' interpretations (interobserver variability) and between observations of a single angiographer spaced out over time (intraobserver variability) has been shown in a number of studies (Zir, Miller, Dinsmore, et al, 1976; DeRouen, Murray, and Owen, 1977). The Coronary Artery Surgery Study (CASS), for example, which was a large, multicenter study that has had a measurable impact on the practice of cardiology today, showed a disturbing degree of variability in the visual interpretation of coronary angiograms (Fig. 11–19) (Kennedy, Fisher, and Killip, 1982).

A few studies have assessed the accuracy of angiographic estimates of coronary stenosis by comparison with postmortem studies in patients who died shortly after coronary angiography (Arnett, Isner, Redwood, et al, 1979). There is often a marked discrepancy between the visual angiographic estimate and the pathologic appearance of coronary stenoses, although some of the discrepancy may be due to technical limitations of these studies. In general, the visual analysis of high-grade lesions tends to overestimate the measured degree of obstruction, whereas the analysis of low-grade lesions tends to underestimate it. Pathologic examination has also emphasized the irregular nature of the residual lumen within an atherosclerotic plaque (Fig. 11–20). The measured degree of diameter stenosis may be markedly different in different projections.

The physiologic impact of a lesion of 75 percent diameter stenosis or greater is relatively easy to predict, as is the lack of significant impact of lesions of less than 50 percent diameter stenosis. The clinical significance of lesions of

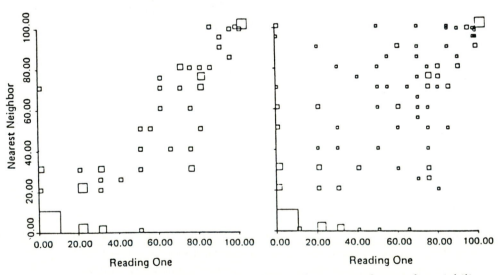

Figure 11–19. Intraobserver (*left panel*) and interobserver (*right panel*) variability in the visual estimation of percent diameter coronary stenosis from the Coronary Artery Surgery Study. (From Kennedy JW, Fisher LD, Killip T. Coronary angiography quality control in the CASS study. In: Bond MG, Insull W, Glogov S, et al, eds. Clinical diagnosis of atherosclerosis: Quantitative methods of evaluation. New York: Springer-Verlag, 1982:475; with permission.)

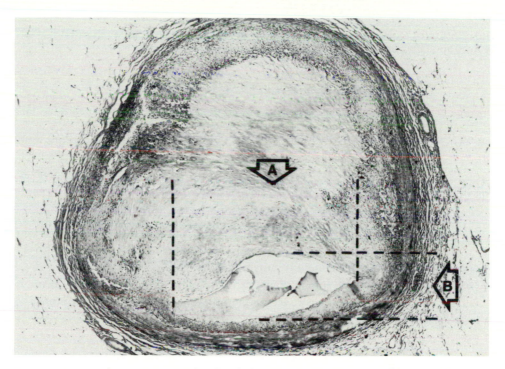

Figure 11–20. Photomicrograph of a diseased coronary artery with a small, irregular-shaped residual lumen. (Some residual casting material remains in the lumen.) The projected size of the lumen varies widely depending upon the angle from which it is imaged (projection A versus B).

intermediate grade, 50 to 75 percent diameter stenosis, is very difficult to predict. Not uncommonly, a patient will be sent for a physiologic test such as exercise stress testing or exercise thallium imaging *after* catheterization to better define the significance of such a "borderline" lesion.

Despite its limitations, the visual inspection of the coronary cineangiogram has some distinct advantages in areas other than measurement of coronary stenosis. An atherosclerotic lesion may be long or complex in shape, may contain areas of ulceration, dissection or clot, or may involve side branches. These features may be more important predictors of the complication rate of coronary balloon angioplasty, for example, than percent diameter stenosis alone, whether estimated visually or measured quantitatively.

In the case of high-grade lesions, a visual estimation of the degree of limitation to contrast flow into the vessel, the TIMI grades (Table 11–2), seems to correlate with outcome in patients with myocardial infarct who were treated with thrombolytic therapy (Wall, Mark, Califf, et al, 1989).

Quantitative Analysis of the Coronary Angiogram

Because the conventional visual method of coronary stenosis analysis is plagued by high variability and poor accuracy, quantitative methods of measuring parameters of coronary stenosis have been developed to overcome these inadequacies.

T A B L E 11–2
Description of Coronary Flow Rate Used in the Thrombolysis in Myocardial Infarction (TIMI) Studies

TIMI Grade	Description
0	No contrast flow beyond the lesion.
1	Contrast flows past lesion but does not fill the distal vessel.
2	Contrast flows past lesion and fills distal vessel, but more slowly than normal.
3	Normal contrast flow to distal vessel.

From The TIMI Study Group. The thrombolysis in myocardial infarction (TIMI) trial. N Engl J Med 1985; 312:932.

Among the simplest noncomputerized methods of quantitation is the use of calipers to measure the minimum lumen diameter and compare it with a caliper measurement of normal lumen diameter on cinefilm frames projected onto a viewing screen. Even this simplistic technique markedly improves the variability in measurement of coronary stenosis, but it is applicable only to the measurement of percent diameter stenosis.

A variety of computer-assisted methods have emerged. Common to each method is the task of definition of the borders of the coronary lumen. These may be manually traced into the computer or determined by various automated and semiautomated algorithms. Automated methods require storage of the cinefilm frame as a digitized image within the computer memory. This may be accomplished either by direct acquisition of the digital image into the computer during the catheterization or by digitization of a frame from the cinefilm. A digital image provides the computer with both the spatial (distance) information necessary to determine diameter stenosis as well as density (brightness) information, which may be used to automate the process of lumen-border detection.

One such system, developed at the Ann Arbor VA Medical Center, has been studied extensively (LeFree, Simon, Sanz, et al, 1988). Using this highly automated technique, inter- and intra-observer variability are very low (LeFree, Simon, Sang, et al, 1988; Skelton, Kisslo, Mikat, et al, 1987). Validation studies have shown that coronary sizes measured using this algorithm are accurate (Skelton, Kisslo, Mikat, et al, 1987), and that there is little difference between the data obtained from direct digital images as opposed to digitized cinefilm (Skelton, Kisslo and Bashore, 1988). Thus, automated methods of coronary stenosis quantitation have the advantages of good reproducibility and accuracy. In addition, the objectivity imposed by an automated algorithm may be beneficial. The immediate availability of these data from direct digital images analyzed during the cath procedure can help direct the decisions during coronary angioplasty, such as correct balloon sizing. A representative output with the various analysis parameters reported is shown in Figure 11–21.

Although the diameter reduction caused by an atheroma is a major feature of the restriction to blood flow, percent diameter stenosis alone is an incom-

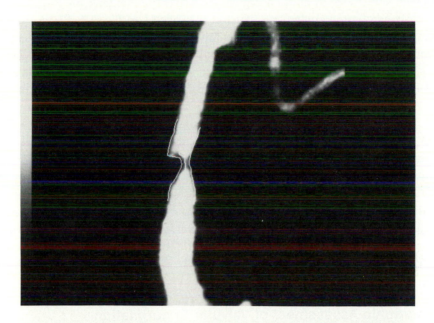

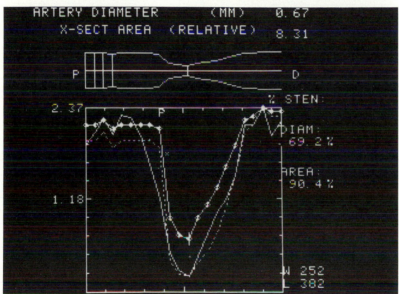

Figure 11–21. Sample computer analysis (*bottom*) of a contrast-enhanced digital image of a coronary stenosis (*top*). The automatically determined edges are shown on the image. Minimum lumen diameter (0.67 mm), percent diameter stenosis (69.2 percent), and percent area stenosis (90.4 percent) are shown in the analysis.

plete description of any coronary lesion. Most plaques and coronary dissections (a common finding after coronary angioplasty) result in eccentric narrowing of the lumen, sometimes to marked degree, such that the diameter measured may depend heavily on the angle from which it is viewed (see Fig. 11–20). Also, the resistance to flow is a function of the length of the lesion and other geometric parameters in addition to the cross-sectional area of the lumen. Finally, if the "normal" segment of artery to which the lesion is compared for measurement of percent diameter stenosis is actually diseased (Fig. 11–22), the degree of luminal restriction will be underestimated.

Analysis of digitized images holds promise for being able to measure some of these other geometric parameters of coronary stenosis. In addition, there are methods of analyzing the contrast flow pattern during injection that give quantitative information about coronary blood flow. Also, for the first time, coronary angiography can provide meaningful physiologic information in addition to information about coronary anatomy. This may become a useful tool in assessing the significance of the "borderline" 50 to 75 percent stenotic lesion as well as the postangioplasty lumen, which is often very complex in shape with dissection or luminal filling defects.

Angiographic Assessment of Valvular Regurgitation

Angiography has long been the standard method for describing valvular regurgitation. Today, the presence of valvular regurgitation can often be accurately assessed by Doppler echocardiography, but there are circumstances in which the

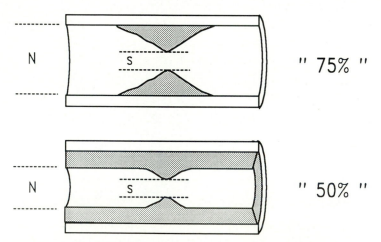

Figure 11–22. The minimum lumen size S is identical in each artery, but the presence of diffuse disease in the lower artery would result in underestimation of the significance of the lesion if compared to the size of the "normal" lumen N. The 75 percent diameter stenosis in the upper artery becomes a 50 percent lesion in the presence of diffuse disease.

Doppler data may be unobtainable or unreliable, so that angiography, along with the other hemodynamic information obtainable at catheterization, may be needed for clinical decision making.

Angiography is most often used to assess aortic and mitral regurgitation, occasionally for tricuspid regurgitation, and very rarely to evaluate pulmonic valve regurgitation.

Technical Considerations

Mitral regurgitation is usually evaluated from the standard left ventriculogram filmed in the 30-degree RAO and 60-degree LAO projections. The contrast injection rate should be that required for a technically good ventriculogram. The image should be framed so that the area of the left atrium will be visible on the film (see discussion of left ventriculography earlier in this chapter). Mitral regurgitation can be artificially produced in three ways: (1) Despite good catheter-tip position for injection in the mitral inflow tract, part of the catheter may be within the mitral apparatus, interfering with mitral closure or allowing direct left atrial injection of contrast. (2) Mitral regurgitation often accompanies ventricular ectopic beats during injection. (3) When the heart rate is particularly slow, the force of power injection in the mitral inflow tract may cause a small amount of *diastolic* regurgitation.

Aortic insufficiency is imaged by injection of contrast in the aortic root just above the aortic valve. The same 30-degree RAO and 60-degree LAO views used for ventriculography may be used, but a steeper RAO angle is usually used so that the aortic root and the descending thoracic aorta are not superimposed on the image. The image should be set up so that much of the left ventricle will be visible during the first part of the film run; during the later part, the image may be panned so that the aortic arch is visible. A contrast volume of 40 to 50 ml injected at 20 to 25 ml per second is usually sufficient. A small preliminary test injection should always be done to avoid power injection into a coronary artery or bypass graft, particularly if aortography is done with something other than a pigtail catheter (such as a Sones or multipurpose catheter). Catheter position 1 to 2 cm above the aortic valve is ideal because a lower catheter position may artificially induce aortic regurgitation.

Tricuspid regurgitation can usually be assessed by echocardiography quite accurately, but right ventriculography may be performed to estimate its severity in some cases. Because the injecting catheter must necessarily cross the tricuspid valve, some degree of tricuspid regurgitation is often induced artificially, but it is almost always a small amount. Right ventriculography should be performed with a similar contrast-injection technique but at a more shallow RAO angle then left ventriculography. Most catheters with multiple side holes can be used, although standard pigtail, angled pigtail, 180-degree curved pigtail, and Berman angiographic catheters are most suitable. Injection should be in the body of the right ventricle near its apex. Regurgitation of contrast into the IVC may be seen on the lateral view.

Grading the Severity of Regurgitation

A semiquantitative scale for grading the severity of valvular regurgitation is shown in Table 11–3. Generally, the 3+ and 4+ grades are considered clinically significant. When mitral regurgitation is very severe, with contrast not only filling the entire atrium but also refluxing into the pulmonary veins, some angiographers use the term "5+." Other angiographers may use the qualitative terms "mild," "moderate," and "severe," which correspond roughly to 1–2+, 2–3+, and 4+, respectively.

Other Valve Morphology

One should look for other structural features of the valves during routine angiography. The angiogram should be evaluated for valvular anomalies and for leaflet motion, calcification, and thickening. Occasionally, rupture of a papillary muscle or chordae tendinae or dissection of the aortic root may be seen.

Quantitative Computer Methods

In valvular regurgitation, a portion of the blood ejected with each beat (the stroke volume) is regurgitant flow and a portion is forward flow. Stroke volume determined from angiographic left ventricular volume data represents total flow, including both forward and regurgitant flow. The percentage of the total stroke volume (SV_{total}) that is regurgitant flow (SV_{regurg}) is called the *"regurgitant fraction"* (**RF**), and is a quantitative expression of the degree of valvular regurgitation:

$$RF = \frac{SV_{regurg}}{SV_{total}}.$$

T A B L E 11–3
Grading Scale for Valvular Regurgitation

Degree of Regurgitation	Description
1+	Minimal regurgitation is seen.
2+	Moderate opacification of the receiving chamber, and clearing with subsequent beats.
3+	Intense opacification of the receiving chamber that is equal to that in the injection chamber at some point.
4+	Opacification of the receiving chamber occurs that is greater than that of the injection chamber.

In practice, total angiographic cardiac output (CO_{angio}) and forward cardiac output (CO_{fwd}), are measured to determine regurgitant cardiac output (CO_{regurg}). Angiographic cardiac output is calculated as SV_{total} times heart rate. Forward cardiac output is measured by oximetry (Fick) or indicator dilution methods. Thus, the regurgitant fraction can be easily calculated as

$$RF = \frac{CO_{regurg}}{CO_{angio}} = \frac{CO_{angio} - CO_{fwd}}{CO_{angio}}.$$

Other methods of quantitative description of valvular regurgitation are under development. With digital imaging systems, it is possible to measure the radiographic density of contrast from frame to frame within the chamber receiving regurgitant flow. The plot derived from such data is called a "time-density curve." Research data suggest that the degree of insufficiency may be quantitated based on parameters derived from such a time-density curve analysis.

SELECTED REFERENCES

Arnett EN, Isner JM, Redwood DR, et al. Coronary artery narrowing in coronary heart disease: Comparison of cineangiographic and necropsy findings. Ann Intern Med 1979; 91:350.

Bolson EL, Kliman S, Sheehan F, et al. Left ventricular segmental wall motion—a new method using local direction information. Comput Cardiol 1980; 245.

DeRouen TA, Murray JA, Owen W. Variability in the analysis of coronary arteriograms. Circulation 1977; 55:324.

Dodge HT, Sandler H, Ballew DW, et al. The use of biplane angiocardiography for the measurement of left ventricular volume in man. Am Heart J 1960; 60:762.

Kennedy JW, Fisher LD, Killip T. Coronary angiography quality control in the CASS study. In: Bond MG, Insull W, Glagov S, et al, eds. Clinical diagnosis of atherosclerosis: Quantitative methods of evaluation. New York: Springer-Verlag, 1982:475.

Kennedy JW, Trenholme SE, Kasser IS. Left ventricular volume and mass from single-plane cineangiocardiogram: A comparison of anteroposterior and right anterior oblique methods. Am Heart J 1970; 80:343.

LeFree MT, Simon SB, Sanz ML, et al. Quantitative coronary arteriography. In: Mancini GBJ, ed. Clinical applications of cardiac digital angiography. New York: Raven Press, 1988: 219.

O'Callaghan WG, Hinohara T. Changes in left ventricular function after myocardial infarction. In: Califf RM, Mark DB, Wagner GS, eds. Acute coronary care in the thrombolytic era. Chicago: Year Book Medical Publishers, 1988:734.

Sandler H, Dodge HT. The use of single plane angiocardiograms for the calculation of left ventricular volume in man. Am Heart J 1968; 75:325.

Sandler H, Dodge HT, Hay RE, et al. Quantitation of valvular insufficiency in man by angiocardiography. Am Heart J 1963; 65:501.

Sheehan FH, Bolson EL, Dodge HT, et al. Advantages and applications of the centerline method for characterizing regional ventricular function. Circulation 1986; 74:293.

Sheehan FH, Mathey DG, Schofer J, et al. Factors determining recovery of left ventricular function after thrombolysis in patients with acute myocardial infarction. Circulation 1985; 71:1121.

Sheehan FH, Mathey DG, Schofer J, et al. Effect of interventions in salvaging left ventricular function in acute myocardial infarction: A study of intracoronary streptokinase. Am J Cardiol 1983; 52:431.

Skelton TN, Kisslo KB, Bashore TM. Comparison of coronary stenosis quantitation results from on-line digital and digitized cinefilm images. Am J Cardiol 1988; 62:381.

Skelton TN, Kisslo KB, Mikat EM, et al. Accuracy of digital angiography for quantitation of normal coronary luminal segments in excised, perfused hearts. Am J Cardiol 1987; 59:1261.

The TIMI Study Group. The thrombolysis in myocardial infarction (TIMI) trial. N Engl J Med 1985; 312:932.

Wall TC, Mark DB, Califf RM, et al. Prediction of early recurrent myocardial ischemia and coronary reocclusion after successful thrombolysis: A qualitative and quantitative angiographic study. Am J Cardiol 1989; 63:423.

Wynne J, Green LH, Mann T, et al. Estimation of left ventricular volumes in man from biplane cineangiograms filmed in oblique projections. Am J Cardiol 1978; 41:726.

Zir LM, Miller SW, Dinsmore RE, et al. Interobserver variability in coronary angiography. Circulation 1976; 53:627.

CHAPTER 12

Pharmacology

Mark Leithe, MD

Various medications are administered prior to, during, and following cardiac catheterization. This chapter discusses those pharmacologic agents frequently encountered by the catheterization technician and nurse, including anxiety-reducing agents, analgesics, antiarrhythmics, inotropic agents, vasodilators, contrast agents, oxygen, thrombolytic agents, and anticoagulants.

Premedication

In order to safely and effectively perform cardiac catheterization, the cardiac patient should receive medication to relax and to avoid untoward side effects from the catheterization procedure. Most catheterization laboratories use an antianxiety medication such as diazepam (Valium) (3 to 10 mg given orally or intravenously) along with an antihistamine such as diphenhydramine (Benadryl) (25 to 50 mg given orally or intravenously) on call to the laboratory. Some operators also advocate the routine use of atropine (0.5 mg given intravenously) just prior to coronary angiography to prevent bradycardia associated with coronary injection and to prevent the chance of a vasovagal reaction, although this is not the routine in our laboratory. With the advent of nonionic contrast agents, bradycardia is so uncommon that prophylactic administration of atropine need no longer be used. Sublingual nitroglycerine (0.3 to 0.4 mg) is also frequently given just prior to selective coronary artery injection in an effort to reduce the possibility of catheter-induced coronary artery spasm and to maximize the size of the coronary vessels. Finally, anticoagulation with 3,000 to 5,000 units of heparin sulfate given intravenously is frequently used during coronary angiography to reduce the incidence of thromboembolic complications. Due to conflicting data regarding the efficacy of heparin in complication reduction, routine use of this drug is left to the operator's discretion. An outline of commonly used premedications is found in Table 12–1.

Prehydration is often given to patients. Recall that most patients are given nothing by mouth prior to catheterization and that many patients arrive in the laboratory dehydrated. Dehydration is most likely a predisposing factor for development of contrast-media–induced acute renal failure. This is of particular concern if the patient has diabetes mellitus or pre-existing renal insufficiency. In the absence of congestive heart failure, 0.9 normal saline may be infused at 150 to 200 cc per hour at least 6 hr prior to the catheterization procedure and should be continued for 6 hr afterward.

Patients with insulin-dependent diabetes mellitus should receive a reduced dose of insulin on the day of their procedure. An infusion of 5 percent dextrose solution should then be started and one-half of their usual total daily dose of insulin should be given as long-acting (NPH) or intermediate-acting insulin. Blood glucose levels should be monitored closely, and elevated glucose should be managed with subcutaneous short-acting (regular) insulin every 4 to 6 hr.

In patients with known contrast allergy, some precautions are necessary. Acute anaphylaxis is twice as common in atopic individuals, and may occur in patients who have received contrast previously without allergic reaction. Contrast injections in the venous circulation tend to result in acute anaphylaxis more commonly than on the arterial side. To help prevent reactions, steroids and H_1 and H_2 histamine receptor blockers are frequently employed. A suggested premedication regimen used in our laboratory is as follows:

1. Methylprednisone, 60 mg given intravenously 12 hr and 1 hr before the procedure. (Alternatively, 20 mg of oral prednisone may be used.)
2. Diphenhydramine HCL (Benadryl), 25 to 50 mg given intravenously, just before the procedure.
3. Cimetidine (Tagamet), 300 mg given orally every 6 hr beginning 12 to 24 hr before the procedure, and cimetidine, 300 mg given intravenously just before the catheterization.

TABLE 12–1
Medications Frequently Administered Prior to Cardiac Catheterization and Coronary Angiography

Drug	Dose	Route
Diazepam (Valium)	3-10 mg	PO or IV (**Caution:** IV administration may cause significant hypotension)
Diphenhydramine (Benadryl)	25-50 mg	PO or IV
Atropine	0.5 mg	IV
Nitroglycerine	0.2-0.4 mg	Sublingual

Anxiety-Reducing Agents

It is helpful to have the patient in a relaxed state at the time of cardiac catheterization. To achieve this, anxiety-reducing agents, known as benzodiazepines, are often used. Midazolam (Versed), lorazepam (Ativan), or diazepam (Valium) are frequently administered orally or intravenously preceding the catheterization. Benzodiazepines exert a calming effect by depressing noncortical central nervous system function, and they possess a wide margin of safety between toxic and therapeutic doses. Because there is little difference between the effects of the different benzodiazepines, the specific agent may be selected for its own properties of speed of onset and elimination. These agents, especially when administered intravenously, can result in respiratory compromise and systemic hypotension; therefore, one must use them with caution. Oxazepam (Serax), midazolam, and lorazepam may be preferred in the elderly and in patients with hepatic insufficiency owing to their more rapid inactivation in this setting and owing to their less hypotensive effects. Table 12–2 outlines commonly used agents and their doses.

Pain Control

Pain control during catheterization begins with the local infiltration of 10 to 20 cc of 1 percent lidocaine HCL (Xylocaine) or with another comparable local

TABLE 12–2
Doses and Characteristics of Commonly Used Anxiety—Reducing Agents

	Oral Dosage Range (mg)	Parenteral Dosage Range (mg)	Elimination Half-Time (hr)	Metabolites	Speed Onset After Single Dose
Oxazepam (Serax)	10–15	—	5–13	Inactive glucuronide conjugate	Slow
Lorazepam (Ativan)	2–6	1–2	10–18	Inactive glucuronide conjugate	Intermediate
Alprazolam (Xanax)	0.25–0.5	—	12–15	Alpha-hydroxyalprazolam, benzophenone	Slow
Chlordiazepoxide (Librium)	5–25	5–25	5–30	Desmethylchlordiazepoxide (M), demoxepam, desmethydiazepam	Intermediate
Diazepam (Valium)	5–10	3–10	20–50	Desmethyldiazepam, methyloxazepam (Temazepam)	Very fast
Midazolam (Versed)	—	1–2	1–4	1-hydroxymethymidazolam, 4-hydroxymidazolam, 1-hydroxymethyl-4-hyroxymidazolam	Very fast

Modified from Kastrup EK, Olin BR, Schwack GH, eds. Drug facts and comparisons. Philadelphia: JB Lippincott, 1988:993.

anesthetic. Lidocaine stabilizes neuronal membranes and, therefore, prevents the initiation and propagation of pain impulses along nerves. Allergic reactions may occur as the result of sensitivity to either the local anesthetic compound itself or to the preservation methylparaben. If an allergy to lidocaine exists, 10 to 20 cc of 1 percent mepivacaine (Carbocaine) may be used as an alternative.

More severe or protracted pain associated with the procedure sometimes requires the use of oral or intravenous narcotic analgesia. Severe pain during or immediately following the procedure requires the intravenous administration of a diluted solution of meperidine HCL (Demerol) (25 to 50 mg) or morphine (3 to 5 mg). Most often however, pain following cardiac catheterization can be managed by the oral administration of acetaminophen or acetaminophen and codeine combination tablets (i.e., Tylenol #3). Frequently, an antiemetic is given concomitantly with the administration of intramuscular or intravenous narcotics to counteract narcotic-induced nausea and to potentiate narcotic analgesic properties. Examples of antiemetics and their doses include prochlorperazine (Compazine) (10 mg given orally or in 25-mg suppositories) and promethazine (Phenergan) (12.5 to 25 mg given intravenously or orally). Note that morphine tends to be vagotonic (reduces heart rate), whereas meperidine HCL tends to be vagolytic (speeds up heart rate). If bradycardia or conduction block is present, meperidine HCL should be preferred to morphine as the narcotic of choice. Both narcotics can result in vasodilation and may reduce systemic blood pressure.

Antiarrhythmics

In order to perform hemodynamic measurements and angiographic studies safely and effectively, it is sometimes necessary to administer antiarrhythmic medication to patients while they are in the catheterization laboratory. Most commonly, frequent premature ventricular contractions (PVCs) will require a lidocaine (Xylocaine) bolus of 75 mg, which can be followed by three subsequent boluses of 50 mg at 5-min intervals. For extended PVC suppression or for the treatment of sustained ventricular tachycardia, the initial dosing should be followed by an infusion of lidocaine at 1 to 4 mg per minute. If lidocaine fails to suppress the ventricular arrhythmia, other antiarrhythmics such as procainamide HCL (Pronestyl) or bretylium tosylate (Bretylol) may be administered as outlined in Table 12–3. Note that bretylium should not be used for isolated PVCs but should be reserved for sustained ventricular arrhythmias. Bretylium has a bimodal action with an initial release of catecholamines followed by catecholamine blockage. Therefore, one should first closely observe for hypertension, which then may be followed by hypotension after a period of 10 to 20 min.

Occasionally, in the presence of supraventricular arrhythmias, the ventricular rate will require slowing, or the supraventricular arrhythmia will require conversion to sinus rhythm. Most commonly, the ventricular rate during atrial fibrillation or flutter will require slowing with digoxin. In the patient not currently being treated with digitalis, an initial dose of 0.5 to 0.75 mg intravenously can be given. In patients already receiving digitalis, 0.25 to 0.50 mg of digoxin

TABLE 12–3
Doses of Antiarrhythmic Agents Commonly Used during Cardiac Catheterization

Agent	Initial Dose	Maintenance Dose
Lidocaine	Bolus of 75 mg, repeat bolus of 50 mg every 5 min times 3 (lower doses used in presence or reduced cardiac output)	Dilute 2 g in 500 ml 5%D/W and infuse at 1–4 mg/min
Bretylium	5 mg/kg undiluted in a bolus; may be repeated in 15 min at 10 mg/ kg for continued ventricular fibrillation; for ventricular tachycardia, use same doses in a 500 mg/50 cc concentration given over 8–10 min	Dilute 2 g in 500 ml 5% D/W and infuse at 1–3 mg/m
Procain- amide	17 mg/kg if no renal insufficiency; 15 mg/kg if mild renal insufficiency; 13 mg/kg if severe renal insufficiency; loading dose given over 30–60 min	Dilute 2 g in 500 ml 5% D/W and infuse at 3 mg/kg/hr if no renal insufficiency; 2 mg/kg/hr if mild renal insufficiency; 1 mg/kg/hr if severe renal insufficiency
Atropine	0.5–1.0 mg	Up to a total dose of 2.0 mg as needed
Isoproterenol	2–10 µg/min	Same doses infused of a 4 mg/250 ml 5% D/W concentration
Digoxin	0.25–0.75 mg IV	—
Verapamil	5–10 mg IV	May repeat 5–10 mg IV after 30 min as needed
Propranolol	1–2 mg IV slowly	May repeat initial dose after 2 min, up to a maximal dose of 5 mg

may be administered intravenously until heart-rate control is achieved. Ventricular rates in a patient with atrial fibrillation should be maintained at between 60 and 80 beats per minute during the catheterization procedure.

In patients without depressed left ventricular systolic function or other contraindications, a beta blocker (propranolol, labetolol, esmolol) or 5 to 10 mg of verapamil given intravenously may be used in combination with or as an alternative to digitalis for the treatment of supraventricular arrhythmias. The termination of supraventricular tachycardia may be necessary and can be accomplished by the administration of verapamil, digoxin, or propranolol in doses outlined in Table 12–3.

Esmolol (Brevibloc) is especially useful in the treatment of supraventricular arrhythmias because its short-lived action is readily reversed once the drug is discontinued. Its dosage regimen is outlined in Table 12–4. A 1-min loading dose infusion of 0.5 mg per kilogram per minute of esmolol is followed by a maintenance infusion of 0.05 mg per kilogram per minute. If the desired effect is not achieved after 4 min, a full 1-minute loading dose of 0.5 mg per kilogram per minute may be repeated, followed by the increased maintenance infusion of 0.1 mg per kilogram per minute. Each maintenance-infusion rate should be adminis-

TABLE 12–4
Esmolol Infusion Rates Based on an Esmolol Concentration of 10 mg/ml*

Patient Weight (kg)	1–min Loading Infusion (500 µg/kg/min) mL/min	4–min Maintenance Infusion (ml/hr)†			
		50 µg/kg/min	*100 µg/kg/min*	*150 µg/kg/min*	*200 µg/kg/min*
50	2.5	15	30	45	60
55	2.75	16.5	33	49.5	66
60	3.0	18	36	54	72
65	3.25	19.5	39	58.5	78
70	3.5	21	42	63	84
75	3.75	22.5	45	67.5	90
80	4.0	24	48	72	96
85	4.25	25.5	51	76.5	102
90	4.5	27	54	81	108
95	4.75	28.5	57	85.5	114
100	5.0	30	60	90	120
105	5.25	31.5	63	94.5	126
110	5.5	33	66	99	132

* If the desired effect is not obtained following the initial bolus and maintenance infusion, an additional loading infusion of 0.5 mg per kilogram per minute can precede each increase in maintenance infusion. Each maintenance infusion rate is continued for at least 4 min before increasing to the next greater maintenance infusion. Two amps (5 gm) in 500 cc saline yields 10 mg/ml.
† To calculate dose delivered by loading or maintenance infusions in milligrams per minute, divide above infusion rates in milliliters per hour by 6.

tered for at least 4 minutes before a rate increase, and may be preceded each time with a 1-minute loading infusion of 0.5 mg per kilogram per min.

It is critical that any patient with hemodynamic compromise in association with either ventricular or supraventricular tachyarrhythmia have sinus rhythm restored with DC cardioversion prior to pharmacologic therapy. For atrial flutter, DC cardioversion involves the use of 50 to 100 watt-seconds; for atrial fibrillation, 50 to 200 watt-seconds; and for ventricular fibrillation, 200 to 300 watt-seconds. If the patient is conscious, premedication with 5 to 15 mg of diazepam or 2 to 4 mg of midazolam given intravenously should precede the electrical cardioversion.

During cardiac catheterization, patients may develop either bradycardia or asystole. In these cases, 0.5 to 1.0 mg of atropine may be given intravenously. This dose may be repeated up to a total dose of 2.0 mg and may reverse the bradycardic event. In cases of sustained refractory bradycardia, an isoproterenol (Isuprel) drip at 5 to 10 micrograms per minute may be instituted until a temporary pacemaker can be placed.

Inotropic Agents

Occasionally, the patient undergoing cardiac catheterization will develop hypotension or manifestations of congestive heart failure due to worsening left ventricular function. During these episodes, the positive inotropic drugs, dopamine or dobutamine, may be administered to improve pump function. Dopamine in doses of 2 to 5 μg per kilogram per minute causes an increase in left ventricular contraction and an increase in cardiac output. Dopamine in higher doses of 5 to 10 μg per kilogram per minute, however, causes an increase in arterial pressure, heart rate, and peripheral vascular resistance. These latter events can work against the diseased heart by increasing afterload and oxygen demand. Dobutamine, in doses of 2 to 10 μg per kilogram per minute, causes an increase in left ventricular contraction without an increase in heart rate and may reduce peripheral vascular resistance in lower doses, probably making this agent preferable in patients with cardiac ischemia or significant regurgitant valvular disease. Infusion rates for doses of dopamine and dobutamine are given in Tables 12-5 and 12-6, respectively.

Drugs with negative inotropic qualities, such as propranolol and esmolol, are sometimes used to test for the reduction of a resting gradient in hypertrophic obstructive cardiomyopathy. Although most experience has been with propranolol (1 to 2 mg given intravenously), esmolol, with its extremely short duration of action, may be the preferred drug in catheterization interventions. Verapamil has also been shown to be efficacious in reducing the resting gradient in hypertrophic cardiomyopathy.

TABLE 12–5
Doses of Dopamine for Varying Standard Dopamine Concentrations at Flow Rates in Drops per Minute

200 mg/500 cc		400 mg/500 cc		800 mg/500 cc	
mcg/min	*drops/min*	*mcg/min*	*drops/min*	*mcg/min*	*drops/min*
20	3	40	3	80	3
40	6	80	6	160	6
60	9	120	9	240	9
80	12	160	12	320	12
100	15	200	15	400	15
120	18	240	18	480	18
140	21	280	21	560	21
160	24	320	24	640	24
180	27	360	27	720	27
200	30	400	30	800	30
220	33	440	33	880	33
240	36	480	36	960	36
260	39	520	39	1040	39
280	42	560	42	1120	42
300	45	600	45	1200	45
320	48	640	48	1280	48
340	51	680	51	1360	51
360	54	720	54	1440	54
380	57	760	57	1520	57
400	60	800	60	1600	60

TABLE 12–6
Doses of Dobutamine for Varying Standard Dobutamine Concentrations at Flow Rates in Drops per Minute

drops/min	500 mg/500 cc *mcg/min*	1000 mg/500 cc *mcg/min*	2000 mg/500 cc *mcg/min*
3	50	100	200
4	60–70	120–140	240–280
5	80–90	160–180	320–360
6	100	200	400
7	110–120	220–240	440–480
8	130–140	260–280	520–560
9	150	300	600
10	160–170	320–340	640–680
11	180–190	360–380	720–760
12	200	400	800
13	210–220	420–440	840–880
14	230–240	460–480	920–960
15	250	500	1000
16	260–270	520–540	1040–1080
17	280–290	560–580	1120–1160
18	300	600	1200
19	310–320	620–640	1240–1280
20	330–340	660–680	1320
21	350	700	1400
22	360–370	720–740	1440–1480
23	380–390	760–780	1520–1560
24	400	800	1600
25	410–420	820–840	1640–1680
26	430–440	860–880	1720–1760
27	450	900	1800
28	460–470	920–940	1840–1880
29	480–490	960–980	1920–1960
30	500	1000	2000
31	510–520	1020–1040	2040–2080
32	530–540	1060–1080	2120–2160
33	550	1100	2200
34	560–570	1120–1140	2240–2280
35	580–590	1160–1180	2320–2360

Vasodilators

Various vasodilator medications are used in the laboratory for a variety of purposes. Sublingual, topical, intravenous, and intracoronary nitroglycerin are used primarily for coronary vasodilatory effects and subsequent increased coronary blood flow. Intravenous nitroglycerin may also be used for its largely systemic venous dilating properties, which reduce left ventricular filling pressures and, consequently, help resolve congestive heart failure. Nitroprusside, with both systemic venous and arterial dilating effects, is used primarily in conditions where preload and afterload reduction are desirable, such as in congestive heart failure, acute mitral regurgitation, acute ventricular septal defect, or severe systemic hypertension (Table 12–7). Inhalation of amyl nitrite increases the left ventricular outflow obstruction in obstructive hypertrophic cardiomyopathy by reducing afterload and is therefore used as a provocative diagnostic test to increase the resting left ventricular outflow tract gradient in this disease. Calcium antagonists such as nifedipine are also used to evaluate the patient's acute response for possible treatment of congestive heart failure, obstructive hypertrophic cardiomyopathy, and pulmonary hypertension. A 10 mg capsule can be punctured and the contents placed sublingually.

Oxygen Therapy

In situations of myocardial ischemia, severe lung diseases, pulmonary edema, or acute respiratory failure, delivery of oxygen in the catheterization lab may be necessary. Oxygen administration in patients with severe lung disease requires close attention to percentage of oxygen administered. These patients may depend on their "oxygen drive." Normal patients increase the respiratory rate as arterial pCO_2 increases and reduce the respiratory rate as arterial pCO_2 declines. Patients depending on their "oxygen drive" use arterial hypoxemia (low pO_2) as their stimulus for ventilation. The addition of even low doses of oxygen is then perceived as the need to reduce the respiratory rate, and the patient may become

T A B L E 12–7
Doses of Nitroglycerine or Nitroprusside for Varying Standard Concentrations at Flow Rates in Drops per Minute

50 mg/500 cc		100 mg/500 cc		200 mg/500 cc	
mcg/min	*drops/min*	*mcg/min*	*drops/min*	*mcg/min*	*drops/min*
3	5	3	10	3	20
6	10	6	20	6	40
9	15	9	30	9	60
12	20	12	40	12	80
15	25	15	50	15	100
18	30	18	60	18	120
21	35	21	70	21	140
24	40	24	80	24	160
27	45	27	90	27	180
30	50	30	100	30	200
33	55	33	110	33	220
36	60	36	120	36	240
39	65	39	130	39	260
42	70	42	140	42	280
45	75	45	150	45	300
48	80	48	160	48	320
51	85	51	170	51	340
54	90	54	180	54	360
57	95	57	190	57	380
60	100	60	200	60	400

apneic. For this reason, the ventimask, with its ability to deliver an accurate percentage of oxygen, offers an advantage over other masks in this setting. Arterial blood gases should be monitored carefully in patients receiving oxygen therapy. Various oxygen-delivery systems are outlined in Table 12–8.

Radiographic Contrast Agents

All radiographic contrast agents are radiopaque because they contain iodine. The iodine molecule absorbs x-rays and prevents x-ray passage, allowing structures

TABLE 12–8
Various Modes of Oxygen Delivery and Their Characteristics

Type	FiO_2 Capability	Comments
Nasal cannula	Each 1 L/min of flow adds 2–3% to the FiO_2	Comfortable, but use should be limited to low flow rates (i.e., < 4 L/min) True FiO_2 uncertain
Ventimask	Available at 24, 28, 31, 35, 40, and 50%	Less comfortable, but provides a relatively controlled FiO_2 Poorly humidified gas at a maximum FiO_2
High-humidity mask	Variable from 28 to near 100%	Levels > 60% may require additional oxygen bleed-in Flow rates should be 2–3 times minute ventilation Excellent humidification
Reservoir masks Non-rebreathing	Not specified, but around 90% if well fitted	Reservoir fills during expiration and provides an additional source of gas during inspiration to decrease entrainment of room air
Partial rebreathing	Not specified, but around 60–80%	
Face tent	Variable; same as high-humidity mask	Mixing with room air makes actual inspired oxygen concentration unpredictable
T tube	Variable; same as high-humidity mask	For spontaneous breathing through endotracheal or tracheostomy tube Flow rates should be 2–3 times minute ventilation

Used with permission from Orland MJ, Saltman RJ, eds. Manual of Medical Therapeutics. Boston: Little, Brown and Company, 1986:152.

of interest to be contrasted from surrounding structures. Until recently, contrast agents were almost all ionic solutions of organic iodine components such as sodium meglumine diatrizoate (Hypaque and Renografin). Selective coronary artery injections of these agents frequently cause sinus bradycardia (sometimes asystole), ventricular fibrillation, significant hypotension, reduced myocardial contractility, and transient electrocardiographic changes. The cause of the adverse side effects is thought to be a combination of hyperosmolality, sodium content, direct toxicity of iodine and sodium, and the binding of calcium.

The administration of radiographic contrast is associated with a small risk of allergic reactions that range in severity from hives to rare anaphylactic reactions. Nonionic contrast solutions such as iohexol (Omnipaque) and iopamidol (Isovue) and the low-ionic solutions such as ioxyglate (Hexabrix) are associated with a much lower incidence of bradycardia, ventricular arrhythmias, hypotension, allergic reaction, and pain upon injection than the ionic contrast agents. All contrast agents are associated with slight renal toxicity. Recent studies from this institution suggest that nonionic agents offer no advantage over ionic agents in preventing renal toxicity. Dehydration appears to increase renal effects of contrast agents; therefore, patients should be adequately hydrated prior to and following angiography.

Thrombolytic Agents

Because acute thrombus formation has been shown to be the cause of the majority of myocardial infarctions, and because it is clear that the sooner an occluded coronary artery is reopened, the more myocardium is salvaged, the use of clot-dissolving drugs (thrombolytic agents) may be encountered in the cath lab.

These medications—commonly streptokinase (STK), urokinase (UK), single-chain urokinase–type plasminogen activator (scu-PA), and tissue plasminogen activators (t-PA)—may be administered intravenously prior to catheterization or be administered intracoronary at the time of catheterization.

The first of these agents, STK, is produced by beta-hemolytic streptococci. It indirectly activates plasminogen by forming an activated STK-plasminogen complex that converts plasminogen to plasmin. Plasmin is an enzyme capable of dissolving fibrin clot (Fig. 12–1). Because allergic reactions are known to occur, 40 mg of the intravenous steroid methylprednisolone sodium succinate (Solu-Medrol) is used as a premedication. Fever is very common with streptokinase. [Because of the possibility of an anamestic antibody response, the administration of this drug cannot be repeated within a 6-month period.] The other three pathways of plasminogen activation occur naturally in humans and are shown in Figure 12–1. The first pathway is the intrinsic pathway, which can produce various degrees of fibrin degeneration and is kept in check by naturally occurring plasma inhibitors. Urokinase, scu-PA, and t-PA work via the intrinsic system and are operational in the remaining two naturally occurring pathways for plasminogen activation (see Fig. 12–1). Because these agents occur naturally, allergic, fe-

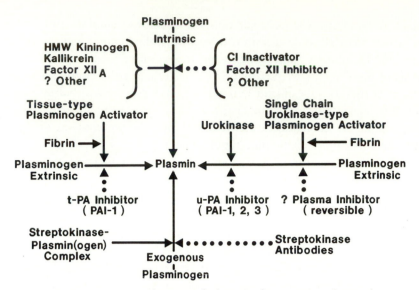

Figure 12–1. Major pathways of plasmin formation. Plasminogen is the precursor of plasma and is found in the blood stream (*top*) as intrinsic plasminogen. Certain thrombolytic agents (single-chain urokinase–type plasminogen activator (*left*) or tissue-type plasminogen activator (*right*) bind to fibrin before activating plasminogen to form plasmin. Streptokinase and urokinase bind directly to plasminogen to form plasmin. A plasminogen-streptokinase complex (*bottom*) can also be given to form plasmin from plasminogen. Plasmin then results in lysis of the clot. (From Califf RM, Mark DB, Wagner GS, eds. Acute coronary care in the thrombolytic patient. Chicago: Year Book Medical Publishers, 1988: 62; with permission.)

brile, or anamestic antibody responses are rare. Tissue plasminogen activators and scu-PA are clot-specific fibrinolytic agents that bind to fibrin and convert fibrin-bound plasminogen to plasmin, which is capable of dissolving fibin clots. The intended advantage of these agents is improved lysis with a reduction in bleeding complications, because t-PA and scu-PA are able to lyse clot without creating a systemic lytic state. Another agent, acylated plasminogen-streptokinase activator complex (APSAC), has also been developed as a clot-specific fibrinolytic agent. To date, however, clinical trials have not shown fewer bleeding complications with these agents versus STK.

The major complications with the use of these agents are associated bleeding events such as bleeding at the site of arterial and venous puncture, gastrointestinal bleeding, and central nervous system bleeding. Contraindications for thrombolytic therapy include recent surgery, lumbar puncture, thoracentesis, recent cardiopulmonary resuscitation, trauma, gastrointestinal bleeding, hemorrhagic diathesis, age over 75, untreated hypertension, or a cerebrovascular event. Intracoronary doses of these agents are given in Table 12–9.

TABLE 12–9
Commonly Used Intracoronary Thrombolytic Agents and Their Doses

Agent	Dose
Streptokinase	250,000–500,000 units
Urokinase	500,000–1,000,000 units
Tissue plasminogen activator	20–30 mg

Anticoagulant Agents

Heparin is generally added to all flush solutions in the laboratory. This naturally occurring substance inhibits clot formation owing to its inhibition of thrombin (a substance responsible for clot formation) by potentiating the action of antithrombin III. Heparin is used following thrombolytic therapy in patients with acute myocardial infarction, in patients requiring anticoagulation for valvular heart disease, and in most patients with unstable angina. Complete systemic anticoagulation is accomplished with a loading bolus dose of 60 units per kilogram intravenously, followed by 15 units per kilogram per hour infused intravenously. The anticoagulated patient should be carefully observed for signs of bleeding. Heparin causes prolongation of the partial thromboplastin time (PTT) and the activated clotting time (ACT). Therapy requires close monitoring of the effects of heparin. Upon cessation of heparin infusion, its effect is no longer detectable after 4 to 5 hr. If more rapid reversal is required, 1 mg of protamine sulfate per 100 units of bolus-administered heparin may be given slowly. The amount of protamine required for reversal of anticoagulation decreases with the amount of time passed from heparin administration. Use of protamine sulfate is associated with a small incidence of allergic reactions, especially in diabetic patients. An ACT of greater than 325 suggests substantial anticoagulation is still present.

At the time of cardiac catheterization, some patients may be receiving warfarin (Coumadin) for chronic anticoagulation. This medication interferes with the hepatic synthesis of vitamin K-dependent coagulation factors VII, IX, and X, and causes a lengthening of the prothrombin time (PT). Generally, warfarin should be discontinued 4 days prior to the procedure, and the PT should be nearly normalized (PT ratio < 1.5) at the time of the study. If rapid reversal of the effects of warfarin is necessary, fresh frozen plasma may be infused for temporary reversal. The subcutaneous administration of 10 to 20 mg of vitamin K may speed the reversal of the anticoagulated state, but this is associated with a small risk of an allergic reaction or hypercoagulable state.

Ergonovine Testing

In some patients, chest pain has been shown to be caused by transient coronary artery spasm in the absence of significant fixed obstruction. Prinzmetal's syndrome, or variant angina, is associated with transient nonexertional pain that often occurs at the same time everyday and with transient ST-segment elevation on EKG. When this condition is suspected, ergonovine maleate, an agent known to elicit coronary vasospasm, can be administered as a provocative test. Following completion of selective coronary injection, ergonovine is injected in doses of 0.05, 0.10 and 0.15 mg at 5-min intervals while the patient is observed closely for changes in EKG, changes in symptoms, and changes in hemodynamics. Prior to the administration of ergonovine, a syringe of nitroglycerin should be drawn up and the operator must be ready for immediate intracoronary nitroglycerin bolus (300 to 500 μg) in case of vasospasm. To assess the presence or absence of spasm, repeat coronary angiography is performed following with infusion of all three doses or immediately upon the development of EKG changes or symptoms. Once this test is completed, the patient may then be given sublingual nitroglycerin to reverse the effects of ergonovine.

Allergic Reactions to Contrast Media and Other Medications

A wide range of allergic reactions to medication (particularly to radiographic contrast materials) may be encountered in the cath lab that range from fever, hives, and skin rashes to facial edema, laryngospasm, or anaphylactic reaction. Mild reactions such as hives or rashes may be treated effectively with intravenous Benadryl (50 mg) or hydrocortisone (100 mg). Treatment of more severe reactions, such as anaphylaxis, requires special attention to circulatory support. Aggressive saline administration during hypotension is the mainstay of therapy. Non–life-threatening severe reactions require the administration of 1 cc of 1:1000 epinephrine subcutaneously, which may be repeated every 15 to 30 min for three doses. Life-threatening anaphylactic reactions require an intravenous bolus injection of 1:10,000 epinephrine every 1 to 5 min up to a total dose of 1 mg. Proper airway management and ventilatory support during these episodes are also necessary. Anaphylaxis results in profound vasodilation. Fluid administration should be paramount in therapy, followed by inotropic support and administration of epinephrine.

SELECTED REFERENCES

Abrams HL. The opaque media: Physiologic effects and systemic reactions. In: Abrams HL, ed. Abrams angiography: Vascular and interventional radiology. Boston: Little, Brown & Co., 1983: 15.

Bertrand ME, LaBlanche JM, Tilmond PY, et al. Frequency of provoked coronary arterial spasm in 1089 consequentive patients undergoing coronary arteriography. Circulation 1982; 65:1299.

Byrd L, Sherman RL. Radiocontrast-induced renal failure: A clinical and pathophysiologic review. Medicine 1979; 58:270.

Flamm MD, Harrison DC, Hancock EW. Muscular subaortic stenosis: Prevention of outflow obstruction with propranolol. Circulation 1968; 38:846.

Green GS, McKinnon CM, Rosch J, et al. Complications of selective percutaneous transfemoral coronary arteriography and their prevention: A review of 445 consecutive examinations. Circulation 1972; 45:552.

Handin RI, Loscalzo J. Hemostasis, thrombosis, fibrinolysis and cardiovascular disease. In: Braunwald E, ed. Heart disease: A textbook of cardiovascular medicine. Philadelphia: WB Saunders, 1988:1758.

Kastrup EK, Olin BR, Schwack GH, eds. Drug facts and comparisons. Philadelphia: JB Lippincott, 1988:993.

Levin DC. Technique of coronary arteriography. In: Abrams HL, ed. Abrams angiography: Vascular and interventional radiology. Boston: Little, Brown & Co., 1983: 485.

Miller RR, Fennell WH, Young JB, et al. Differential systemic arterial and venous actions and consequent cardiac effects of vasodilator drugs. Prog Cardiovasc Dis 1982; 24:353.

Myers GE, Bloom FL. Cimetadine (Tagamet) combined with steroids and H-1 antihistamines for the prevention of serious radiographic contrast material reactions. Cathet Cardiovasc Diagn 1981; 7:65.

Nattel S, Zipes DP. Clinical pharmacology of old and new antiarrhythmic drugs. Cardiovasc Clin 1980; 11:221.

O'Reilly RA. Vitamin K antagonists. In: Colman RW, Hirsch J, Marder VJ, et al, eds. Hemostasis and thrombosis: Basic principles and clinical practice. Philadelphia: JB Lippincott, 1982:955.

Rosenberg RD. Heparin-antithrombin system. In: Colman RW, Hirsch J, Marder VJ, et al, eds. Hemostasis and thrombosis: Basic principles and clinical practice. Philadelphia: JB Lippincott, 1982:962.

Rosing DR, Kent KM, Borer JS, et al. Verapamil therapy: A new approach to the pharmacologic treatment of hypertrophic cardiomyopathy. I. Hemodynamic effects. Circulation 1979; 60:1201.

Schwab SJ, Hlatky MA, Pieper KS, et al. Contrast nephrotoxicity: A randomized prospective trial of ionic and nonionic radiographic contrast. N Engl J Med 1989; 320:149.

Stoner JD, Bolen JL, Harrison DG. Comparison of dobutamine and dopamine in treatment of severe heart failure. Br Heart J 1977; 39:536.

CHAPTER 13

Common Disease States

Katherine B. Kisslo, RDMS, and Thomas M. Bashore, MD

Aortic Stenosis

Aortic stenosis is defined as narrowing of the aortic valve orifice due to either congenital or acquired disease. The stenosis causes increased pressure in the left ventricle (LV) and an accompanying systolic pressure gradient across the aortic valve. Figure 13–1 illustrates an aortic gradient in a patient with aortic valvular stenosis. The normal aortic valve orifice area is 2.5 to 4.9 cm^2. Severe aortic stenosis is present when the orifice is 0.8 cm^2 or smaller.

Etiology

Aortic stenosis may be caused by a number of factors:

1. A congenitally malformed aortic valve, which may be bicuspid, unicuspid, or dome-shaped.
2. Calcific (senile) aortic stenosis, which results from the deposition of calcium within the cusps of a trileaflet aortic valve. This deposition is likely secondary to mechanical stress over time and degeneration of the cusp tissue. It is generally a disease of the elderly.
3. Rheumatic heart disease, which may result in scarring and fusion of the aortic valve leaflets. This is usually accompanied by associated mitral valve involvement.
4. Prosthetic aortic valves, which create some obstruction depending on the type (ball-in-a-cage, porcine, bileaflet, "tilting-disc" type, and so forth). Central occluding devices (ball or disc) create the greatest obstruction.

5. Other less common conditions may stiffen the aortic valve and result in obstruction, but they are so uncommon as to be clinically irrelevant in a routine practice situation.

Pathophysiology

Chronic increased afterload (pressure overload) on the LV causes left ventricular hypertrophy in accordance with the Laplace relation (stress = pressure × radius/ wall thickness). Ultimately, LV dysfunction occurs as the heart muscle weakens and fails.

Physical Findings and Symptoms

Turbulence of blood across the stenotic valve results in a systolic crescendo-decrescendo (loud, then soft) murmur. The stiff aortic valve fails to open appropriately, and its closure sound (A_2) may be reduced. Early in the course, the mobile yet stiff valve will make a popping sound when it opens (ejection click). Because the blood leaves the heart more slowly than normal and because the total amount of blood flow may be reduced, the pulse pressure at the carotids may be diminished.

Symptoms include congestive heart failure (due to poor LV compliance and the poor stroke volume being ejected), angina (due to LV hypertrophy and coronary underperfusion of the inner lining of the heart), and syncope (due to arrhythmia or failure of the LV to pump an adequate stroke volume in response

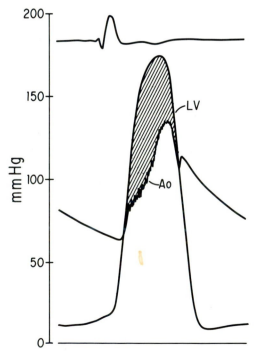

Figure 13–1. Pressure gradient in aortic stenosis. The pressure in the left ventricle (LV) is higher in systole than the aortic (Ao) pressure. The *shaded area* represents the gradient.

to the peripheral needs; this is particularly seen with exertion when the LV senses the pressure is too high and LV baroreceptors dilate peripheral vessels.)

Other Diagnostic Tests

A number of tests are used to diagnose aortic stenosis, including Doppler echo-cardiography, which is used to evaluate aortic valve motion and structure, left ventricular size, function, wall motion, and wall thickness, and to estimate aortic valve gradient; fluoroscopy and chest radiographs, which allow the evaluation of the degree of valve calcification (because calcification in the aortic valve will appear radiopaque) and heart size; ECG, which can determine the presence of left ventricular hypertrophy or whether calcium has eroded into the conduction system and created variable degrees of heart block; and radionuclide angiography, which gives the ejection fraction and overall wall motion.

Diagnosis in the Cath Lab

Hemodynamic Evaluation

Pressure on either side of the aortic valve must be measured in order to calculate the aortic gradient. The left ventricular to aortic pressure gradient may be expressed in several different ways (Fig. 13–2).

The peak-to-peak gradient refers to the difference between the maximal pressure in the LV and the maximal pressure in the aorta. This peak-to-peak difference rarely occurs at exactly the same instant in time; however, it is the easiest to measure because it can be obtained by measuring the peak left ventricular pressure and "pulling back" the catheter to subsequently record the peak aortic pressure.

The peak instantaneous pressure gradient is the maximum pressure difference when the LV and aortic pressures are measured at the same time. This occurs on the upslope of the aortic pressure tracing. It is usually greater than the peak-to-peak gradient, and is analogous to the maximum gradient calculated by Doppler echocardiographic methods. Some of the differences between Doppler echocardiographic and cardiac cath pressures are because most cardiac cath physicians are accustomed to using the peak-to-peak gradient, whereas the Doppler reports the peak instantaneous gradient.

The mean gradient is the average pressure difference between the LV and the aorta during the entire time the aortic valve is open (the systolic ejection period). This is the gradient that is used to calculate valve area. It is impossible to "eyeball" this value; it must be planimetered (traced) in some manner.

The pressures needed to obtain an aortic gradient may be recorded by several different methods:

1. Separate catheters may be placed in the aorta and in the LV, and the pressures recorded simultaneously.
2. A double micromanometer-tipped catheter may be positioned such

that one of the transducers lies in the aortic root and the other in the LV. This method produces the most accurate, noise-free recording of these pressures.

3. An arterial sheath pressure may be used to represent aortic pressure for comparison with the LV pressure. This method requires that the sheath pressure recordings be set back in time to compensate for the delay in the transmission of the pressure wave from the aorta to the sheath (Fig. 13–3).

4. A pullback pressure tracing may be recorded as the catheter is pulled back from the LV to the aorta. This method gives only a peak-to-peak gradient and does not allow for the accurate determination of a simultaneous gradient.

   On rare occasions, when the aortic valve cannot be crossed retrograde with a catheter, transseptal catheterization may be necessary to enter and record LV pressure. This is most common when certain prosthetic valves are in the aortic position.

The calculation of aortic valve area is generally done with the formula developed by Gorlin and Gorlin in 1951. This formula is based on fundamental hydraulics, and requires knowledge of the flow across the aortic valve and the

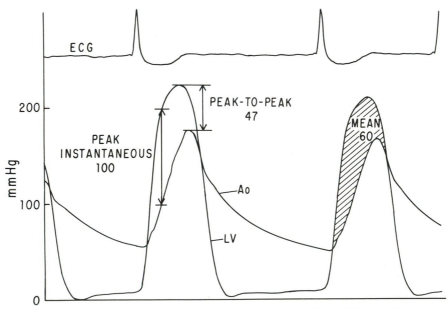

Figure 13–2. Ways of expressing aortic pressure gradient. The peak-to-peak gradient (47 mm Hg) is the difference between the maximal pressure in the aorta (Ao) and in the left ventricle (LV). The peak instantaneous gradient (100 mm Hg) is the maximal pressure difference when the pressures are measured in the same instant in time between the Ao and LV (usually during early systole). The mean gradient (*shaded area*) is the average pressure difference during systole (60 mm Hg).

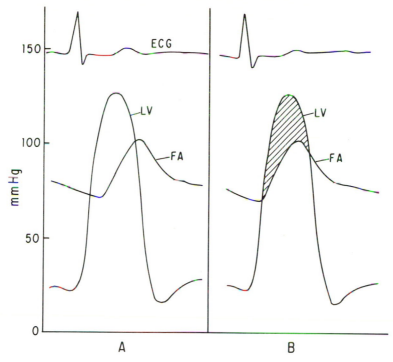

Figure 13–3. Delay in arterial pressure tracing. *A,* The femoral artery (FA) pressure is delayed in time compared to the left ventricular (LV) tracing. *B,* The FA must be set back so that the upstrokes of the two pressure tracings match in order to estimate what the mean gradient across the aortic valve would be (*shaded area*).

mean pressure gradient. In the equation, flow is expressed in the number of seconds in a minute that flow occurs across the valve. The systolic ejection period is defined as the time from aortic valve opening until its closure. Flow is calculated by dividing the cardiac output by heart rate times the systolic ejection period. The equation is as follows:

$$\text{aortic valve area} = \frac{\text{CO/(systolic ejection period)(HR)}}{44.3 \times \sqrt{\text{mean gradient}}},$$

where CO is cardiac output, HR is heart rate, and 44.3 is an empiric constant. A simplified formula for the calculation of aortic valve area has been reported by Hakki:

$$\text{aortic valve area} = \frac{\text{cardiac output}}{\sqrt{\text{mean gradient}}}.$$

For either of these methods, the measurement of cardiac output must be part of the catheterization procedure. Whatever output that crosses the valve is required; thus, if aortic regurgitation is present, angiographic, rather than the Fick or thermodilution cardiac output must be used. If both aortic regurgitation and mitral regurgitation are present, the aortic valve area cannot be determined and only the gradient should be reported.

Angiographic Evaluation

An aortic root injection of contrast media should be performed in patients with aortic stenosis to evaluate the valve structure (number of aortic cusps), to look for poststenotic dilatation, and to determine the degree of aortic insufficiency that is present (if any). A left ventriculogram will allow the evaluation of LV size and contractile performance and assess whether mitral regurgitation is also present.

Aortic Insufficiency

Aortic insufficiency is defined as leakage of blood backward across the closed aortic valve during ventricular diastole.

Etiology

Aortic insufficiency may be caused by a number of factors:

1. Primary aortic cusp disease due to a congenitally malformed valve, rheumatic disease, calcific aortic valve disease, endocarditis, or sinus of Valsalva aneurysm.
2. Aortitis (inflammation of the aorta and valve cusps) due to syphilis, ankylosing spondylitis, or giant cell arteritis.
3. Dilated aortic anulus and root due to Marfan's syndrome, Ehlers-Danlos syndrome, annuloaortic ectasia, cystic medial necrosis, hypertension, or pseudoxanthoma elasticum.
4. Loss of commissural support due to trauma, ventricular septal defect, or aortic dissection.
5. Prosthetic aortic valve (malposition, ring detachment).

Pathophysiology

In *acute aortic regurgitation,* the LV is unable to accept the sudden increase in diastolic volume without a dramatic decrease in LV diastolic pressure. This condition puts the LV under substantial strain, increases the filling pressure, and results in pulmonary congestion. Because the LV is normal in size, most of the chamber volume is used to produce a forward stroke volume that returns to the LV during the next diastole. Thus, the stroke volume that reaches the body is decreased, the systemic pulse pressure is narrowed, and the heart rate is elevated in an attempt to compensate for the low forward stroke volume (remember that cardiac output = heart rate × stroke volume).

In *chronic aortic regurgitation*, the LV adapts to the increased volume over time by wall hypertrophy as well as chamber dilatation. The dilated LV can produce a large stroke volume, which results in a wide pulse pressure. Thus, even though a lot of blood may leak back into the LV during diastole, there is still enough forward stroke volume to meet peripheral demands. Compensatory hypertrophy occurs. The LV end-diastolic pressure is frequently normal because the LV has dilated and can accept this extra volume without increasing filling pressure. See Figure 13–4 for a comparison of the hemodynamics of acute versus chronic aortic insufficiency.

Physical Findings and Symptoms

One of the physical findings of aortic insufficiency is a diastolic decrescendo "blowing" murmur, caused by the regurgitant flow across the aortic valve. In chronic aortic insufficiency, there is increased amplitude of the peripheral pulse

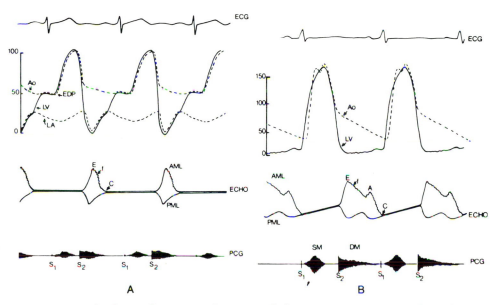

Figure 13–4. The hemodynamics of acute and chronic aortic regurgitation. *A,* Acute aortic regurgitation (AR) results in a marked rise in the left ventricular end-diastolic pressure (LVEDP). The aortic (Ao) pulse pressure is normal, the left atrial (LA) pressure is elevated, the mitral valve closes prematurely (C-point) on echo, and the phonocardiogram (PCG) shows a short, soft diastolic murmur that results from the AR. *B,* In chronic AR, the LVEDP may be normal, there is a wide aortic pulse pressure with a reduced aortic diastolic pressure, the mitral valve closes normally at the onset of LV systole, and the AR murmur is obvious. (From Morganroth J. 1977; with permission.)

due to the increased stroke volume ejected from the heart with each beat. The LV apex is markedly enlarged and hyperdynamic.

Symptoms are usually fatigue from LV failure (low output) and pulmonary congestion (high LV filling pressures).

Other Diagnostic Techniques

Echocardiography is used to evaluate the aortic valve, aortic root and LV size and function. Color flow Doppler can estimate the amount of regurgitation. Radionuclide angiography can assess the ejection fraction and wall motion at both rest and exercise. The chest radiograph reveals heart size and whether pulmonary congestion has occurred. The electrocardiogram is used to assess whether LV hypertrophy is present and to evaluate the heart rhythm.

Diagnosis in the Cath Lab

Hemodynamic Evaluation

Most studies of aortic insufficiency in the cath lab deal with patients with chronic aortic insufficiency. In those patients, the pulse pressure is quite wide because the increased stroke volume results in an increase in aortic systolic pressure, and the aortic regurgitation results in a low diastolic aortic pressure. LV end-diastolic pressure is generally nearly normal in chronic aortic insufficiency but markedly elevated in acute aortic insufficiency. No aortic gradient is demonstrable unless aortic stenosis is also present.

Angiographic Evaluation

An aortogram should be performed to quantitate the degree of aortic insufficiency and to look for associated aortic root abnormalities (see Chapter 11). The amount of aortic regurgitation can be estimated by noting the degree of opacification of the aortic root relative to the opacification of the LV. The amount of aortic insufficiency is considered

> 1+, if minimal regurgitation is seen in the LV;
> 2+, if moderate LV opacification, but clearing of the contrast during subsequent systoles is observed;
> 3+, if intense LV opacification occurs equal to that of the aorta at some point; and
> 4+, if LV opacification occurs greater than that of the aorta.

A left ventriculogram will allow for quantitation of LV size and performance and for determination of the angiographic volumes. An estimate of the amount of aortic insufficiency can also be made by combining angiographic stroke volume (includes aortic insufficiency regurgitant volume back into the LV), and the forward stroke volume measured by Fick or thermodilution. Because angiographic stroke volume would be expected to be greater than total forward stroke volume in aortic insufficiency, a regurgitant fraction can be derived as follows:

$$\text{regurgitant fraction} = \frac{\text{angiographic stroke volume} - \text{forward stroke volume}}{\text{angiographic stroke volume}}.$$

Mitral Stenosis

Mitral stenosis is defined as narrowing of the mitral valve orifice that causes an increase in left atrial (LA) pressure and an accompanying diastolic pressure gradient across the mitral valve. The normal mitral valve area is 3.0 to 6.0 cm^2. Severe mitral stenosis is believed to be present when a valve area is reduced to between less than 1.5 to 1.0 cm^2.

Etiology

Mitral stenosis may be caused by a number of factors:

1. The most common cause of mitral stenosis (MS) is as a consequence of rheumatic fever. It results in thickening and shortening of the chordae tendinae and gnarling of the leaflets, which leaves them immobile. Cusp fusion is evident. Over time, calcium can build up. Rheumatic mitral stenosis most commonly produces symptoms in young to middle-aged women.
2. Severe mitral anular calcification can result in functional narrowing of the mitral orifice. Mitral anular calcification is most commonly seen in elderly women, but it can be seen in many disease states as well.
3. A congenitally malformed mitral valve can cause stenosis (i.e., parachute mitral valve). Only one papillary muscle may be present.
4. Prosthetic mitral valve dysfunction can result in mitral stenosis. Calcification of bioprosthestic (tissue) valves or thrombosis of mechanical valves are the most common causes.

Pathophysiology

Mitral stenosis results in an increase in LA pressure and, consequently, in LA size. The pressure increase plus the involvement of the atrial tissue eventually result in atrial fibrillation. Mitral stenosis reduces the LV filling rate and the LV diastolic volumes are often low or normal. Pulmonary hypertension eventually occurs not only due to the elevated LA pressure backing up into the lungs, but also to pulmonary arteriolar constriction and obliterative changes in the pulmonary vascular bed. A representative pressure gradient in mitral stenosis is shown in Figure 13–5.

Physical Findings and Symptoms

Because the LA pressure is higher than the LV pressure during diastole, the mitral valve is pushed open wide even at the end of diastole. Rather than drifting shut just before ventricular systole begins, the stenotic mitral valve slams shut from the wide-open position and S_1 is accentuated. When the closed mitral valve opens, it also "pops" open with an accompanying sound (the opening snap) in early diastole. Because blood flow across the valve is turbulent in diastole, a mitral murmur (diastolic rumble) is heard.

Symptoms of mitral stenosis are similar to those of pulmonary congestion. This is particularly true with exertion or at higher heart rates, when the abbreviated diastolic filling time requires an even higher LA pressure to adequately fill the LV during each cardiac cycle. Right-heart failure from pulmonary hypertension and RV pressure overload, and hemoptysis (coughing up blood) from ruptured pulmonary vessels under high pressure may also occur in the later stages of the disease.

Other Diagnostic Tests

Echocardiography is used to image valve morphology, to evaluate LA size and LV size and function, and to measure mitral valve area. Doppler echocardiography

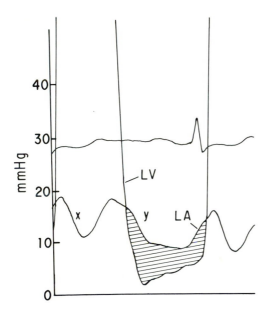

Figure 13–5. Prssure gradient in mitral stenosis. The pressure in the left atrium (LA) exceeds the pressure in the left ventricle (LV) during diastole, resulting in a diastolic pressure gradient (*shaded area*).

can quantitate mitral valve gradient and estimate valve area by a method called the "pressure half-time" or by direct planimetry of the orifice of the valve. The chest radiograph may show increased LA size and evidence for pulmonary congestion or pulmonary hypertension. When the LA enlarges, it pushes the left mainstem bronchus upward, and this is often seen in the chest radiograph. The ECG reveals LA enlargement and evidence for right ventricle hypertrophy. It is used to evaluate heart rhythm, because atrial fibrillation commonly occurs.

Diagnosis in the Cath Lab

Hemodynamic Evaluation

The mean pressure gradient across the mitral valve in diastole must be measured. This should be done by tracking the LA pressure versus the LV diastolic pressure. To obtain LA pressure, a transseptal puncture must be done in order to enter the LA from the right side of the heart. Because the pulmonary capillary wedge (PCW) pressure adequately reflects LA pressure in most instances, the PCW pressure may be used as a substitute for LA pressure. When the PCW pressure is used, the wedge tracing may have to be set back in time a small amount to compensate for the delay in the pressure transmission through the pulmonary venous and capillary beds. All pressures should be recorded at an expanded scale (i.e., 0 to 40 mm Hg) to allow for maximum display of the gradient (see Fig. 13–5).

Cardiac output must be measured to allow for calculation of the area of the mitral valve orifice. The effective area of the mitral valve orifice (using the PCW versus the LV) is calculated by the Gorlin formula:

$$\text{mitral valve area} = \frac{CO/(\text{diastolic filling period})(HR)}{44.3\,(0.85)\,\sqrt{\text{mean gradient}}},$$

where CO is cardiac output, HR is heart rate, and 0.85 is an empiric constant derived from the original Gorlin evaluations.

Right ventricular systolic and diastolic pressures can be used to assess RV function in conjunction with the mitral gradient.

Angiographic Evaluation

A left ventriculogram is used to evaluate LV size and function and to quantitate the degree of mitral regurgitation present (if any). The inflow pattern of blood without contrast helps outline the inflow filling pattern from the LA to LV across the mitral valve. Calcium can be similarly observed, and its location (anular versus leaflet) discerned. Aortic insufficiency is often present as an associated lesion in rheumatic heart disease; therefore, an aortogram is usually done to quantitate any aortic insufficiency that might also be present.

Mitral Insufficiency

Mitral insufficiency is defined as leakage of blood across a closed mitral valve during ventricular systole. The normally functioning mitral valve apparatus requires the proper alignment and function of not only the mitral leaflets, but also the mitral anulus, the chordae tendinae, and the papillary muscles. Mitral regurgitation can result whenever any component of this apparatus is abnormal.

Etiology

A number of factors may cause mitral insufficiency:

1. Rheumatic mitral valve disease results in scarring and deformation of the leaflets, which may then become incompetent.
2. In mitral valve prolapse (myxomatous degeneration of the valve leaflets), the leaflets may be too large or chordae too long to coapt properly.
3. Papillary muscle dysfunction may be a result of coronary artery disease or primary myocardial disease. Mitral regurgitation occurs as a result of inadequate papillary muscle contraction or misalignment of the papillary muscles.
4. Endocarditis or a vasculitis (such as lupus) can create a hole in the mitral leaflet.
5. Ruptured chordae tendinae are usually associated with mitral valve prolapse, but they can be due to trauma or endocarditis.
6. Mitral anular dilatation and LV dilation with misalignment of the mitral apparatus may occur in dilated cardiomyopathy.

Pathophysiology

The consequences of mitral regurgitation are a reflection of both the magnitude and the acuteness of the process. When acute mitral regurgitation occurs, the LA is still normal in size and is unable to accept the increased volume without a markedly elevated pressure resulting. A large V wave occurs that can be seen in the PCW tracing and, at times, is reflected in the pulmonary arterial pressure (Fig. 13–6). The LV ejection fraction increases because the blood is ejected into both the aorta and the LA. The LV thus empties more completely.

In chronic mitral regurgitation, the LA has enlarged over time and is able to absorb the effect of the regurgitant jet without markedly elevating LA, PCW, or pulmonary pressures. Over time, there is a gradual increase in LV end-diastolic volume and a loss of LV contractile function; eventually, heart failure occurs. When the RV fails from pulmonary hypertension, tricuspid regurgitation may occur, and the heart becomes huge on chest radiograph (cor bovine).

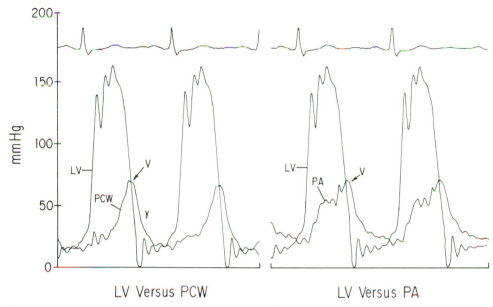

Figure 13–6. Mitral regurgitation and poor left atrial compliance.*Left panel,* The left ventricular (LV) pressure and the pulmonary capillary wedge (PCW) pressure are shown. Note the large regurgitant V wave. *Right panel,* The marked V wave is even transmitted to the pulmonary artery (PA) and is seen to be superimposed on the PA tracing.

Physical Findings and Symptoms

A high-pitched holosystolic murmur may be heard at the apex radiating to the axilla. The murmur is due to the turbulence of blood flowing across the leaking mitral valve in systole. Longstanding mitral regurgitation can lead to pulmonary hypertension, atrial fibrillation, and congestive heart failure.

Other Diagnostic Tests

Echocardiography is used to image the valve leaflets and rule out structural abnormalities. Left ventricular chamber size and function can be determined. Doppler echocardiography can provide a gross estimate of the amount of mitral regurgitation present. The chest radiograph may show massive cardiomegaly as noted above. The electrocardiogram may reveal LV hypertrophy and an enlarged LA. Eventually, atrial fibrillation may occur.

Diagnosis in the Cath Lab

Hemodynamic Evaluation

As shown in Figure 13-6, a large V wave may be present in the PCW pressure (or LA pressure). The Y-descent (reflecting LV filling) remains rapid, however, unless some mitral stenosis is also present. Right-heart and pulmonary pressures will eventually become elevated.

Angiographic Evaluation

During the left ventriculogram, the degree of mitral regurgitation is graded by evaluating how much contrast leaks back into the LA during systole (see Chapter 11). The left ventriculogram is also used to determine LV ejection fraction and the LV volumes. The quantitation of mitral regurgitation follows guidelines similar to those for aortic regurgitation. The following criteria are usually used to estimate the degree of mitral regurgitation:

1+, if there is trace regurgitation.

2+, if there is opacification of the LA that clears with subsequent diastole.

3+, if there is equal opacification of the LA and LV at some point.

4+, if there is greater opacification of the LA than the LV.

A regurgitant fraction can also be determined in a manner similar to that of aortic insufficiency. Total stroke volume can be determined using the angiographic stroke volume. Forward stroke volume (to the periphery) can be defined by thermodilution or Fick method. The difference between the angiographic stroke volume and the forward stroke volume is the regurgitant stroke volume. This is the amount that goes backward into the LA. The regurgitant fraction is the ratio of this regurgitant stroke volume to the angiographic stroke volume.

Hypertrophic Cardiomyopathy

Hypertrophic cardiomyopathy is defined as marked hypertrophy of the heart, especially the interventricular septum. The disease is usually congenital, and it goes by numerous other names, such as hypertrophic obstructive cardiomyopathy (HOCM), asymmetrical septal hypertrophy (ASH), and idiopathic hypertrophic subaortic stenosis (IHSS).

Etiology

Genetic hypertrophic cardiomyopathy is the most commonly seen type. A variety of forms of disproportionate septal hypertrophy are associated with abnormal septal myocardium on pathologic examination. One form primarily involves the LV apex.

Acquired hypertrophic cardiomyopathy is usually associated with systemic hypertension, especially in the elderly. It is occasionally seen with other forms of valvular disease.

Pathophysiology

The hypertrophied septum results in narrowing of the LV outflow tract. This creates an obstruction below the aortic valve; hence, the term: idiopathic hypertrophic subaortic stenosis (IHSS). The mitral leaflet forms the lateral wall of the LV outflow tract and either actively participates in the obstruction or is drawn into the outflow tract by the negative pressure created as the velocity of blood flow increases through this area in systole (Venturi effect). The markedly thickened LV results in elevated LV end-diastolic pressure, and mitral regurgitation is frequent. The LV chamber is usually small, and because of this, the ejection fraction may be very high (> 80 percent).

The dynamic nature of the LV outflow gradient distinguishes this obstruction from aortic valve stenosis. Anything that reduces systemic pressure (reduces afterload), reduces LV chamber size (reduces preload), or increases contractility (increased inotropy) will increase the gradient. The opposite also occurs. If afterload or preload is increased or contractility is reduced, the amount of outflow obstruction will decrease and the gradient will be reduced. Thus, provocative tests are frequently performed in the cath lab to demonstrate the dynamic nature of the subaortic gradient (see below).

Physical Findings and Symptoms

The heart is enlarged and dynamic. The murmur of aortic stenosis is present, but there is no delay in the carotid. In fact, a bisferious, or double-peaking, carotid pulse may be present due partially to mid-systolic obstruction of blood flow. The symptoms in hypertrophic cardiomyopathy are generally those of pulmonary congestion and relate to the high LV end-diastolic pressure. Syncope and sudden death occur in certain subsets of patients.

Other Diagnostic Tests

The echocardiogram may reveal marked asymmetrical septal hypertrophy relative to the posterior LV free wall. The septum is usually greater than 1.3 times the posterior wall in thickness by echocardiography. The mitral valve may be drawn into the LV outflow tract during systole—a phenomenon known as systolic anterior motion (SAM). The contractile pattern is usually hyperdynamic. The ejection fraction may be high as shown by radionuclide angiography (≥ 80 percent). The chest radiograph reveals only mild cardiomegaly in most cases, and the ECG varies widely, occasionally demonstrating marked LV hypertrophy, occasionally appearing to be almost normal.

Diagnosis in the Cath Lab

Hemodynamic Evaluation

Provocative maneuvers are used to demonstrate the dynamic nature of the LV outflow tract gradient. The Valsalva maneuver (bearing down and preventing venous return to the heart) results in less LV filling (reduces preload), and the LV chamber becomes smaller. Afterload can be reduced using amyl nitrite (Fig.

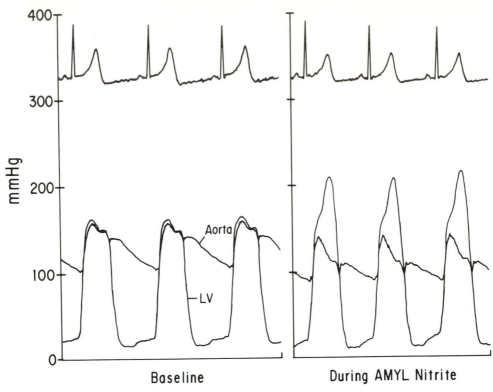

Figure 13–7. Idiopathic hypertrophic subaortic stenosis (IHSS) with amyl nitrite. *Left panel*, there is almost no systolic pressure gradient between the left ventricle (LV) and the aorta at baseline. After the inhalation of amyl nitrite (*right panel*), the fall in the aortic pressure causes a large pressure gradient to develop and the LV pressure to increase.

13–7), or contractility can be increased with isoproterenol, with similar results. All of these maneuvers result in an increase in the subaortic gradient.

Careful analysis of the location of the gradient confirms that the obstruction is below the aortic valve (Fig. 13–8) and not at the level of the valve. It is important to demonstrate a "chamber" just below the aortic valve where there is no aortic gradient (yet one is still measuring LV pressure). Placing the catheter further into the LV then results in a gradient being recorded. Normally, the beat following a premature ventricular contraction (PVC) would be expected to result in an increase in the pulse pressure in the aorta due to increased contractility, reduced afterload, and increased filling. In hypertrophic cardiomyopathy, however, these factors result in a net increase in obstruction and a reduced stroke volume. The resultant reduction in the pulse pressure after a PVC is referred to as "Brockenbrough's phenomenon" (Fig. 13–9), and is just the opposite of what one would expect in normals or in patients with valvular aortic stenosis. The early ejection of blood and then the creation of an outflow obstruction may also result in notching of the aortic pressure (the "spike-and-dome" tracing).

PULLBACK LV TO SUBAORTIC CHAMBER TO AORTA

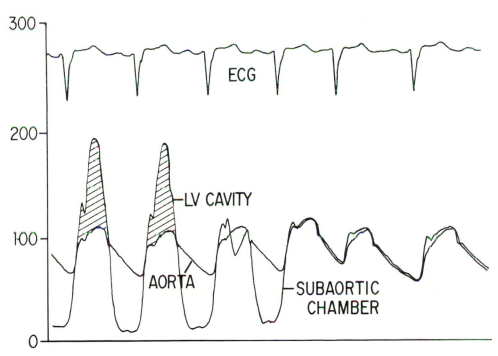

Figure 13–8. Gradient below the valve in idiopathic hypertrophic subaortic steno-sis (IHSS). Using a double-transducer catheter, a gradient deep in the left ventricle (LV) can be found (*shaded area*). As the catheter is withdrawn into the subaortic chamber (just below the aortic valve), the distal transducer is still in the LV but no aortic gradient is seen. Continuing to withdraw the catheter results in both transducers in the aorta (at right). The important finding is that a pressure can be measured in the LV with no gradient just below the valve despite a high gradient deeper in the LV.

Angiographic Evaluation

The left ventriculogram may reveal mitral regurgitation, and careful observation of the mitral motion may reveal systolic anterior excursion. The most striking feature is the high LV ejection fraction. Occasionally, the ventricle appears to empty entirely during systole (empty ventricle). Hypertrophy may not always be confined to the septum, because apical forms are also observed at times. Aortic regurgitation may be present owing to valvular injury from the underlying su-baortic jet.

Dilated Cardiomyopathy

Dilated cardiomyopathy may be defined as diffusely abnormal contraction of the left ventricle with a dilated LV chamber.

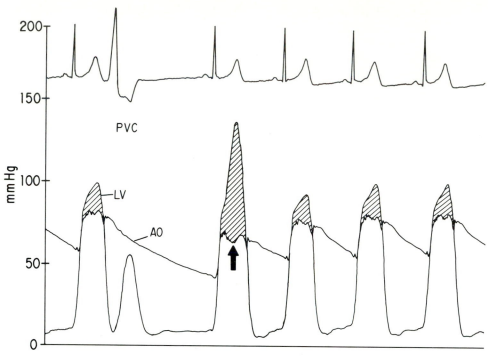

Figure 13–9. Brockenbrough phenomenon in hypertrophic cardiomyopathy. The Brockenbrough phenomenon is the failure of the post-PVC aortic pulse pressure to increase (as would occur normally). As shown, after the PVC, a long pause occurs that results in a fall in the aortic pressures (reduced afterload). The contractility of the post-PVC is increased, and the combination of reduced afterload and increased contractility causes greater outflow obstruction. Therefore, the stroke volume of the post-PVC beat is less, and the pulse pressure falls. A "spike-and-dome" configuration is also seen on this beat (shown at *arrow*).

Etiology

Cardiomyopathies are often of unknown (idiopathic) etiology. Many believe that viral illnesses may be a precipitating factor. Occasionally, cardiomyopathy is seen after administration of certain drugs (especially cancer chemotherapy agents), following pregnancy, or after longstanding systemic hypertension. Some patients with coronary artery disease develop an ischemic cardiomyopathy as well.

Pathophysiology

The LV is markedly dilated. The LV walls are thin, and the ejection fraction is reduced (usually < 30 percent). Mitral regurgitation is frequent. The forward stroke volume may be low, and the blood pressure may be similarly reduced. The dilated LV eventually results in an inability to pump enough blood forward without increasing the LV end-diastolic pressure to such an extent that pulmonary congestion occurs.

Physical Findings and Symptoms

The LV is large, and a filling sound (S_3) may occur after the mitral valve opens. Mitral regurgitation may be heard. Pulmonary congestion and fatigue are common. Wasting and cardiac cachexia occur in the late stages.

Other Diagnostic Tests

The echocardiogram reveals a dilated hypocontractile LV and an enlarged LA. Mitral regurgitation may be present by Doppler. The radionuclide angiogram reveals a reduced ejection fraction with a dilated LV. The chest radiograph shows the large LV, the LA, and evidence for pulmonary congestion. The ECG may reveal LV hypertrophy and an increase in size of the LA. Atrial fibrillation is common. The ECG may also reveal evidence for prior myocardial infarction if coronary disease is present.

Diagnosis in the Cath Lab

Hemodynamic Evaluation

The LV end-diastolic pressure is usually elevated, as is the PCW pressure and pulmonary pressures. A V-wave from mitral regurgitation may be present on the PCW tracing.

Angiographic Evaluation

The LV angiogram reveals a dilated, poorly contractile LV. Mitral regurgitation with a large LA is common.

Myocardial Biopsy

Myocardial biopsy may be useful in selected cases to determine the etiology, especially if an acute inflammatory process is suspected (see Chapter 9).

Pericardial Tamponade

Pericardial tamponade results when fluid accumulates between the two layers of pericardial sac. Normally, less than 50 cc of serous fluid is present. If fluid accumulates, the chambers of the heart become compressed when the pericardial pressure rises, and normal diastolic ventricular filling in both early and late diastole is impaired.

Etiology

Pericardial tamponade may be caused by the following factors:

1. Trauma.
2. Open heart surgery.

3. Pericarditis, which may be due to infection, drug-induced vasculitis, collagen diseases, acute myocardial infarction, uremia, and other causes.
4. Tumor and hemorrhage.
5. Other, less common etiologies.

Pathophysiology

When about 150 cc of fluid accumulates in a normal pericardium, tamponade may occur. Intrapericardial pressure rises as fluid accumulates and becomes exponential (Fig. 13–10) after about 50 cc. This rapid rise explains why cardiac compression can occur rapidly once a certain amount of fluid has accumulated and why removal of even a small amount of fluid with a pericardial needle can rapidly restore normal hemodynamics.

A paradoxical pulse may occur owing to filling of the RV and "crowding out" of the LV during inspiration. A paradoxical pulse means that the LV pumps less blood to the systemic circulation during inspiration than expiration, resulting in a fall of the systemic blood pressure during this period. Blood pressure then rises again during expiration when the increased lung pressures reduces filling of the RV and the lungs empty out to increase filling of the LV.

Because the stroke volume is reduced, heart rates are increased. The high pressure in the RA is reflected in distended jugular neck veins. The rise in intrapericardial pressure prevents the two ventricles from filling adequately. Therefore, the problem in tamponade is not impairment of systolic function, but the inability to properly fill the ventricles during diastole due to compression from the high intrapericardial pressure.

Physical Findings and Symptoms

Chest pain is the most common symptom felt by patients with acute pericarditis. A pericardial "rub," the result of the inflamed pericardial surfaces rubbing to-

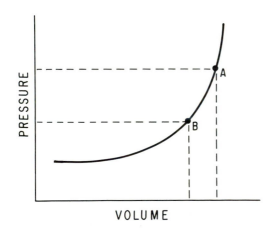

Figure 13–10. Pericardial pressure-volume curve. The rise in pericardial pressure is exponential with an increase in volume. Therefore, removal of even a small volume during tamponade (point A to point B) results in a dramatic decrease in intrapericardial pressure.

gether, may be present on auscultation. When tamponade occurs, the jugular venous distension and paradoxical pulse described earlier may appear.

Other Diagnostic Tests

The echocardiogram reveals an "echo-free" space around the heart that is consistent with the presence of fluid. Compression of individual chambers may also be observed. The chest radiograph reveals cardiomegaly, with the heart shadow taking on a "water-bottle" configuration. Pulmonary congestion is not usually seen because the problem is one of filling of the right and left sides of the heart. The ECG may reveal evidence of epicardial injury (ST elevation) acutely or reflect the swinging heart within the pericardium by noting "electrical alternans," or a rhythmic varying in the size of the QRS wave. The type of fluid can be determined by placing a needle in the pericardium and draining its contents (see Chapter 9). Other imaging techniques such as computerized transaxial tomography or magnetic resonance imaging, may also be helpful.

Diagnosis in the Cath Lab

Hemodynamic Evaluation

The compression of the heart results in elevation of the pressures in each cardiac chamber. Indeed, the mean RA pressure will equal the mean LA pressure, and the RV end-diastolic pressure, LV end-diastolic pressure, and the PA end-diastolic pressure will be the same. This is referred to as "equalization of pressures," and it occurs in both constriction and tamponade (Fig. 13–11).

Because RV and LV filling is blunted, the Y-descent (filling wave) in the atrial tracings are usually blunted and the X-descent (atrial relaxation) appears to be greater than the Y-descent (ventricular filling) (Fig. 13–12). Removal of pericardial fluid immediately establishes normal hemodynamics.

Angiographic Evaluation

Angiography has only a minor role to play in diagnosing tamponade. An RA injection in the anteroposterior view may reveal the shadow of pericardial fluid outside the normally thin RA lateral wall. During coronary angiography, the coronary arteries that are usually observed on the extreme of the heart shadow may be seen buried within the heart shadow owing to the fluid surrounding the heart.

Constrictive Pericarditis

Constrictive pericarditis results from scarring and compression of the heart due to fibrosis and fusion of the layers of the pericardium to the heart surface.

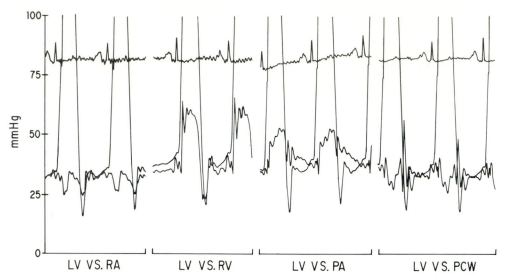

Figure 13–11. Equalization of diastolic pressures in constrictive pericarditis. When the pressure in the left ventricle (LV) is tracked versus those in the right atrium (RA), pulmonary artery (PA), and pulmonary capillary wedge (PCW), the diastolic pressures are similar. In the second panel, the right ventricular (RV) diastolic pressure is half of the RV systolic pressure. In this patient, all diastolic pressures are markedly elevated.

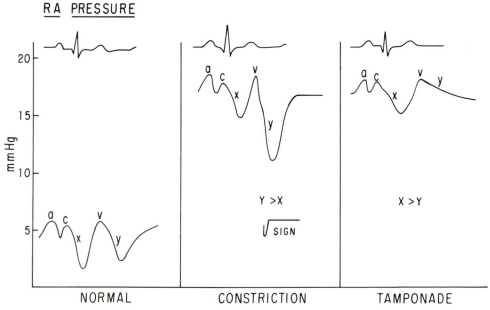

Figure 13–12. Right atrial pressures with normal hemodynamics, pericardial constriction and tamponade. In constriction and tamponade, right atrial pressures are higher than normal. The Y-descent is increased in constriction (note the "square-root sign" after the Y-descent). In tamponade, the Y-descent is slower.

Etiology

Constrictive pericarditis may be caused by the following factors:

1. Following inflammatory pericarditis (especially tuberculosis) or after open heart surgery.
2. Radiation therapy.
3. Other etiologies.

Pathophysiology

The constriction from the pericardium puts the heart in a vise-like grip that does not allow normal diastolic filling to occur. Systolic contraction is generally unaffected.

Physical Findings and Symptoms

The inability to fill the RV results in markedly elevated right-sided pressures and elevated neck veins. The increased RA pressure may cause hepatic congestion, ascites, and peripheral edema. Patients note fatigue due to low cardiac output, and they experience marked edema in later stages.

Early filling of the ventricles is rapid owing to the high atrial pressures, and an early diastolic filling sound (pericardial knock) may be heard on auscultation. Filling quickly ceases, however, as the limiting cloak of the pericardium prevents the heart from dilating in mid to late diastole.

Other Diagnostic Tests

The echocardiogram may suggest pericardial thickening, associated pericardial effusion, or diastolic filling abnormalities. The chest radiograph may reveal a small heart, and calcium in the pericardium may be evident. At times, pericardial calcium may be extensive. The electrocardiogram is generally nondiagnostic.

Diagnosis in the Cath Lab

Hemodynamic Evaluation

As shown in Figure 13–12, the hemodynamics of tamponade and constriction may be remarkably similar except for the manner in which the ventricles fill. In constriction, one can envision the heart as lying in a cement vault. The heart can initially relax normally, but as it fills, eventually it slams against the walls of the vault and can fill no more. Early diastole is the only time that filling can occur and, because atrial pressures are high, early filling is rapid and brisk. This is reflected as a rapid Y-descent of the atrial pressure tracings and a rapid early filling waveform in the ventricular pressure. Once the "walls" of the pericardial vault are reached, however, filling stops and the pressure rapidly rises. This re-

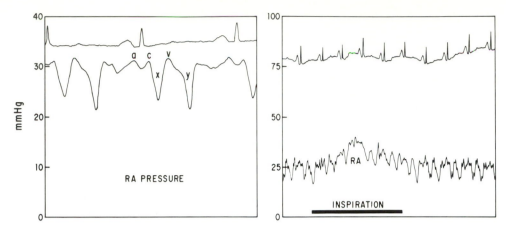

Figure 13–13. Kussmaul's sign in pericardial constriction. *Left panel*, Note the pronounced Y-descent in the right atrial (RA) pressure, which is consistent with constriction. *Right panel*, With inspiration, the RA pressure fails to fall or even rises because of impairment of RV filling. This phenomenon is called "Kussmaul's sign."

sults in a "square-root sign" type of filling pattern that is reflected in both the atrial and ventricular diastolic filling patterns.

The Y-descent in the atrial pressure is thus much greater than that of the X-descent (the opposite is true in tamponade). The restricted filling of the RV results in the normal inspiratory decrease in RA pressure being lost. Indeed, the RA pressure may either not drop or may rise during inspiration—a phenomenon known as "Kussmaul's sign" (Fig. 13–13).

Angiographic Evaluation

The angiographic signs of constriction are subtle and not generally helpful in making the diagnosis. If accompanying fluid is present, some of the same features as seen with tamponade may be observed.

SELECTED REFERENCES

Bland EF: Rheumatic fever: the way it was. Circulation 1987;76:1190–1195.
Markiewicz W, Rorovick R, Ecker S: Cardiac tamponade in medical patients: Treatment and prognosis in the echocardiographic era. AJC 1986;111:1138–1142.
Rahimtoola SH: Perspective on valvular heart disease: An update. J Am Coll Cardiol 1989;14:1–23. (Review)
Shabetai R: Pericardial and cardiac pressure. Circulation 1988;77:1–5.
Wigle ED, Sasson Z, Henderson MA, Ruddy TD, Folup J, Rakowski H, Williams WG: Hypertrophic cardiomyopathy. The Importance of the Site and Extent of Hypertrophy. A Review. Prog Cardiovasc Dis 1985;28:1–83.

Basic Electrophysiology

Michael J. Barber, MD, PhD

In 1968, a description of a percutaneous catheterization technique to record electrical activity from the bundle of His was reported in an intact dog heart. Subsequent studies in 1968 and 1969 refined these techniques and ultimately led to the first report of a catheter recording of the His bundle electrogram in humans. Over the next several years, intracardiac recordings were performed in human beings and evaluated the timing of various cardiac events (i.e., atrial, His bundle, and ventricular activation). These studies confirmed observations made over the previous 50 to 60 years in animal models and enabled a new group of cardiologists, the electrophysiologists, to begin to evalute the functional aspects of the electrical conduction system and the effects of pharmacologic agents, pathophysiologic states, and autonomic influences on the human heart and its conduction properties.

Perhaps the most significant advance occurred in 1971, when Dr. Hein J.J. Wellens first described the technique of programmed electrical stimulation whereby electrical stimuli were applied carefully to the heart. This technique, when used in conjunction with the rapidly developing refinement of intracardiac recordings, allowed cardiologists to evaluate in greater detail the functions of the cardiac conduction system and specialized cardiac tissues (sinoatrial and atrioventricular nodes), as well as to evaluate the propensity and mechanisms for patients to develop cardiac dysrhythmias.

Although a comprehensive review of electrophysiology and electrophysiologic techniques is beyond the scope of this chapter, it is important that all people involved in aspects of invasive cardiology understand at least the principles and fundamentals of cardiac dysrhythmias and their evaluation. In this section, we discuss the basic principles of cardiac electrophysiology and describe the various techniques, materials, and approaches used to evaluate patients with cardiac dys-rhythmia. For those interested in a more in-depth description and explanation of electrophysiologic studies, several references are provided at the end of this chapter.

Basic Electrophysiology

Cardiac function requires that the contractile apparatus of the heart be electrically activated and that this electrical activation progress in an organized fashion such that the heart muscle itself can eject blood (see Chapter 7). The electrocardiogram (ECG) is a simple recording of this sequence of electrical activation, reflecting the depolarization (activation) and repolarization (relaxation) of the heart muscle. Because the body can conduct electrical current, the forces of depolarization and repolarization may be sensed by small electrodes attached to the arms, legs, and chest and connected to the ECG machine.

Briefly, before any understanding of cellular electrophysiology can be gained, one must first understand the principles of recording the ECG. In a routine 12-lead ECG, each of the 6 limb leads (I, II, III, aV_R, aV_L, aV_F) and 6 chest leads (V_1 through V_6) are utilized as an "exploring" electrode to evaluate specific "subregions" of the heart.

Two arrangements of electrodes are used to explore the electrical activity of the heart. The first of these arrangements utilizes the comparison of electrical potential between two individual electrode leads. This is called a "bipolar-lead system." Leads utilizing a bipolar system (I, II, III) compare electrical activity between two distinct locations on the body, as shown in Table 14–1. By convention, an electrical signal that travels toward the positive electrode of a bipolar lead will generate a positive, upward deflection on the ECG (Fig. 14–1). Conversely, an electrical signal moving away from the positive lead (or toward the negative lead) will generate a negative, downward deflection on the final tracing.

TABLE 14–1
Standard 12-Lead Electrocardiogram System

Bipolar Leads	Positive Lead	Negative Lead
I	Left arm	Right arm
II	Left leg	Right arm
III	Left leg	Left arm
Augmented Leads		
aV_R	Right arm	—
aV_L	Left arm	—
aV_F	Left leg	—

Precordial leads (unipolar; referenced to the body)

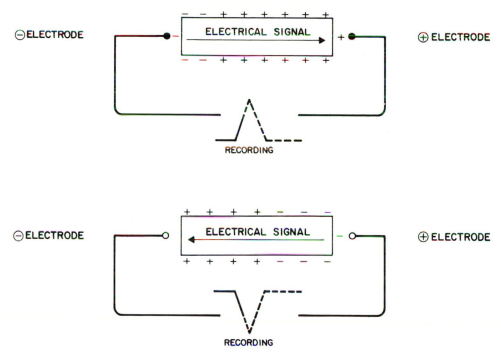

Figure 14–1. Schematic representation of the eletrical signal generated using a bipolar-lead recording system. As the electrical signal (wave of depolarization) approaches the positive electrode, an upward deflection is seen, as shown by the recording tracing. This tracing reaches a peak and then returns to baseline as the signal passes the electrode. Conversely, an electrical signal moving away from the positive electrode generates a negative deflection.

The second electrode arrangement used to explore the electrical activity of the heart compares the electrical potential seen by a single exploring lead to the electrical potential generated when an average of the total body electrical potential is measured by two or more "reference" electrodes. These reference electrodes allow the exploring electrode (also called a "unipolar electrode") to look at a more localized area of myocardial activation (i.e., the area located directly under the electrode), and assist in evaluating subregions of the heart. Unipolar leads include the augmented limb leads (aV_R, aV_L, aV_F) as well as the precordial leads (V_1 through V_6). Again, by convention, an electrical signal traveling toward the unipolar electrode will generate an upward, positive deflection, whereas an impulse traveling away from the unipolar lead will be recorded as a negative, downward deflection.

To understand the electrical forces that generate the ECG, we will first look at an isolated electrical event in a single cell. This is called an "action potential", and it is the summation of these individual electrical events that ultimately results in the production of a recordable 12-lead ECG. In ventricular muscle, utilizing microelectrode recording equipment, an action potential may be recorded from a single cell. A schematic of such an action potential is seen in Figure 14–2.

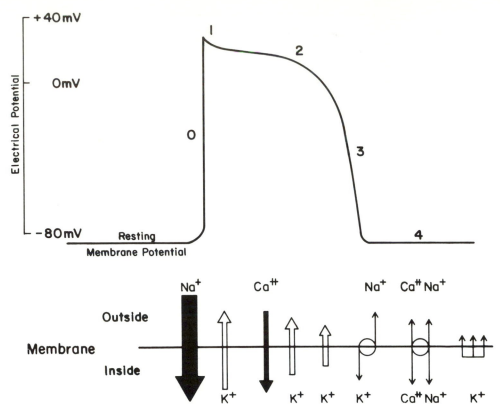

Figure 14–2. Schematic representation of an action potential recorded from ventricular muscle during normal activation. *Arrows* indicate the direction and relative number of ions flowing during each phase of the action potential. Bidirectional flow represents activity of the sodium-potassium or sodium-calcium pumps in the cell membrane. Na^+ = sodium ions. K^+ = potassium ions. Ca^{++} = calcium ions. 0, 1, 2, 3, 4 = phases of the cardiac action potential.

Each action potential is the result of controlled movements of sodium, calcium, and potassium ions into and out of the cell. Under resting conditions, the concentration of sodium ions outside of the cell is approximately 15 times the intracellular concentration. Conversely, the intracellular concentration of potassium ions is approximately 35 times the concentration of potassium located outside the cell. These tremendous concentration gradients are actively maintained by the sodium-potassium pump, and it is this pump that generates the "resting" membrane potential. The lack of sodium inside the cell results in the negative nature of this membrane potential (i.e., at rest, the potential is about − 80 mV). The pump is constantly moving sodium to the outside of the cell while moving potassium back into the cell.

With activation of the cellular membrane, channels (holes) located in the membrane and usually closed to sodium-ion movement open rapidly. This results in unrestricted flow of ions (cellular depolarization), and sodium rushes into the cell while potassium flows out of the cell. This massive influx of positive sodium ions causes the cell's electrical potential to rapidly increase from its negative resting value of -80 mV to a positive value of 30 mV. With this rapid change in the electrical potential of the cell, stores of intracellular calcium normally bound to membranes and unavailable are released into the cell and become available for participation in cardiac contraction. Additionally, with the change in cellular potential, channels controlling the flow of calcium outside the cell open up and allow even more calcium to enter the cell. All of this calcium becomes available to increase contraction of the muscle cell.

As the flow of ions slows and approaches equilibrium, the ion pumps (sodium-potassium and sodium-calcium) gradually restore the resting cellular potential (repolarization of the cell as shown in Fig. 14–2), and the muscle contraction initiated by the ion changes reverses and relaxation ensues.

Figure 14–3 schematically demonstrates the relationships between the action potential of a single ventricular cell, a generalized myocardial contraction, and a surface ECG tracing. Prior to ventricular activation, there is activation of the atria. Contraction of the atria precedes that of the ventricles. The P wave of the surface ECG represents depolarization and subsequent contraction of the atria. The electrical impulse travels through the atria to the atrioventricular node, where it subsequently passes to the ventricles. With the onset of depolarization of the ventricular cells, a rapid wave of electrical activity sweeps over the ventricle.

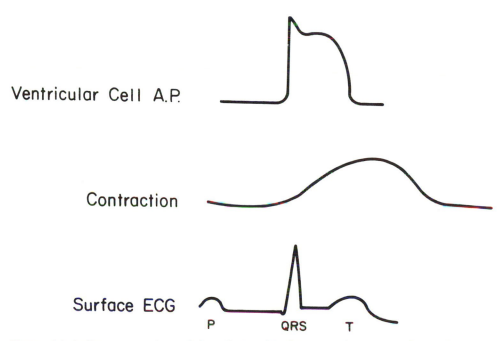

Figure 14–3. Representation of the relationship between the ventricular action potential (A.P.), ventricular muscle contraction, and the surface electrocardiogram (ECG).

As can be seen, the rapid depolarization phase of ventricular cells corresponds to the QRS complex as seen on the surface ECG. The QRS complex represents the "sum" of the electrical activity of all individual ventricular cells during depolarization. With the completion of depolarization comes the plateau phase of the action potential (see Fig. 14–2). Although ion movements during this phase are occurring at the cellular level, very little net current flows. As a result, this time is perceived on the surface ECG as a period of electrical quiescence and results in the isoelectric portion of the tracing between QRS complex and the T wave. With the onset of cellular repolarization, a T wave is generated. Upon completion of repolarization, the resting membrane potential is reestablished and the cells become quiescent until the next impulse is initiated for conduction.

Relation of the Intracavitary Electrogram to Cellular Activation and the Surface ECG

With the inception of electrophysiologic recording, catheter electrodes have been the standard by which electrical signals from cardiac muscle are recorded. Similar to the bipolar electrodes on the ECG, an intracavitary electrogram is recorded using a bipolar electrode system. In this case, however, instead of the electrodes being located on the arms or legs of the patient, they are separated by 5 to 10 mm at the end of a catheter (Fig. 14–4). This catheter can be advanced under fluoroscopic guidance to make contact at the desired location in the heart and record local electrical activity. Similar to the bipolar arrangement of the ECG, one electrode of the pair is defined as the positive electrode (cathode); this is usually the distal electrode. The other electrode is referred to as the negative electrode (anode); this is usually the proximal electrode. The positive electrode of the bipolar lead generates a positive, upward deflection when a signal approaches.

A number of different types of catheters are available for intracavitary use, but all provide the ability to record from a localized region of the heart. Theoretically, the local electrogram generated by recording from a catheter electrode reflects the electrical activity of the myocardium immediately adjacent to the catheter. As a result, the electrogram should record a more localized, discrete electrical event and, when compared to the ECG, should be of briefer duration and narrower morphology. An example of the relationship and morphology of local intracavitary electrograms from the right atrium, His bundle, and the right ventricle compared to the surface ECG is shown in Figure 14–5.

Basic Equipment

Performance of an electrophysiologic study requires a laboratory adequately equipped for such testing. It is not the intention of this chapter to provide a complete and detailed list of such equipment. Rather, it is our goal to briefly

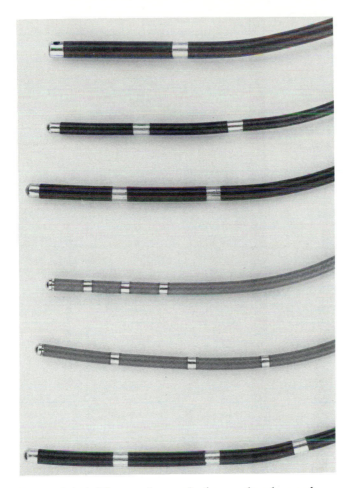

Figure 14–4. The sensing end of several catheter electrodes commonly used in the electrophysiology lab. From *top* to *bottom*: 6 French quadripolar, 5 French quadripolar, 5 French quadripolar (narrow spacing), 6 French tripolar, 5 French tripolar, and 7 French bipolar catheters. Except for the 5 French narrow-space catheter (5 mm), the interelectrode distance for all catheters is 10 to 12 mm.

introduce the reader to the general organizational scheme of the laboratory and to provide information as to the type of equipment necessary to perform electrophysiologic evaluations.

The general organization of the electrophysiology laboratory is detailed schematically in Figure 14–6. As with any laboratory involved in patient care, the laboratory should be well lit and clean. Routinely, four or five electrocardiographic leads should be displayed on a monitor continuously throughout the

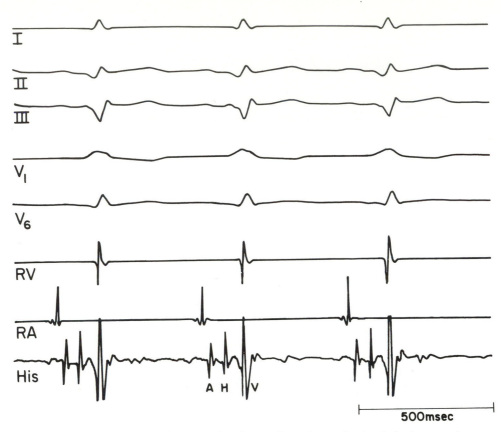

Figure 14–5. Retouched photograph of actual tracings obtained during an electrophysiologic study. From *top* to *bottom* are leads I, II, III, V₁ and V₆ of the electrocardiogram, an electrogram recorded from the right ventricular apex (RV), a right atrial electrogram (RA) recorded near the SA node, and a His bundle electrogram. Deflections labeled on the His bundle recording represent local atrial (A), ventricular (V), and His bundle (H) activity.

study. These leads usually consist of leads I, II, III, V₁, and V₆. The patient also should be connected to a defibrillator system with a separate monitor attached. This facilitates synchronized and asynchronized cardioversion attempts in the event that a serious cardiac dysrhythmia is initiated (this is a frequent occurrence in the eletrophysiology lab).

Frequently, during the course of an electrophysiology study, a complete 12-lead ECG is required. Because it is not practical to continuously monitor 12 channels of information for an entire electrophysiology study, a separate ECG machine should be present in the lab and the patient connected to the machine prior to beginning any evaluation. Then, in the event of a significant arrhythmia, a 12-lead ECG can be obtained readily with essentially no effort. Finally, an integrated recording system capable of producing a permanent hard copy (chart recorder) as well as a taped result (high-quality FM tape recorder) of the study is

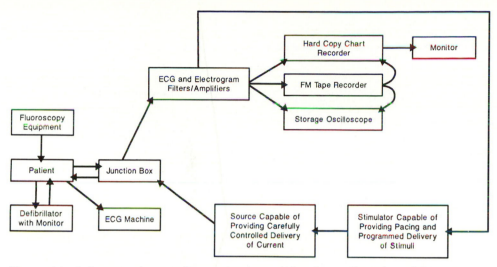

Figure 14–6. Suggested general organization of the electrophysiology laboratory.

necessary. A storage oscilloscope introduced into the system provides the ability to rapidly analyze small changes in the recorded electrograms and facilitates interpretation of the data. Finally, in order to perform the actual electrophysiologic protocols, a high-quality, multifunction stimulator capable of pacing and introducing various types of electrical stimuli is fed into an amplifier system for delivery of constant well-controlled levels of current to the electrodes.

Patient Preparation

Once the stimulation/recording system is functional, an electrophysiologic study may be performed. Intracardiac positioning of catheter electrodes requires vascular access similar to techniques described earlier for cardiac catheterization (see Chapter 8). The patient should be connected to the recording equipment immediately upon arrival in the eletrophysiology lab. The proposed access site is then prepped and draped in a sterile fashion. Access is usually obtained on the venous side because most recording and stimulation protocols are performed from right atrial, His bundle, and right ventricular sites. In most cases, a modified Seldinger technique is utilized after the skin over the right femoral vein has been anesthetized with either procaine or lidocaine local anesthesia. In some instances, the left femoral vein, right or left subclavian veins, or the median basilic vein may be utilized. Additionally, arterial access also may be necessary if left ventricular programmed stimulation is indicated.

Once access into the vessel has been accomplished with an 18-gauge thin-walled needle, a short, flexible J-guidewire is inserted through the needle. Over the guidewire, a dilator/sheath combination is advanced (Fig. 14–7) into the vein.

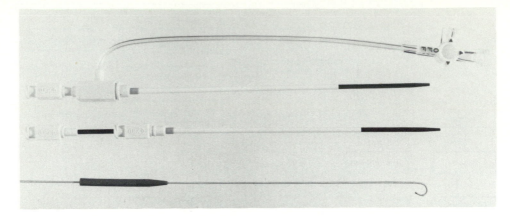

Figure 14–7. Photograph of a 7 French sheath/dilator system with side port for infusion of fluids (*top*), a 6 French sheath/dilator combination (*middle*), and a flexible J-guidewire used to facilitate venous access during an electrophysiology study.

The wire and dilator are removed, and the desired catheter electrode (see Fig. 14–4) is introduced through the sheath. The catheter then is advanced under fluoroscopic guidance to the desired location for recording the appropriate electrogram. Often, a second, or even third, catheter is introduced through the femoral vein to record from other locations in the heart. Under these circumstances, insertion of the catheters is performed in a similar fashion with the venous puncture sites separated approximately 1 cm cephalad or caudal to the original site of venous entry.

Sites of Electrogram Recording in the Heart

Routine electrophysiologic studies may require recordings from any combination of the four cardiac chambers as well as the His bundle (Fig. 14–8). The right atrium (RA) is easily accessible utilizing venous cannulation. The most common site for recording and stimulating in the RA is located in the posterolateral wall of the RA at the junction of the superior vena cava. This location is in the region of the sinus node and may be utilized to stimulate the heart from its "normal" site of impulse origin.

Recording directly from the left atrium (LA) can be more difficult. This chamber may be approached in a number of ways, including transeptally from the RA or retrogradely from the left ventricle by crossing the mitral valve. Most commonly, the LA is approached indirectly by positioning the catheter electrode in the coronary sinus. The os (opening) of the coronary sinus vein is located in the RA on the lower atrial septum near the tricuspid valve. Using fluoroscopic guidance, the electrode catheter is positioned in the os of the coronary sinus and

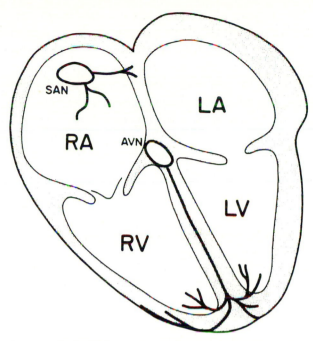

Figure 14–8. Schematic representation of the heart showing the four cardiac chambers as well as the general location of the sinoatrial (SAN) and atrioventricular (AVN) nodes. Emerging from the AVN is the His bundle, which subsequently divides into the left and right bundle branches.

carefully advanced into the coronary sinus vein. The coronary sinus lies between the LA and the left ventricle, and by advancing the catheter retrogradely, it reaches the left ventricular border. In this area, it records both LA and left ventricular electrical activity. Other, less practical techniques to record from the LA include positioning the catheter in the main pulmonary artery or passing a special esophageal electrode to a position in the esophagus, where it will record from the posterior LA. These last two techniques are of limited value because they often require electrical current levels that are uncomfortable for the patient if the atrium is to be paced.

All areas of the right ventricle (RV) are easily accessible utilizing any venous access site. Routinely, the electrode is passed through the tricuspid valve and positioned in the apex or outflow tract of the RV at a point just below the pulmonic valve.

Recording and stimulating from the left ventricle (LV) is not a routine part of most electrophysiologic studies, as discussed previously. When LV stimulation is necessary, the ventricle most often is entered in a retrograde fashion with the catheter passed from the femoral artery, through the aorta and aortic valve. Once in the LV, stimulation and recording can be performed from any site. Occasionally, the LV may be entered by a transseptal cannulation entering the LA from the RA and advancing the catheter through the mitral valve to the LV.

The final common location for intracardiac recording is in the region of the His bundle. To accomplish this, the catheter (usually a tripolar catheter) is advanced to the RA and into the RV across the tricuspid valve. Once the catheter has entered the RV, it is slowly withdrawn using clockwise rotation of the catheter. This clockwise rotation keeps the recording electrodes in contact with the ventricular septum and within the area where the His bundle is located. The His bundle recording assists during electrophysiologic study in the evaluation of the function of the cardiac conduction system.

Complications of Electrophysiologic Studies

Electrophysiologic studies are safe, with the reported rate of significant complications ranging from 0.6 to 2 percent (see Chapter 6). Although this low rate of complications makes the risk of undergoing electrophysiologic evaluation acceptable, significant problems may arise. The most common reported complications of electrophysiologic studies include the development of local hematomas or deep venous thrombosis, although these are rarely associated with significant problems. Other less common but potentially more serious complications include the risk of infection, pulmonary embolus, cardiac perforation, cardiac tamponade, intractable cardiac arrhythmias, heart block, pneumothorax (with subclavian vein access), and, rarely, death. Although problems do not occur often, they can be serious, and require that each patient be carefully and individually evaluated prior to study. Additionally, alerting the patient to the risks of the study (i.e., obtaining informed consent) prior to performing any evaluation is necessary.

Indications for Electrophysiologic Study

Electrophysiologic studies have been used for approximately 20 years to evaluate various types of cardiac arrhythmias. Over this period, data have been obtained that can aid the physician in determining when an electrophysiologic study should or should not be performed. In 1985, the North American Society of Pacing and Electrophysiology (NASPE) appointed a committee to review these data and establish guidelines to assist in determining whether an electrophysiologic study needed to be performed (Akhtar, Fischer, Gillette, et al, 1985). Although electrophysiologic testing is indicated in patients with bradyarrhythmias, tachyarrhythmias (supraventricular and ventricular), complex ventricular arrhythmias, syncope, cardiac arrest, sinus node dysfunction, and conduction system block, as well as to evaluate the effectiveness of drug therapy, contraindications do exist. We will briefly present some indications and contraindications for electrophysiologic study, but we refer the reader to the NASPE guidelines for a complete discussion.

Bradyarrhythmias

Inadequate cardiac output due to a slow heart rate may lead to symptoms of weakness, tiredness, dizziness, presyncope, or syncope. Bradyarrhythmias may result from several etiologies, including dysfunction of the sinus node resulting in a slow heart rate, atrioventricular heart block resulting in slow ventricular response, conduction block in the His-Purkinje system resulting in a slow or absent ventricular response, or abnormal autonomic tone to the heart resulting in bradycardia.

In all cases, if symptoms and the presence of marked bradycardia, atrioventricular block, or slow ventricular response can be correlated, the need for electrophysiologic study is probably eliminated, and a pacemaker should be considered without further delay to treat the bradyarrhythmia. If symptoms cannot be correlated with ECG changes or it is unclear exactly what the ECG changes are demonstrating, an electrophysiologic evaluation should be pursued.

These studies should focus on evaluating the function of the sinus node, the conduction properties of the atrioventricular node and His-Purkinje system, the potential for an adequate ventricular "escape" rhythm to occur during periods of bradycardia, and the influence of the autonomic nervous system on the heart. Upon completion of these studies, the data may be used to determine the need for further therapy, (i.e., medication, pacemaker).

Supraventricular Tachycardias

Cardiac output is a function of the heart rate multiplied by the stroke volume of the ventricle. In the case of bradyarrhythmias, in spite of the fact that stroke volume generally increases at slower heart rates, if the rate is too slow, adequate compensation cannot occur and symptoms (fatigue, weakness, syncope, and so forth) of low cardiac output result. Similar problems can arise with the tachyarrhythmias. In this case, the ventricle is not allowed an adequate amount of time to fill completely and the ventricular stroke volume decreases. There is a fall in the cardiac output in spite of an increased heart rate, and symptoms similar to those just described may result.

The supraventricular tachycardias consist of arrhythmias with their origin above (supra-) the ventricle and include atrial flutter, atrial fibrillation, sinus tachycardia, ectopic atrial tachycardia, or atrioventricular nodal re-entrant tachycardia. Additionally, accessory atrioventricular pathways—also known as "atrioventricular bypass tracts" and most commonly associated with the Wolff-Parkinson-White syndrome—may lead to a supraventricular tachycardia.

Often, careful analysis of the surface electrocardiogram alone or in conjunction with an esophageal electrogram recording during the arrhythmia can reveal the mechanism of the supraventricular tachycardia. If the mechanism can be determined from these methods, electrophysiologic study may not be necessary and treatment can be managed using antiarrhythmic drugs while monitoring the patient closely. In a select group of patients, however, electrophysiologic study will help determine the appropriate diagnosis and treatment of the arrhythmia. The indications for invasive study vary, but they usually include the following: tachycardias associated with significant symptoms, tachycardias associated with an excessively rapid heart rate (greater than 200 beats per minute), or refractoriness of a known tachycardia to conventional therapy. Occasionally, it also is necessary to perform an electrophysiologic study to distinguish a supraventricular tachycardia with abnormal ventricular conduction (aberrancy) from ventricular tachycardia.

Ventricular Tachycardia

In spite of a thorough evaluation of the surface ECG during a period of tachycardia, it is often impossible to be certain whether a patient has a supraventricular tachycardia with aberrant ventricular conduction or ventricular tachycardia. Because prognoses of these two tachycardias are quite different, it is essential that the correct diagnosis be made. Electrophysiologic testing can identify the origin of the arrhythmia when induced in the electrophysiology lab.

Before electrophysiologic studies and programmed electrical stimulation were available, patients with recurrent ventricular tachycardia were begun on empiric antiarrhythmic therapy and closely monitored for recurrence of the dysrhythmia. If the tachycardia recurred, the medication was changed and the patient again closely followed until a "successful" drug regimen was achieved. Although this type of therapy theoretically had its benefits, high failure rates, the potential side effects of drugs that may not suppress the tachycardia, and the unpredictable risk of making the tachycardia worse (this is called "proarrhythmia" and may occur in 5 to 15 percent of all patients) make this form of treatment unacceptable.

It is now recommended that all patients undergo a baseline electrophysiologic study prior to initiating any drug therapy for ventricular tachycardia. The baseline study enables the physician to use programmed electrical stimulation to determine whether the tachycardia is inducible and how easily it can be brought on. Once baseline data are obtained, drug therapy can be initiated and repeat, serial testing performed as necessary until a drug that successfully prevents induction of the ventricular tachycardia is found. This may require two to six electrophysiologic studies before an adequate response is achieved.

Cardiac Arrest

Patients who survive an out-of-hospital cardiac arrest that is not associated with a definable event such as myocardial infarction, pulmonary embolus, electrolyte disorder, drug overdose, or trauma have a 40 to 50 percent chance of suffering a similar event within the first year after the initial episode. If, after careful evaluation, no etiology for the cardiac arrest can be found, these patients should undergo an electrophysiologic evaluation similar to patients with ventricular tachycardia. If ventricular tachycardia or ventricular fibrillation is induced, then serial electrophysiologic testing should be performed in an attempt to find an antiarrhythmic drug to control the dysrhythmia. All patients with an out-of-hospital cardiac arrest, also called "sudden death," must undergo programmed electrical stimulation of the left ventricle if right ventricular programmed stimulation does not reveal an etiology for the arrest.

Ventricular Tachycardia after Myocardial Infarction

The role of electrophysiologic testing in patients who have ventricular arrhythmia after myocardial infarction is, as of this time, evolving. Most physicians would agree that ventricular fibrillation or polymorphic ventricular tachycardia (more than one QRS morphology seen during the tachycardia) at the time of infarction is probably of little clinical significance and does not require further evaluation. Sustained, monomorphic ventricular tachycardia (one QRS morpholgy) in association with a myocardial infarction carries a worse prognosis and merits electrophysiologic evaluation after the patient has recovered from the infarction. Sustained or nonsustained ventricular tachycardia that occurs after completion of the myocardial infarction requires electrophysiologic evaluation utilizing programmed electrical stimulation and serial drug testing as necessary.

Acute Pharmacologic Therapy of Arrhythmias

Over the past 15 to 20 years, there has been an upsurge in the development of antiarrhythmic drugs. Original investigative work focused on the control and therapy of supraventricular tachycardias, whereas the thrust of antiarrhythmic research over the last 10 years has centered on therapy for ventricular arrhythmias. There are several excellent reviews and book chapters that discuss, in detail, the management of chronic supraventricular and ventricular dysrhythmias. Although chronic treatment and control of arrhythmias is the goal of all electrophysiologists, for the nonelectrophysiologist, a basic knowledge of how to control and stablize arrhythmias acutely initiated in the catheterization or electrophysiology laboratories is all that is required. Some examples of arrhythmias that require acute pharmacologic or electrical intervention follow.

Bradycardia

Sinus bradycardia exists in adults when the rate of discharge from the sinus node falls to less than 60 beats per minute. Electrocardiographically, this rhythm is characterized by a normal P-wave morphology, a constant PR interval measuring between 120 to 200 msec, and an associated QRS with each P wave. Sinus bradycardia may result from excessive vagal activity, from decreases in sympathetic tone, including carotid sinus hypersensitivity, vomiting, intracranial tumors or bleeding, or during acute (inferior) myocardial infarction. Hypothermia, hypothyroidism, and sepsis also may cause sinus bradycardia. It should be noted that sinus bradycardia may be present in normal, healthy individuals, so its presence does not necessarily reflect a pathologic state.

As discussed previously, bradycardia is only significant if the decrease in heart rate results in a significant fall in cardiac output and resultant hypotension. Sinus bradycardia, as such, usually requires no therapy unless symptoms accompany the dysrhythmia or ventricular arrhythmias are associated with the slow heart rate.

Initial therapy consists of 0.5 to 1.0 mg of atropine given intravenously and repeated at approximately 5-min intervals as necessary to a total dose of 2.0 mg. In some instances, atropine is ineffective in increasing the sinus rate, and patients may require the initiation of an isoproterenol infusion (1 to 2 μg per minute, intravenously) to stabilize their rhythm at an acceptable level. Rarely, a temporary transvenous pacemaker may be required to support the patient until his rhythm stabilizes. In most cases, a temporary pacemaker is inserted via venous access into the right ventricular apex under fluoroscopic guidance. In some instances, however, atrial pacing may be preferable in order to preserve the atrioventricular relationship of contraction. If bradycardia persists, no drug is generally suited for chronic management of bradycardia, and consideration of a permanent pacemaker is necessary.

Heart Block

Bradycardia in the form of an inadequate number of ventricular contractions with a resultant decrease in cardiac output may be seen with block of the atrial impulse in the atrioventricular node; this is called "heart block." Heart block is a disturbance of impulse conduction that may be transient or permanent as the result of anatomical or functional impairment of the atrioventricular node. Because conduction through the atrioventricular node is extremely sensitive to modulation by vagal tone, sympathetic tone, cardiac drugs, myocardial ischemia, and ion-concentration changes, varying severity in the degree of conduction disturbance through the node may be seen. Atrioventricular node heart block is categorized by the severity of this altered conduction, and therapy for heart block is adjusted dependent upon the type of block.

Essentially, there are three "degrees" of heart block. During first-degree heart block, conduction time through the atrioventricular node is prolonged (PR interval greater than 200 msec), but all impulses are conducted, and the PR interval remains relatively constant. Because all atrial impulses are conducted to the ventricle, bradycardia will exist only if the sinus node decreases its rate of discharge below 60 per minute. As a result, this type of heart block requires no therapy except as indicated for sinus bradycardia. It is important to note, however, that these patients can progress to a higher, more severe degree of heart block, and should be observed carefully.

Second-degree heart block occurs in two forms—Mobitz type 1 (Wenckebach) and type 2. Type-1 second-degree heart block is characterized by a progressive lengthening of the PR interval that reflects an increasing atrioventricular conduction time until the atrial impulse is delayed to such an extent that it is not conducted to the ventricle. With failure to conduct, the atrioventricular node recovers, and the process repeats itself. This type of heart block is often associated with acute (inferior) myocardial infarction. It is transient, benign, and does not require intervention in the form of drugs or temporary pacing. In contrast, type-2 second-degree atrioventricular block presents with a constant PR interval that remains stable up to the time that block of the atrial impulse is seen. The block may occur on an occasional or repetitive basis and, unlike type-1 second-degree heart block, has a more ominous prognosis. Type-2 second-degree block may progress unpredictably to complete heart block (see below) or may result in the block of several atrial impulses in a row. This may be associated with symptoms or loss of consciousness. The presence of type-2 second-degree atrioventricular block in the setting of an acute (anterior) myocardial infarction is associated with a high mortality rate, generally due to pump failure, and may require temporary or permanent pacing. In general, type-2 second-degree atrioventricular block is not treated with drugs, although isoproterenol or atropine may be tried under acute conditions if clinically indicated.

Third-degree atrioventricular block, also called "complete heart block," is present when no impulses are conducted from the atria to the ventricles. As a result, a subsidiary ventricular pacemaker usually located immediately below the region of block takes over as the rhythm generator. Unfortunately, the ventricular escape rhythm often is less than 40 beats per minute and is associated with symptoms of inadequate cardiac output (fatigue, angina, presyncope, syncope). Complete heart block may be caused by a number of factors, including hypersensitivity to carotid sinus stimulation, electrolyte disturbances, infection, cardiac valvular disease, cardiac surgery, drug toxicity, coronary artery disease, or myocardial infarction. If complete heart block develops acutely, atropine or isoproterenol may be employed to support the patient while a temporary pacemaker is being placed. Atropine will reverse or improve complete heart block due to increased vagal effects on the atrioventricular node, whereas isoproterenol, acting as a synthetic catecholamine, may increase the rate of discharge of the ventricular focus. Isoproterenol should not be used, or used only with extreme caution, in patients who have heart block on the basis of an acute myocardial infarction because the catecholamine effects may worsen the myocardial ischemia.

Supraventricular Tachycardias

Several types of supraventricular tachycardias may be seen and recognized in the acute setting. It is important to emphasize that unless a patient is hemodynamically unstable, symptomatic (angina, dyspnea), or otherwise compromised, it is most important to attempt to treat the precipitating cause of the tachycardia and then to treat the arrhythmia itself. Often, correction of the initiating event will cure the arrhythmia. In the unstable patient in whom the tachycardia is contributing to the problem, appropriate therapy should be employed.

Perhaps the most common supraventricular tachycardia seen is atrial fibrillation. This arrhythmia is characterized by the absence of discernible P waves on the ECG and disorganized atrial activity. In untreated patients, the rate of conduction of the atrial impulses is variable and results in a ventricular response that is irregular at a rate of 100 to 180 beats per minute. As described earlier, a rapid ventricular rate may actually lead to a decrease in cardiac output and associated symptoms. In addition, owing to the loss of atrial contraction which may contribute as much as 20 percent to the cardiac output, even patients with a well-controlled ventricular response rate may have symptoms. Atrial fibrillation is seen in patients with rheumatic heart disease, mitral valvular disease, pulmonary emboli, pericarditis, thyrotoxicosis, cardiomyopathy, hypertension, coronary artery disease, and myocardial infarction. Injection of the sinoatrial nodal artery with contrast dye during coronary angiography also may precipitate atrial fibrillation.

If the sudden onset of atrial fibrillation is associated with acute cardiovascular decompensation, electrical cardioversion is the treatment of choice. In the absence of cardiovascular compromise, the initial drug of choice is digitalis administered by an intravenous or oral route. Digitalis has its primary effect on the atrioventricular node and slows conduction such that the ventricular response to atrial fibrillation is decreased. Digitalis has a slow onset of action, and, occasionally, a beta-blocker (propranolol, esmolol) is employed in conjunction with digitalis. These two drugs, however, often do not convert the patient back to normal sinus rhythm, and, after an adequate trial of therapy, oral quinidine is added. If, after several days of combined digitalis/quinidine therapy, atrial fibrillation persists, consideration of elective cardioversion is made. It should be pointed out that atrial fibrillation is often well tolerated and may not require conversion to sinus rhythm.

Atrial flutter is less common than atrial fibrillation, and it is defined as an atrial rate of 250 to 300 beats per minute. It is characterized on ECG by the presence of regular, rapid P (flutter) waves, which give the isoelectric interval of the ECG a "sawtooth" appearance. The atrial impulses are generally conducted through the atrioventricular node to the ventricle in a regular fashion, resulting in one ventricular depolarization for every two or three flutter waves. This results in a ventricular response rate of approximately 100 to 150 beats per minute. The causes of atrial flutter include rheumatic heart disease, cardiomyopathy, pulmonary emboli, pericarditis, acute alcohol ingestion, or ischemic heart disease.

In atrial flutter, unlike atrial fibrillation, the atria contract and may contribute to the cardiac output, but the rhythm is generally unstable and often reverts to sinus rhythm or degenerates to atrial fibrillation. In contrast to atrial fibrillation, synchronous direct-current cardioversion is often utilized as the initial therapy for atrial flutter. After sedating the patient, low-energy (25 to 100 J) shocks can be administered and frequently will convert the patient to sinus rhythm. If the patient cannot be successfully cardioverted or if cardioversion is contraindicated, rapid atrial pacing utilizing a temporary atrial pacing wire may be employed. Alternatively, in patients with a stable blood pressure, verapamil given in intravenous boluses of 5 to 10 mg (total dose not to exceed 20 mg) followed by an intravenous infusion of 5 μg per kilogram per minute may be used to slow the ventricular response. In patients with recent onset of atrial flutter, verapamil may convert the rhythm to normal sinus but rarely restores sinus rhythm in patients with chronic atrial flutter.

If atrial flutter cannot be controlled with the therapy just described, digoxin should be given to slow the atrioventricular conduction and subsequently the ventricular response. Frequently, atrial flutter will change to atrial fibrillation with administration of digoxin and, if underlying causes of the atrial flutter are corrected, normal sinus rhythm may occur by withdrawing the digoxin. If digoxin alone does not convert the atrial flutter or control the ventricular response, propranolol, quinidine, procainamide, disopyramide, or verapamil may be added.

Supraventricular tachycardia includes those arrhythmias arising from the sinus node, atria, and atrioventricular node. Athough it is not entirely accurate to categorize qualitatively all of these arrhythmias under the same heading, therapy for these acute supraventricular tachycardias is often similar, and precise diagnosis is frequently not possible utilizing the 12-lead ECG alone. Three important points to remember when considering whether to treat a supraventricular tachycardia acutely include the following: Does the rhythm need to be treated acutely? Is this a supraventricular tachycardia or atrial fibrillation/flutter? Does the possibility of a pre-excitation syndrome (i.e., Wolff-Parkinson-White) exist? If, after all available information is examined, it is felt that the patient has a supraventricular tachycardia that requires therapy, then the following regimen is recommended.

Supraventricular tachycardia can originate from the sinus node, the atria, or the atrioventricular node. Etiologies of supraventricular tachycardias include organic heart disease, myocardial infarction, pulmonary emboli, chronic lung disease, metabolic derangements, drug toxicity, and acute alcohol ingestion. The goals of therapy are to slow the generation of impulses at the origin of the tachycardia and/or slow the ventricular response. Although most supraventricular tachycardias are well tolerated, symptoms such as dyspnea, angina, palpitations, light headedness, syncope, weakness, and nausea may exist.

If the patient is hemodynamically stable, verapamil in 5- to 10-mg doses (total dose not to exceed 20 mg) may be administered intravenously. Alternatively, maneuvers that increase vagal tone may be employed as first-line therapy in the treatment of supraventricular tachycardia. These include coughing, gagging, Valsalva maneuver, Mueller maneuver, ice water to the face (dive reflex), gentle ocular pressure, and carotid sinus massage. All of these augment the vagal output and may convert the supraventricular tachycardia to sinus rhythm.

If vagal maneuvers and verapamil therapy fail, use of intravenous beta-blockers such as propranolol or esmolol may be tried. The beta-blockers must be used cautiously in patients with heart failure, chronic lung disease, or a history of asthma because they may exacerbate these conditions and depress cardiac function. If beta-blockers are contraindicated, one may wish to consider the need for direct-current cardioversion. Although other medications are available (procainamide, quinidine, disopyramide), these are generally reserved as therapy to prevent recurrence of the arrhythmia and have only limited application in the acute treatment of supraventricular tachycardias. If Wolff-Parkinson-White syndrome is thought to be the source of the patient's tachycardia and medical therapy is indicated, chronic therapy with flecainide is most commonly employed.

Ventricular Tachycardia

The origins of ventricular tachycardia are usually the specialized tissue of the conduction system distal to the bifurcation of the His bundle, the ventricular muscle itself, or a combination of both tissues. The diagnosis of ventricular tachycardia is suggested when a series of three or more wide QRS complexes is seen on ECG or monitor. Associated with the wide QRS complexes may be atrioventricular dissociation (P waves unrelated to the QRS) or retrograde P waves (impulses from the ventricle that are conducted to the atria backwards through the atrioventricular node such that the atria are activated in a direction opposite to their normal activation). Ventricular ectopy, in and of itself, may be normal and not require immediate therapy, but ventricular tachycardia almost always requires evaluation. Again, as with the other arrhythmias we have discussed, evaluation of the patient is required to determine whether acute intervention is necessary. Ventricular tachycardia induced while positioning a pigtail or other type of catheter in the LV has no clinical significance.

Ventricular tachycardia that does not cause hemodynamic deterioration, congestive heart failure, dyspnea, angina, or other symptoms may be managed medically. The first-line drug for ventricular tachycardia in the actue setting is lidocaine. Lidocaine is administered as a series of boluses (75 mg, 75 mg, 75mg) over 5 to 10 minutes followed by an intravenous infusion (1 to 4 mg per minute). If lidocaine is successful in terminating or controlling the tachycardia, the infusion should be maintained and causes of the ventricular tachycardia sought. If maximum doses of lidocaine fail to control the arrhythmia, procainamide (intravenous bolus of 1 g given over 10 to 20 min followed by an infusion of 2 to 6 mg per minute) or bretylium (intravenous bolus of 350 to 700 mg given over 10 to 20 min followed by an infusion of 0.5 to 2.0 mg per minute) may be administered. Although both drugs are effective, they may cause significant hypotension and resultant deterioration in the patient's clinical status. All intravenous drugs should be administered with caution over several minutes, and vital signs should be checked frequently.

If the ventricular tachycardia does not respond to medical therapy or if hypotension, angina, heart failure, confusion, or loss of consciousness develop, the arrhythmia should be treated immediately with direct current cardioversion. If the patient is alert, low-energy (100 to 200 J) synchronized cardioversion may be attempted after adequate sedation. High-energy (200 to 400 J) synchronized cardioversion is performed in the severely compromised or unconscious patient. If the patient is not connected to a defibrillator, a sternal blow with the closed fist, also called "thump-version," may be attemped while waiting for the defibrillator. Striking the chest may cause a premature ventricular contraction that can interrupt the re-entrant pathway of the tachycardia and result in reversion to sinus rhythm. It also should be noted that a chest thump may not affect the tachycardia, may accelerate the tachycardia, or convert the tachycardia to ventricular fibrillation.

In a small population of patients, medication or cardioversion may only temporarily interrupt the tachycardia. Patients with recurrent or incessant ventricular tachycardia may require that a temporary pacing catheter be inserted into the RV. This catheter allows the physician to artificially introduce premature ventricular contractions into the ventricular tachycardia in an effort to interrupt the arrhythmia cycle. Similarly, if the tachycardia is sensitive to changes in the heart rate, the temporary pacemaker may be used to pace the heart and suppress the tachycardia until reversible conditions contributing to the maintenance of the ventricular arrhythmia are corrected.

Ventricular Fibrillation

Ventricular fibrillation occurs in a variety of settings, including during myocardial infarction, antiarrhythmic drug administration, attempted cardioversion of ventricular or supraventricular tachycardia, periods of hypoxia, drug overdose, and coronary arteriography. It can be recognized on ECG and cardiac monitor by the absence of well-defined QRS complexes, which are replaced with irregular electrical activity of varying contour and amplitude. This arrhythmia represents a severe derangement in the heart beat and is uniformly fatal within 3 to 6 min after onset if no efforts are made to correct the situation.

Treatment of ventricular fibrillation is simple and consists of immediate, and, if necessary, repeated, unsynchronized direct-current cardioversion at high-energy levels (200 to 400 J). Cardiopulmonary resuscitation in the form of ventilation and chest compressions should be performed only if immediate defibrillation cannot be effected. If a defibrillator is readily available, as little time as possible should be lost prior to the administration of the cardioversion shock(s).

Unlike many other arrhythmias, ventricular fibrillation mandates the treatment of the arrhythmia first, followed by the search for conditions contributing to the arrest. After reversion of ventricular fibrillation to sinus or other acceptable rhythm, it is essential to monitor the patient continuously and to watch for recurrence of arrhythmia. Administration of lidocaine, procainamide, or bretylium may prevent recurrence of arrhythmia, and correction of metabolic abnormalities, including electrolytes, pH, and oxygenation, helps prevent further episodes of ventricular fibrillation. A search for conditions contributing to the arrhythmia should include evaluation for an acute myocardial infarction, pulmonary embolus, or drug ingestion.

Electrophysiologic Evaluation of Arrhythmias

As with therapeutic options, different arrhythmias require different approaches in the electrophysiology laboratory to evaluate and elucidate the mechanism as well as direct the mode of therapy for the specific arrhythmia. In this section, we present discussions of representative studies that are routinely performed in the electrophysiology laboratory to evaluate arrhythmias.

General Principles

The electrophysiologic study for a specific arrhythmia should consist of an organized approach to the analysis of the problem. For the electrophysiologic study to be meaningful to the observer, certain concepts and methods must be understood. These include the measurement of intracardiac conduction intervals, the methodology of programmed electrical stimulation, and the correlation of the intracardiac recordings to the surface ECG.

Figure 14–5 demonstrates simultaneous electrical recordings obtained from a surface ECG (lead II) tracing, the high RA near the sinus node (HRA), the area of the bundle of His (HBE), and the RV apex. Notice the timing of electrical events. As you would expect, the area of the sinus node (HRA tracing) is activated first during normal sinus rhythm. This is followed by activation of the atria in their entirety (P wave). At some point during atrial depolarization, the impulse travels to the lower RA and approaches the atrioventricular node. Near the node, the atrial tissue is activated, resulting in a local electrogram as shown on the His bundle recording (A deflection on HBE tracing). Activity through the atrioventricular node itself is too small to be detected by conventional electrophysiologic recording techniques; therefore, the next area of activation seen during the normal conduction of the impulse is that of the His bundle (H deflection on HBE tracing). The time between the A deflection of the HBE tracing and the H deflection is called AH interval and reflects conduction through the atrioventricular node. The next activity generated is that of the impulse spreading over the ventricles. This occurs rapidly in the normal heart and is associated with the QRS complex on the ECG. Evaluation of conduction through the His-Purkinje conducting system is made by measuring the interval between the onset of the His deflection (H) and the earliest onset of ventricular activation as seen on the surface ECG leads or the ventricular electrogram (V) in the His bundle recording. This conduction time is called the HV interval. During ventricular depolarization (RV tracing), activation of the region of the RV apex results in the generation of the local ventricular electrogram. During an electrophysiologic study, prior to stimulation or drug administration, these tracings and their associated intervals are obtained. Values for normal intervals in adults are shown in Table 14–2.

Evaluation of Sinus Node Function

Disorders of sinus node function are becoming increasingly recognized as a cause of syncope of cardiac origin. Approximately 30 percent of all permanent pace-

TABLE 14–2
Normal Intervals in Adults

PR	120–200 msec
QRS	60–120 msec
QT	310–430 msec
RR	600–1000 msec
AH	45–140 msec
HV	25–55 msec

makers implanted are for specific treatment of bradyarrhythmias due to sinus node dysfunction.

As humans age, the number of functional sinus nodal cells decreases. Additionally, histologically, the area of the sinus node demonstrates increased amounts of fibrosis. Both of these conditions may contribute to the deterioration of sinus node function and inability of the node to maintain an adequate heart rate. The first step in evaluating whether sinus node dysfunction exists is to obtain a 12-lead ECG. In a substantial number of patients (10 to 15 percent), a significant abnormality can be identified. If a random ECG is normal or unrevealing, the patient should undergo prolonged (24 to 48 hr), continuous ECG monitoring. Although this may enable the physician to determine the cause of the patient's symptom, most episodes of symptoms or significant bradycardia are, unfortunately, unpredictable and not seen on 24-hr holter monitor. Some medical centers offer an extension of this technology in the form of continuous outpatient monitoring utilizing a "loop" monitor or a telephone monitor. The theory of both of these systems is that the patient, when he has an episode of his symptoms, can contact the hospital after the fact and play back the most recent portion of his recording. If no events occur, these monitors simply erase and record over the old information, replacing it with new information. The patient determines when the recordings should be reviewed by a physician based on his own clinical condition and symptoms. These techniques have the advantage of constant surveillance. If a symptomatic bradycardia or sinus node dysfunction can be documented by any of the preceeding screening tests, this may exclude the need for further invasive testing. If these tests are unsuccessful in revealing an etiology of the patient's problems, an exercise test may contribute information concerning etiology of the problem. As a final diagnostic measure, electrophysiologic testing is employed.

A standard electrophysiologic study to evaluate sinus node function requires monitoring of several surface ECG leads as well as recordings from the atria, His bundle, and ventricles. Once baseline intervals have been measured, evaluation of the sinus node includes assessment of sinus automaticity (impulse formation) and sensitivity of the node to changes in autonomic tone.

Suppression of sinus node automaticity by driving the heart at a rate faster than the inherent rate of the node is called "overdrive suppression." To evaluate the degree of suppression, the high RA is paced via the electrode catheter for 30 sec at a constant heart rate just above that of the sinus rate. At the end of 30 sec, pacing is abruptly terminated, and the interval between the last paced beat and the first sinus beat is measured. This is called the "sinus node recovery time" (SNRT), and it reflects the ability of the sinus node to recover from over-drive pacing. The heart is allowed a rest period, and pacing is again instituted, this time at a faster rate. The SNRT is serially measured after pacing rates ranging from 80 to 200 beats per minute. With each test, the recovery time is corrected for the baseline heart rate and a corrected sinus node recovery time (CSNRT) determined. In all cases, the sinus node should demonstrate a spontaneous impulse within 1.5 sec after cessation of the pacing drive train, and should have a CSNRT of less than 525 msec. A SNRT of greater than 1.5 seconds or a CSNRT of greater than 525 msec reflects abnormal sinus node function.

Sinus node sensitivity to changes in autonomic tone can be evaluated in a number of ways. Carotid sinus massage with ECG and electrogram monitoring may reveal patients with hypersensitivity of carotid sinus reflexes. Stimulation of the carotid sinus by rubbing the neck activates parasympathetic (vagal) discharge to the heart, which causes slowing of the heart rate. Occasionally, this maneuver may result in profound slowing of the heart and subsequent "sinus arrest" with pauses in excess of 3 sec. Such a response is abnormal and may be responsible for the patient's symptoms.

Upon completion of the baseline procedures, pharmacologic testing may be performed. Propranolol (8 to 12 mg, intravenously) is used to assess the role of the sympathetic nervous system in preventing bradycardia because it blocks sympathetic neural input to the sinus node. This leaves the parasympathetic nervous input to the node unchecked and enables the physician to repeat SNRT and carotid sinus massage testing in the absence of sympathetic interference. If desired, atropine (1 to 3 mg, intravenously) also may be administered to block parasympathetic input to the sinus node and evaluate the degree of sinus node dysfunction in the absence of vagal interference.

Evaluation of Atrioventricular Node Function

Theoretically, abnormalities in atrioventricular conduction may result from disturbances in any region of the heart; therefore, precise localization of the site of conduction disturbance is of extreme benefit to the physician. Obviously, failure of the impulse to be conducted through any one of the regions separating the atria from the ventricles will result in atrioventricular block. These regions include the atrioventricular node, His bundle, and His-Purkinje conduction system. In the case of atrioventricular block, all of the above-mentioned regions require evaluation, but for the purpose of this chapter, evaluation of atrioventricular nodal function will be discussed.

The atrioventricular node accounts for the major portion of the time delay in normal atrioventricular transmission. The range for normal AH intervals varies from 45 to 140 msec (see Table 14–2) but it can be profoundly influenced by changes in autonomic tone. The influence autonomic tone has over atrioventricular nodal function should be evaluated during the course of every study that is examining abnormalities in conduction.

Routine analysis of atrioventricular node function requires that electrograms from the RA, His bundle, and RV be recorded. The study begins with atrial-pacing protocols similar to those described for the sinus node. Atrial pacing provides a method by which the functional ability of the atrioventricular node to conduct impulses from the atria to the ventricles may be determined. Atrial pacing is most commonly performed from the high RA and is begun at a rate just slightly faster than the inherent rate of the sinus node. The pacing rate is then progressively increased while monitoring the AH and HV intervals. The normal response of the atrioventricular node to increasing heart rate is gradual lengthening of the AH interval until type-1 second-degree (Wenckebach) block occurs in the atrioventricular node. In most normal individuals, this appears at heart rates ranging from 120 to 180 beats per minute. Throughout the pacing protocol, the HV interval should remain stable. It is emphasized that, in normal hearts, block occurs in the atrioventricular node and demonstrates characteristics of type-1 second-degree block. The presence of higher degree atrioventricular block is abnormal.

It also is useful to evaluate the atrioventricular node by measuring the effective and functional refractory periods of the node. As described above, refractoriness is defined as resistance or lack of response to a stimulus. The refractory period of tissue is the time following a response (depolarization) to a stimulus when the muscle or conducting tissue has inadequately recovered to the point that a second response (depolarization) is possible. In other words, a brief period follows the initial response to a stimulus during which a second response is impossible in spite of attempted stimulation. This refractoriness is due to incomplete recovery of the cardiac cells to their resting membrane potential and inability of the cells to be excited until adequately repolarized. Refractoriness also reflects the ability of the atrioventricular node to conduct an impulse and whether this ability is normal or blunted.

Atrial pacing can be repeated in the presence of autonomic manipulations to determine the sensitivity of the atioventricular node to neural input. As described previously, carotid sinus massage stimulates the parasympathetic input to the node; this slows atrioventricular nodal conduction. Carotid sinus massage performed while pacing from the atrium may uncover profound vagal influences on the atrioventricular node and reveal the development of significant heart block that otherwise would not be seen. These findings may assist in determining whether a pacemaker is required. Additionally, atropine may be used to assist in the evaluation of the vagal influences on the atrioventricular node by blocking conduction of parasympathetic nerves to the node. Propranolol blocks sympathetic input to the atrioventricular node and allows the observer to evaluate atrioventricular nodal conduction in the absence of catecholamine interference. Finally, isoproterenolol infusion can be used to facilitate conduction through the atrioventricular node during atrial pacing and supply data concerning the "best" possible function of the node.

Electrophysiologic study of the atrioventricular node then consists of evaluation of nodal function in the baseline state and during physiologic (carotid sinus massage) and pharmacologic manipulations to ascertain the "best" and "worst" conduction properties of the node. In addition, blood pressure data and clinical symptoms should be monitored. If, during any of these tests, the patient develops significant bradycardia with associated hypotension or clinical symptoms, the manipulations can be repeated while the patient is temporarily paced from the ventricle alone, the atrium alone, and during sequential atrial and ventricular pacing. If pacing abolishes the hypotension and/or clinical symptoms, a permanent pacemaker should probably be considered.

Evaluation of Supraventricular Tachycardia

Supraventricular tachycardias induced in the electrophysiology laboratory include atrial fibrillation, atrial flutter, sinus node re-entrant tachycardia, atrial re-entrant tachycardia, atrioventricular re-entrant tachycardia, and supraventricular tachycardia secondary to an accessory pathway. The development and refinement of intracardiac recording and programmed electrical stimulation have resulted in a greater understanding of the physiologic mechanisms responsible for these tachycardias. The two basic mechanisms responsible for supraventricular tachycardias are automaticity and re-entry.

Automaticity, or an automatic rhythm, results when cells undergo accelerated spontaneous depolarization (see Fig. 14–2) and reach their threshold for activation at a rate faster that the sinus node. Although automaticity is well accepted as an etiology of arrhythmias, it is difficult to evaluate because it can be neither predictably initiated nor terminated. A re-entrant arrhythmia involves an entirely different physiologic substrate, because the tachycardia can exist only in the presence of variably conducting regions of the heart. In order for the re-entry to manifest itself, there must be two distinct pathways or regions in that heart that form the complete circuit of conduction and allow the presence of continuous (re-entrant) electrical activity. This continuous electrical activity results in a "tail-chasing" scenario and enables the supraventricular tachycardia to sustain.

During electrophysiologic study to evaluate supraventricular tachycardia, recordings from the RA, RV, His bundle, and LA (via the coronary sinus vein) are necessary. While recording from these sites, programmed electrical pacing protocols from the RA and RV are performed. Additionally, refractory period determinations in the RA, RV, and atrioventricular node are measured. If the tachycardia is initiated, attempts to modify and/or interrupt the arrhythmia are made. These techniques include programmed atrial and ventricular stimulation during tachycardia, vagal maneuvers, atropine/propranolol administration, isoproterenol infusion, and verapamil therapy. Treatment of the supraventricular tachycardia is based upon the results of the electrophysiologic study.

Evaluation of Ventricular Tachycardia/Fibrillation

Ventricular tachycardia and ventricular fibrillation are relatively common arrhythmias, and they require complete electrophysiologic evaluation. As described previously, empiric therapy is often unsuccessful (and even dangerous); therefore, serial electrophysiologic testing is done to enhance the accuracy of drug therapy.

Most commonly, electrogram recordings from the RV are all that are necessary for an adequate evaluation of ventricular tachycardia, but often a second electrode is inserted and a His bundle recording obtained. Refractory periods are determined during sinus rhythm and at several (at least three) paced heart rates. While pacing the heart at a fixed stimulus rate (S_1), a premature ventricular stimulus (S_2) is applied after 8 to 10 S_1 stimuli (this is called a "stimulus drive train"). The S_2 stimulus is slowly moved closer to S_1, beginning in late diastole and progressing until it will not initiate a premature ventricular complex—refractoriness. Once refractoriness is achieved at a given pacing rate, other drive-train rates are tested as per a routine protocol, and refractoriness is measured at these rates. If a single premature stimulus does not elicit the tachycardia, the pacing protocols are repeated, this time with the addition of a second (S_3) premature stimulus at the end of the S_1 drive train. The double premature stimuli (S_2S_3) are moved in toward the S_1 again until refractoriness to these two stimuli is obtained. This is repeated at all heart rates previously examined. Finally, a third premature ventricular stimulus (S_4) is added to the protocol at the end of the drive train, and triple premature ventricular contractions $(S_2S_3S_4)$ are administered. These extrastimuli again are moved progressively closer to the final stimulus of the S_1 drive train until refractoriness is achieved. This progressive addition of extrastimuli moved closer and closer to the drive train stresses the heart and, if it is susceptible to a tachycardia, will initiate it. These pacing procedures are performed from at least two RV sites if no ventricular tachycardia is produced.

With the induction of ventricular tachycarcdia, a 12-lead ECG is obtained to aid in diagnosing the site of origin of the tachycardia. Once an ECG is recorded, the ventricular tachycardia is interrupted either by programmed stimulation from the ventricle, pacing from the ventricle, antiarrhythmic drugs, or in cases of hypotension and syncope, direct-current cardioversion (200 to 400 J). It is now obvious why the ECG machine should be readily available and the patient always connected to the defibrillator whenever an electrophysiologic study is performed.

Summary

In patients with disturbances in cardiac rhythm, electrophysiologic studies can assist the physician in the diagnosis, therapy, and control of the arrhythmia. Although an electrophysiologic study should not take the place of a careful history and physical examination, noninvasive evaluation, or exercise testing, it certainly is an indicated procedure in many instances and often may provide a definitive diagnosis when other investigative efforts fail.

In patients with documented tachycardias of undiagnosed or uncertain etiology, electrophysiologic testing facilitates identification of the arrhythmia and possible mechanisms involved in the genesis of the disturbance. Correct diagnosis of the tachycardia can decrease the chances of the patient having serious hemodynamic compromise or potentially life-threatening complications of the arrhythmia. Additionally, through careful evaluation or serial electrophysiologic testing, appropriate therapy can be directed. In patients with bradyarrhythmias, electrophysiologic studies can assist in determining the cause of the bradycardia and aid in predicting whether the patient will need further support in the form of pacemaker placement. In atrioventricular conduction disturbances, this technique is useful in identifying patients at risk for progression of conduction disorders. Also, patients with severe underlying conduction system disease who, without appropriate therapy, would be susceptible to symptomatic bradycardia, weakness, dizziness, syncope or death can be identified.

SELECTED REFERENCES

Akhtar M, Fischer JD, Gillette PC, et al. NASPE ad hoc committee on guidelines for cardiac electrophysiologic studies. Pace 1985; 8:611.

Hammill SC, Sugrue DD, Gersh BJ, et al. Clinical intracardiac electrophysiologic testing: Technique, diagnostic indications and therapeutic uses. Mayo Clinic Proc 1986; 6:478.

Josephson ME, Seides SF. Clinical and cardiac electrophysiology: Techniques and interpretations. Philadelphia: Lea & Febiger, 1979.

Prystowsky EN. Electrophysiologic-electropharmacologic testing in patients with ventricular arrhythmias. Pace 1988; 11:225.

Rosen MR. The links between basic and clinical cardiac electrophysiology. Circulation 1988; 77:251.

Salerno DM. Review: Antiarrhythmic drugs: 1987 (two parts). J Electrophysiol 1987; 1:217, 356.

Wellens HJJ. Electrical stimulation of the heart in the study and treatment of tachycardias. Baltimore: University Park Press, 1971.

Zipes DP. Management of cardiac arrhythmias: Pharmacological, electrical and surgical techniques. In Braunwald E, ed. Heart Disease. Philadelphia: WB Saunders, 1984: 648.

INDEX

307

Shaver..